MAKING MEDICAL DOCTORS

MAKING MEDICAL DOCTORS:

Science and Medicine at Vanderbilt Since Flexner

TIMOTHY C. JACOBSON

The University of Alabama Press

Tuscaloosa

Library of Congress Cataloging-in-Publication Data

Jacobson, Timothy C., 1948–
  Making medical doctors

  Includes bibliographies and index.
    1. Vanderbilt University. Medical Center—History.
2. Vanderbilt University. School of Medicine—History.
I. Title. [DNLM: 1. Vanderbilt University. Medical
Center. 2. Vanderbilt University. School of Medicine.
3. Schools, Medical—history—Tennessee. W 19 J17m]
RA982.N26V365 1987   610'720768'55   86-6991
ISBN 0-8173-5243-0 (pbk. : alk. paper)

British Library Cataloguing-in-Publication Data is available.

To RB

Contents

PART THREE: ON TECHNIQUE

PART FOUR: CHALLENGE AND RESPONSE

Illustrations

Acknowledgments

To Vernon E. Wilson and Roscoe R. Robinson, past and present Vice-Chancellors for Medical Affairs at Vanderbilt, go the thanks due to generous patrons; to Paul C. Nagel the thanks for bringing us together; to Rudolph H. Kampmeier thanks for letting me come to know one of Vanderbilt's "new men." To Gerald George go the thanks due a friend with a good place to write.

Preface

This book is about the union of science and medicine. Its general subject is that institution where science and medicine most dramatically came together: the modern medical school and center. Its particular subject is the medical school and center of Vanderbilt University, which in the 1920s was rebuilt as a model for medical education and research. Some of the names and circumstances that attended its origin are unique to Vanderbilt. Many of the ideas and ambitions that have shaped its evolution are not. The book's point is implicit in its structure and depends on forging two kinds of linkages, both of which transcend local matters.

The first is the linkage across space: literally from Vanderbilt to Baltimore, New York, and Europe, the sources of the ideas and the money that made the local story happen as it did. James H. Kirkland would not have been who he was without Abraham Flexner; Abraham Flexner who he was without Frederick T. Gates, Henry S. Pritchett, and the other foundation masters; G. Canby Robinson who he was without the Johns Hopkins medical institutions, William Osler, and a select corps of European masters. Such connections shape the narrative of the first two parts of the book: "Question of Possibility" and "Design for Permanence."

The second is the linkage across time, which is addressed first in the Introduction and then predominates in Part Four, "Challenge and Response," which deals with recent decades. Here the point simply is that what these men did or hoped to do—and how it came undone—matters to us today. The political equation of power and dependence governing the way science and medicine work has changed, as Vanderbilt's story clearly shows. And it changes still. The intellectual equation relating medicine as science to medicine as service changes too, in ways some of which were foreseen by Flexner's generation and some of which at that time could not possibly have been imagined. These are the changes that we today must sort out, and we will be vastly aided in that job if we remember something of those others before us who also once passed this way.

To Part Three, "On Technique," remains the task of capturing the experience of a special, and now vanished, generation of doctors. The way these doctors, who reached maturity and the height of their influence between the two world wars, actually did medicine, surgery, and science made them who they were. It also makes them of enormous interest to us both because we no longer do these things in the same way (and seem no more satisfied as a result) and because even in today's and tomorrow's vastly changed medical world their shadow is and will remain apparent. The way they did things is important because of the power of the ideas behind their technique; that power endures and shapes our own progress.

The entire book explores a metaphor central to their vision and that of the laymen like Flexner and Kirkland who helped give it substance. In the evolution of medical education and research, the solitary act of climbing the peaks of progress and prestige led eventually downward to a broader, more public plain where less glamorous contests would be fought and decided. This book seeks the experience that defined the character of the medical leaders who scaled those rarefied heights and that conditioned the hopes, frustration, and confusion of those whom, perhaps too well, they sought to serve. The historical record that it follows leads finally to the question of how the promise of progress could be turned upon itself to induce among those who had clamored for it suspicion and resentment for those who had provided it.

MAKING MEDICAL DOCTORS

Introduction

The convergence of inductive science and the healing arts in the nineteenth and twentieth centuries produced what we know and praise today as modern medicine: a vast and sophisticated armamentarium to cure disease, ease pain, and save life. Science thus conceived and applied has helped medicine advance enormously. It has also enabled the doctors to secure self-esteem, social legitimacy, and dominion over medicine's marketplace. Science and medicine, it seemed, were truly meant for one another, their union destined to be long and placid. It is turning out to be long; it has not always been placid.

Science in medicine did not triumph all at once or simply by virtue of its ever-greater insight into disease and how to cure it. Rather, the culture of science slowly changed the context in which medicine was done. It changed the way the people who practiced medicine, and their patients, thought about health and therapeutics. It changed the way they thought about medical knowledge and where it came from, once from the sickroom but later from the laboratory especially. And it changed the way they chose to transmit knowledge to the next generation of doctors.

The union between science and medicine was worked out over many years by many people who saw in it different things. Along the way tensions abounded. If, for example, the purpose of medicine was to heal and the purpose of science to know, then their union supposed that the things science came to know would signify for the things medicine needed to heal. Often they did, but not always and not necessarily. Healers who ministered to sick people sometimes resented laboratory staff who did not. Laboratory workers whose discoveries mocked old concepts could be impatient with practitioners

I

whose problems were less tidy and who accepted new revelations sometimes slowly.

The strains were strains arising among those who lived under the same roof and served the same master but who spent their days differently. The strains have not as yet brought and are not likely to bring the house down, but their extent suggests they may be permanent. They were clearly evident in the relationship between the academic doctors in the leading research laboratories and medical schools and doctors in the practicing profession. They were also manifest within the medical schools, which were themselves monuments to the union of science and medicine. Among those monuments, none was conceived, constructed, and run more deliberately than Vanderbilt's medical school, whose intellectual architect, G. Canby Robinson, made a supreme effort to reduce the tensions and enhance the possibilities. His plan for doing that and what followed from it are the immediate subject of this book. Behind that story lies another, implicit in the relationship of science in medicine to the social and cultural texture of the world it has come to inhabit. That story has to do with knowledge, supply, demand, and expectations.

As doctors and patients responded to the promise of science in medicine, patrons soon followed. The meeting of money and medicine in the early twentieth century was no accident, and the bounty lavished on schools like Vanderbilt by the great philanthropies bespoke an attitude characteristic of the captains of industry who had produced it. Long before the turn of the century, the story was that John D. Rockefeller did not make mistakes: whenever and wherever he invested, others scrambled, hungry for the crumbs from his table, hoping their meager share would pay off half as richly as his usually did. Backing winners was a matter of intuition and experience, and in the wide-open world of Gilded Age capitalism where entrepreneurial talent of a high order met with abundant human and natural resources, the winnings could be handsome. It was a habit of mind that carried over into activities less mercenary than financial and industrial empire building but where the prospects of success if not profit still governed. The dispersal of great wealth, like its acquisition, reflected the desire for tangible though no longer pecuniary return on investment. The getters turned givers were driven in their new endeavor much as they always had been: to act, to win, and to matter. This they shared with the new medical scientists whom they patronized and whose own new-found ability truly to make a difference determined them to act and to win in what they saw as a battle against disease. Thus sanctioned by spirit and by interest, their marriage promised to be a long and happy one.

Its first offspring bore all the marks of its vigorous and ambitious parents.

The reformed, endowed medical schools of the 1920s and 1930s brought large resources and talent to the service of what all knew would be great things. Though by later standards some of the advances then wrought in medical knowledge and clinical care seem modest, at that time they had an effect far beyond their medical merits alone. Confidence in scientific medicine invested both the profession of academic medicine and the practicing profession with important symbolic value for those they served. The possibility of an ever-improved condition, though it would prove elusive, fed appetites accustomed to progress generally. Important discoveries generated demand for more advances until a perception of progress had become the presumption of progress.

Richly supported by outside resources, the new medical schools enjoyed much freedom to respond largely to inner scientific imperatives. Asking important questions, finding important answers, and demanding of the learners as much as they demanded of themselves, dedicated scientists in the new laboratories and clinics performed prodigies of research and teaching. On the anvil of their experience an image was fashioned by the blows of long hours and hard work. It pictured a fraternity of scholars and healers doing what conscience and intellect dictated. As it flattered the medical staff, so it clothed with new mystery the wonderful work they did and raised considerably the awe with which others came to regard them. Though many of them were modest and only too aware of the failings of their profession, it was an image easy enough to acquiesce in and one that in time would bestow the mantle of authority and certainty on a craft that was in fact changing and experimental. The image owed much to a confluence of means, knowledge, and will and seemed for a moment happy and uncomplicated. But to the extent that it was uncomplicated it was also unstable, and as the chemistry changed in the 1940s two elements in particular—the autonomy of the medical schools and the doctors they trained, and the demand for the knowledge they developed and transmitted—grew more and more incompatible.

Wartime and the troubled peace that followed altered many earlier perceptions of possibility. Modern medical care came to be one of the assumed components of the good life, and as demand for it went up so did external pressures on the medical staff and institutions that were supposed to meet it. Changing demand for medical service plus the expensive nature of the facilities required for modern medical research and teaching led to increased government involvement in research and education, first as self-styled servant of demand for more medical knowledge through subsidies for research, and later as would-be master of supply of medical personnel through aid to medical schools for education. Compared with other countries, American medicine's flirtation with government subsidy seemed tame and in keeping with the nation's generally more ambiguous stance toward the welfare state. But however tentative the mandate for government action to satisfy rising demand for modern medicine, it added to quality another consideration that to some threatened to overshadow it. Costs rose, and with them came new pressures for and questions about accountability to political authority.

Through it all, neither the widely held perception of scientific medicine as an absolute good nor the desire to have it more abundantly changed. Both ideas were embodied in the reformed medical schools of the twenties and thirties, and by the fifties, sixties, and seventies they had a profuse growth of various private third-party insurers and public assistance schemes aimed at spreading the risk and assuring access to medicine's bounty. Though critics might complain about the inertia of antiquated professional attitudes and institutional arrangements and condemn the bedlam of programs and policies that allegedly resulted, few could fail to be impressed in general by the massive mobilization of national resources—public and private—to give the people what they wanted. The arguments were over how, not whether, the wonders should be dispensed.

Despite the consensus about ends, continuing uncertainty over the proper means plus anxiety over ever-rising costs has led to considerable anger and frustration. As yet the basic presumption about the fundamental good of the product remains unclouded, with doubt focusing rather on its providers, to whom blame has been easy to attach. As a result, seldom if ever has any profession that indisputably produces so much of what so many say they want found itself so embattled. It is not, however, merely a question of rearranging some of the components of "the system"—of tinkering with the way the providers provide or are compelled to provide the knowledge and the care stemming from it. If there are flaws in costly scientific medicine, they may have more to do with the perception of the initial promise than with the provision of the final product. And they may be flaws that were present all along, becoming apparent only recently under the pressure of high costs and threats of outside control.

The promise of progress made long ago in the early days of medical reform has not been empty, and it holds perhaps as much today as it did then. Progress is not grinding to a halt. But it is important to understand what that promise was and what it was not. It said that science in medicine, given freedom and funding, could cure disease, ease suffering, and save life. That is, it could do the same things that medicine before science had claimed and tried to do. Many of its conceptions of health and disease and of how the human body worked obviously were different; its aim was not. It would pursue that aim through hard work, clear thinking, occasional discovery, and careful clinical application. Its successes would depend on chance and the growth of its knowledge, one an imponderable and the other a process of accretion, itself tentative and subject to error and constant revision. Science in medicine did not promise perfect health or a cure around every corner, though for a while it seemed to produce that. Indeed, the deeper it probed human biology the more it discovered it did not know and the more questions it found wanting of answers.

Yet the promise was not often or widely so interpreted. Among practitioners and patients alike, science's early dramatic successes inflated expectations that next year too another great revelation would ensue, enabling vastly improved treatment of this disease or that. Though much was accomplished, in the mind of an impatient people ever more anxious over an alleged right to medical care, it could never be enough. There was being established a level of entitlement, a standard of provision that presumed continued progress but which itself was difficult to scale down if progress did not materialize. For that, science in medicine was not alone responsible. Levels of entitlement and standards of provision were going up, often unreasonably, in other areas of society as well. The old art of healing had always been bound up with its cultural context, and so the science of medicine is today in this respect particularly.

Thus angered over the good health we want and consider our due but which our doctors cannot guarantee, we accuse those we have appointed to supply it and in whose wonderful skills we put our faith. How to resolve that dilemma is a matter of personal choice and public policy and belongs to the future. How the history of Vanderbilt University illuminates the path traveled en route there is the subject of what follows.

Prologue: Three Men and a Celebration

I

One small legacy of the Civil War stands today in a medium-sized southern city: a medium-sized university that bears the Dutch name of the founder of the New York Central Railroad. Vanderbilt is a monument to a national exercise in remorse and to the determination of former enemies once again to be friends. Its beginnings belong to a time of physical and spiritual reconstruction in which the South and the nation took up exciting new plans for the building of a better world. That late-nineteenth-century world is popularly remembered by the symbols it left (railroads, great industrial cities, the western frontier) and by the reputation of those who shaped it—robber barons in a Gilded Age whose crimes still bring shudders, or captains of industry in an age of enterprise whose feats still inspire wonder.

Universities loom smaller among the icons of those times, even though some important ones appeared then, Vanderbilt among them. Their day in the sun belonged to a future when knowledge itself would become an industry. Their glory then was just the hope of the founders' dreams: visionaries, the founders are commonly called. But what vision moved the Dutch-named founder of the New York Central Railroad, whose million dollars southern churchman and kinsman by marriage Holland N. McTyeire had coaxed to establish a university in Nashville, remains a question. Behind his wire-rimmed spectacles few glimmers of idealism were known to lighten shrewd calculations of profit and loss, least of all idealism about universities. But Cornelius Vanderbilt probably understood that reconciliation of old sectional foes called for deeds as well as for words, and he probably understood that as time passed, appropriate monuments to common endeavor

7

might in the minds of the South's notoriously proud and provincial people soften the image of an old battlefield enemy. Schools and colleges rather than railroads and cotton mills, themselves easily seen as a new northern imperialism, seemed right. Patriotism surely moved him to hear the entreaty of his southern relatives and to extend a gesture to the South in the name of good will and understanding. Beyond that, Cornelius Vanderbilt likely did not speculate. His career was a studied series of decisions made largely without philosophical agony, whether they involved railroads or universities.[1]

Whether Commodore Vanderbilt himself ever saw much difference between such things mattered little anyway. He did not live to see much of what his gift built, and his descendants' interest in his university oscillated considerably. Rather, the school he helped to start fell to the guidance of people of different mettle whose aims and interests he knew little of, yet people as talented in administration and scholarship as he had been in commerce and finance. Their numbers were not large, but their strength did not require large numbers. Like the Commodore who in his day also had had little company, they knew what they wanted and, more than most, were in the habit of achieving it.

Half a century after Vanderbilt's beginnings, their success could be read in much brick and mortar in what had once been a cornfield and, more than that, in the solid accomplishment of two generations of teachers and students. Their failures, fewer by comparison, were less well recalled. The Commodore had gone, but others had followed, bestowing the largess of other Yankee fortunes on this southern school. Bishop McTyeire had gone and so had the churchly connection that he represented, but had been replaced by others who, while sharing his faith, more willingly separated religion from education while professing loyalty to both. Much had changed, and the word in 1925 was that more laboratories and freer inquiry would be Vanderbilt's answer to pundits who gleefully paraded the image of a benighted South before northerners of less good will than Cornelius Vanderbilt.[2]

Small wonder then that for the university's fiftieth anniversary there assembled in Nashville by invitation an array of the great and the near-great, in this field and that, to dignify the half-century watershed. The proceedings of their celebration were enthusiastically reported by the local press and carefully preserved by the university itself. That record reads like the records of most such birthday parties: ebullient, congratulatory, filled with good will. The gathering predictably occasioned an outpouring of homilies about solid foundations ("retrospect") and shining futures ("prospect"). That much is common and familiar—heard no doubt long before and certainly many times long since. But something remains that is not any longer familiar in those words and in that pose, something that helps measure the distance in mind as well as in time traveled since then. This is because in addition to marking a semicentennial, October 1925 also marked the opening of the new Vanderbilt Medical School and Hospital, the most modern in the South and among the most advanced in the nation. The presumptions that attended that beginning loom large in what followed and haunt us still. Therefore, it is good to consider them here, at the beginning, and in the boldly assertive idiom that then seemed so fitting.

The new Vanderbilt Medical School and Hospital so proudly shown off that October of 1925 had sprung from the minds and labors of three men whose ideas and hopes it embodied and who were on hand to witness its commencement. Two were laymen, one a physician: James H. Kirkland, native southerner, born a year and a half before the Civil War began, and chancellor of Vanderbilt since 1893, a post he held longer than anyone else; Abraham Flexner, then secretary of the General Education Board established by John D. Rockefeller, Sr., and author fifteen years before of the famous report on medical education that bears his name; G. Canby Robinson, medical educator, administrator, and dean, whose immediate responsibility it had been to build and staff the new school and then to run it. Of the three, Flexner was guest along with many others, Kirkland and Robinson harried hosts. Flexner and Kirkland made speeches; Robinson emceed and probably played the anxious guide to the multitudes that had come not just to celebrate old times at Vanderbilt but to inspect his new medical creation. There is no record of meetings among the three men that October, but it was not a time for private talks. Their lives had become entangled years before and would remain so for some time to come. The relations among them were complicated and, as is frequently the case with talented and ambitious people with similar interests, they found themselves serving one cause but for sometimes different reasons. October 15–18, 1925, however, called forth simpler emotions and, for a moment at least, it was their role merely to celebrate genuine accomplishments for which all modestly took too little credit. They had arrived at that common place along several routes, which in the end buttressed one vision of modern medicine and, beyond that, of scientific knowledge and its utility.

Kirkland was a liberal and thus most marked for disappointment. His life divides almost equally between two centuries: born in 1859 on the eve of one great war, he died in 1939 on the eve of another one. In between he saw the building, rebuilding, and consolidation of the nation's power and the increasing prosperity of its people. As a native of the poor South he approved of such material things and, though his talents led him down different paths, he might well have prospered making steel or building railroads instead. He became one of the country's leading educational entrepreneurs and a master grantsman before that word ever entered the language. During his long years as head of Vanderbilt he guarded, nursed, and added to its endowment and set high standards of financial management. He understood better than many people how money works and how much of it a university consumes. Though he ran a school and not a business, his mind ran to frequent calculations of profit and loss, of risk and return, toward the end of building a fortune not his own. The energy and talent that he brought to that job easily matched the energy and talent of some of the more famous getters and builders who were his contemporaries: John D. Rockefeller, Sr., Andrew Carnegie, James J. Hill, George Eastman, and others. He understood such men and apparently they him, if the large sums shifted from their accounts to his are a fair measure of such understanding. With them he shared a need to accomplish, to matter, and to leave a mark—less in his case as a monument to self than as assurance that for his labor progress had accrued to his fellows.

Kirkland was comfortable enough with his times, which is characteristic of the sort of old-fashioned liberalism he embodied. By a few things— religious faith, intellectual integrity, family life—he set great store. So anchored, he viewed change as an open field for free will to produce right living and good works. He believed in God, family, country, the South, and Vanderbilt, roughly in that order, and in them all he read that progress was not merely possible but indeed tomorrow's probable forecast. A shrewd judge of probabilities for all his career, he willingly and wisely invested the hard work needed to realize the promise of his faiths, and he expected the same in faith and works from others. His understanding of progress belonged as he did to his time and was informed by that large view of the world and man's place in it for which Kirkland's generation was the last collective representative. Temperate in all things and disarmingly respectable, that generation welcomed ordered change in the serene conviction that history was progressively yielding improvement, contentment, and concord.

Likewise serene, Kirkland's adult life happily mirrored the security of that faith. During a career lasting more than half a century, he held only two jobs: professor of Latin at Vanderbilt and chancellor. He was happily married, had one daughter, a house on campus, an apartment in the suburbs, a cottage in Canada; he retired at age seventy-five and died at seventy-nine. Much of the documentary evidence plus the reminiscences of those who knew him invite the fittingly forthright and cheerful biography that was in fact not long in being written (the year after his death, Kirkland's long-time friend and admirer, Vanderbilt English professor Edwin Mims, published his glowing

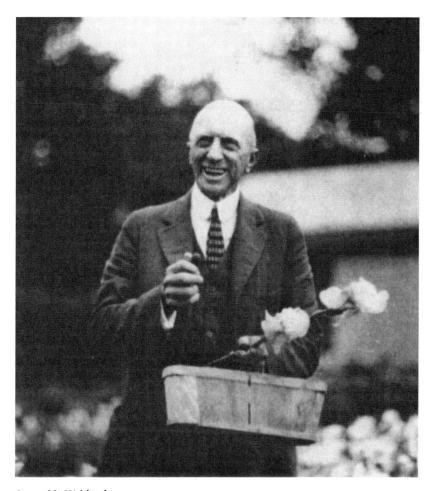

James H. Kirkland

portrait, *Chancellor Kirkland of Vanderbilt*). After nearly fifty years it might well be done again. Much that might engage a new biographer would also interest a wide range of readers, for Kirkland's life touched a larger world than Vanderbilt, though to many he seemed synonymous with it. His life story fully treated would tell more than a little of his times. The records of his life are reasonably abundant and reveal something of his character, which bears on the subject of this particular book.[3]

Kirkland believed, in addition to the stewardship of wealth, in the stewardship of talent and energy. Wealth was never his to give; talent was. True to his Methodist soul, he applied his to the holy cause of making the world into something God might once again be proud of, and where his fellows might be aided along paths of right living. Proud of service, he viewed it as a public charge of which there should be adequate public record. When he died, he was at work on a history of Vanderbilt meant surely less as monument to himself than as record—simply that—of how the job of building Vanderbilt had been done at that time by those who had been there to do it. It would have been a fitting last testament for a man who was what he did. Though not all of what he did concerns us here, something of his background and training does matter in our view of that man who in the autumn of 1925, then at the pinnacle of his career, shepherded the dignitaries around his fifty-year-old campus with its sparkling new medical school. In that most recent and most expensive addition he took much satisfaction and pride. It represented for him more years of hope and labor and patience than it did for anyone else, though he was himself not a physician.

The South where Kirkland was born became in 1861 a battleground for conflicting claims of liberty and union. So fierce was that battle and so comprehensive was the new settlement that reconstructing those momentous issues of 1860 and 1861 required considerable historical imagination in later generations of reunited Americans. Few, years later, chose to dwell any more on the constitutional issues that had been involved, and in the end the Civil War for most southerners and other Americans distilled to only two things: suffering and romance. It came to that for a man born in Spartanburg, South Carolina, on its eve, whose brother's blood was shed by it, whose home life and place were touched by it, and whose father died in the course of it. Later in life Kirkland seldom dwelled upon it, but this much we know: Kirkland's father, William, a Methodist preacher and missionary to the slaves on South Carolina's rice plantations, died suddenly in March 1864, at age fifty. Brothers Joseph, Allen, and William left college and entered the Confederate army. Allen was wounded late in the war and sent home just in time to see federal soldiers in the streets of Spartanburg. William was imprisoned for nine months in the North and died a young man. Joseph died in 1871. Mother Virginia, like countless other war widows, fell to the the heavy task of supporting the balance, and the boy James saw it all.

Kirkland's family suffered like many did, less than some, more than others. It saw firsthand the real and immediate meaning of moral arguments about slavery and the coercion of wayward commonwealths. Out of that fire, it would be tempting to say, the survivors (young James among them) emerged chastened or, in the words of Kirkland's biographer, "eager hearted, self-reliant, alert in mind, serious in purpose, celestial voices prophesying a life dedicated to some high aims."[4] Perhaps. Kirkland became some of those things and he certainly had some high aims. But of his beginnings it can only be said that the future chancellor and builder of medical schools grew up in circumstances none would choose—circumstances that taught heroism, self-sacrifice, and endurance (the things later and so artfully enshrined in romance) but also folly, capriciousness, disease, and smallness of purpose. How much of such things Kirkland actually gleaned from those years is unknown, but for a man of the temperament that he later showed himself to be, it might fairly be inferred from his tempestuous southern upbringing that he might then have begun to develop the sober perspective that was evident later when, taking the measure of different sorts of people and events, he proved so often to back the winners and guess the future rightly.

His own more immediate future, however, led far from that rural southern beginning, and it points to the second part of his youth that bears on the man who presided over the university's celebration in 1925. In the 1870s Kirkland studied and excelled in classics at Wofford College, a small denominational school in Spartanburg, a place of no particular distinction but no worse than much the South then offered. There Kirkland discovered and was discovered by Charles F. Smith (whose family had been Kirkland's neighbors in Spartanburg), a young scholar recently returned from Harvard and, more importantly, from Germany, and by William M. Baskervill, Smith's acquaintance in Germany and a pioneering English philologist. Kirkland finished a master's degree in 1878 and then taught school and tutored Latin, Greek, and English at Wofford, in preparation for that ritual completion of the late-nineteenth-century scholar-to-be's education: the pilgrimage to Germany.

He sailed in 1883, following in an already long line of his countrymen who flocked to the universities of the Second Reich and their great scholars and teachers. He was in good company. Smith had preceded him in 1880 to finish work on his own doctorate; Baskervill had been there, as had Woodrow Wilson, William James, and many others. They went to learn from the undisputed masters of the trade an approach to scholarship, a method of research, and implicitly at least an understanding of knowledge and its usefulness. Unmatched as an educational migration by anything until the great reverse movements from Europe to North America of more recent times, the pilgrimage carried young scholars in many fields seeking the best training that could be had in law, history, religion, psychology, languages, and medicine. Before it more or less terminated with the outbreak of the Great War in 1914 and the subsequent tumble in Western esteem for most things German, two other men in particular managed to follow the same well-worn path across the sea, two men who with Kirkland would share German training and the limelight at Vanderbilt in October 1925: Abraham Flexner and G. Canby Robinson.

After preliminary stops in Edinburgh, London, Holland, and the Rhineland, Kirkland settled in Leipzig, where after a short eighteen months he received his degree. What he learned in the process was likely shared by many other students there and elsewhere and in many fields. Kirkland read languages, specializing in Anglo-Saxon, Old English, Old German, and Sanskrit. He became a philologist, though the general skills he acquired mattered more than what he said in a long and best forgotten thesis on an obscure Anglo-Saxon poem called "The Harrowing of Hell." For hard, plodding German professors he performed hard, plodding, and frequently boring work. He learned respect, if not reverence, for the facts, for bodies of information thoroughly mined and then arranged in such way as to hide as much as possible the presence of the arranger. He learned to be a careful scholar, according to a canon then ascendent, under which the first generation of truly professional academic scholars was being trained. That canon produced a school of prodigious fact gatherers. Careful research, close attention to the text, and the most reluctant of authorial intrusion characterized their training and the scholarly method it taught. Its practitioners viewed themselves as guardians of mysteries unfit for ordinary people, to be shared with only a few and then only after much work and assorted rites of passage. They produced much, and much that was by that standard very good. Yet it would be hard to convince a later generation that much of the substance of what these scholars produced was not obscurantist and the method whereby they produced it not to a degree intellectually crippling.

Yet for half a century at least (much longer in some places and in some disciplines) to that new and exciting style the learned and would-be learned raised sharp salute, and as they passed from learner to teacher they trained their own eager recruits in the same drill. To them, scientific (that is to say, all proper) scholarship was inductive, proceeding from the specific—the discrete observables sought out and gathered up with infinite care—to the general, or if not the general at least to some point that seemed the sum of the many parts. So it was in countless seminars, lectures, and laboratories throughout Europe and the United States. As it turned out, the search for the truth through the search for the facts yielded sometimes more facts than truth. But for many practitioners that evidently was enough, perhaps because in time they came to believe that the facts and the truth were the same thing.

Some, no doubt, were collectors at heart. Others quite certainly became collectors as a result of education, admonition, and habit.

To that club Kirkland in Leipzig paid his dues, becoming a full member in 1885 when he received his doctorate, an event fittingly praised by his greatest fan, his mother, and duly reported in the hometown newspaper.[5] His correspondence with her from Germany reveals an eager young scholar, devoted to his subject, convinced utterly of its importance, and ambitious to make his mark in it. He was then in his middle twenties, and though grateful to his German mentors, he was ready nonetheless to be out from under their eye to pursue his own lines of work. For that he went to Berlin for more Anglo-Saxon and to Geneva where he planned to study romance philology and French. But there he was stricken for three months with typhoid fever, pleurisy, and various complications, three months that altered for good his plans for further study. Early in 1886 he left Switzerland for the Riviera and a tour of Italy with a group of American friends, and then he returned to Leipzig in preparation for his departure from Europe. He had been gone three years and in them had packed a solid German education, elements of the grand tour, and ample chance for meeting Europeans themselves, from scholars to landladies. He accomplished with ease the large leap from Wofford College, the small southern denominational school, to the rarefied atmosphere of the German universities. He returned home, anxious as most young students are about the immediate course of a career long planned, worked, and hoped for. His plan worked. He was promptly elected to the chair of Latin at Vanderbilt, there to put to hard use on the children of the poor rural South his freshly minted learning.

Kirkland knew much about being a scholar. He had learned great respect for detail, factual accuracy, thoroughness, and other assorted Teutonic virtues. But to regard the James Hampton Kirkland, who nearly four decades later led his university's fiftieth birthday celebration and who helped open its new medical school, is to be struck with at least one irony that could not have been apparent when the much younger man returned from Germany to take up, so he thought, the scholarly life. For he practiced that life only six years before becoming chancellor, a job he held for forty-one. He never wrote another book and never produced any more research that his old German professors would have greatly admired. The Anglo-Saxon and the Sanskrit were largely left behind as his life moved in other directions.

To be trained in philology in a late-nineteenth-century German university was not to be prepared for the management of even the relatively small numbers of people and sums of money that belonged to late-nineteenth-century Vanderbilt. Not that the mismatching of formal training with later occupation is in itself especially odd, but in Kirkland's case it bears witness to something that he may well have pondered quietly but never spoke aloud. He spent much of himself, in the middle years of his career, in the building and planning of the first modern medical school in the South. It was a job that he, the layman, shared with many physicians, many of whom were with him that October 1925. That school, and many of those doctors, G. Canby Robinson included, were fiercely dedicated to a new ideal of academic medicine and medical education, the model for which was the Johns Hopkins University, its medical school and hospital, and through it the academic and scientific universe of imperial Germany. The approach was very scientific and very inductive; it began with ascertaining the facts and working from there. Generalization, if it occurred at all, was light. As a younger man, Kirkland too had followed those precepts—though they may have poorly prepared him for the sort of work he would eventually do: to administer, manage, and act. Yet they must at least have taught him the intellectual language, the mental attitude of the academic doctors with whom he would later work and argue. Trained as a scientific scholar, Kirkland became something quite different: a mover of people and of money, moved himself both by a large vision of what the end should be (for him, the advancement of educational opportunity for the people of the South) and by close and constant calculation about the most probable ways to get there. He managed others trained as he had been, but who actually did what they had been trained to do. He must have seen in those around him every day the shadow of what he might have become. Whether he looked with remorse at the road once so shining but quickly foresaken, or with relief at the narrowness and devious turnings from which he had been saved, remains private and hidden safely away.

The record tells what he did and through it what he was. Kirkland was a liberal at the end of an era in which that moderate faith became more and more difficult to sustain. Moderately pious, moderately patriotic, moderately patient, enormously diligent, enormously hard-working, and enormously respectable, he believed in progress and justice and right living. Or he believed in the pursuit of such things, which was what he did. His expectations were and remained modest, at a time when those of many around him were not. As a manager, it was his job to tailor the demands and expectations of talented and ambitious individuals to his own best calculations of probable return. It was a job that suited his moderate temperament but that at times strained even his large resources of patience and compromise. While sober probabilities governed day to day this man whose life divided in years if not in ideas so evenly between the nineteenth and the twentieth centuries, it was large possibilities that ever informed his view of things to come, liberally redeeming the hard reality of what had to be.

Also present to celebrate a birthday and a beginning was another shrewd calculator of probabilities and possibilities, also a nonmedical man, though one whose name probably was as widely recognized by physicians as any of their own kind. In 1925 Abraham Flexner was fifty-nine years old and, like Kirkland, at the peak of his career. His route there, though, differed markedly from his friend's, the chancellor's, whose career was such a model of regularity and stability. Confessedly an opportunist, Flexner was the study of a man who had busied himself over a broad range of the world's affairs, and with more intelligence and with greater success than many of his most talented fellows. He is remembered today largely for the famous exposé of American medical education that came to bear his name.[6] But like the things for which so many of the famous are remembered, that report leaves much unsaid. The story behind it is an often-told tale, its enormous impact a product of timing, luck, the skill of its author, and the confluence of interest between a profession and several major philanthropies. Vanderbilt's medical school—the one being dedicated in October 1925—was a major monument to it. Parts of the report bear especially on the dilemma of modern medicine described above and will receive some close scrutiny in the pages that follow. But for now, the man Flexner, rather than his report, commands our attention, for like the man Kirkland, this individual and his spirit stamped this place as few others have. It was fitting that he had come in person to mark its commencement.

With Kirkland, his good friend, Flexner shared a southern boyhood straight from the pages of a self-help novel. It was a good boyhood for a successful man to write about later in his autobiography.[7] He was born in 1866 in Louisville, the sixth of nine children, to Moritz and Esther Abraham Flexner, Jewish immigrants, he from Bohemia and she from the Rhineland. Moritz Flexner (rather like his sixth child much later and for different reasons) did many things. He was a peddler, a small-time businessman, a venturer in the wholesale hat business—and a loser in the Panic of 1873 when he forfeited a small fortune and most hope for its recovery. That hope, though, in the nine years of life that remained to him, he transferred to his children, and had his life been longer, pride in their success would have been his recompense. Flexner's mother, trained as a seamstress in Paris, had immigrated in 1855 and married Moritz Flexner a year later in Louisville. Together they raised a family and kept a home that Abraham would later recall with much warmth and affection. The intellectual opportunity that it and Louisville offered in the 1870s and 1880s was modest, but not so the intellectual endowment of the Flexner offspring. Abraham reported that his adolescent reading consisted of Plutarch, Bunyan, Hawthorne, Thoreau, Carlisle, and *The Spectator;* that the schools, though generally impoverished, boasted a few inspiring teachers; and that the local library, which supplied him with after-school employment for two years, offered among its ten thousand volumes ample space for his eyes and mind to run. He remembered living conditions typical for that day and place: the chocolate-colored water of the Ohio River and the flow from polluted pumps where everyone drank; the typhoid, whooping cough, diphtheria, and tuberculosis that left doctors and patients alike helpless. He remembered the animosity for damn yankees that fellow Kentuckians, reluctant to join the Confederacy during the war, so fiercely displayed after it.

He also remembered what it was like to be poor, and many years later he saw in that condition an advantage that as a young man he would not have recognized. Had he lived to read Flexner's autobiography, Kirkland (who had seen the same things only a few years before and in another southern state) would surely have applauded. In fact, it was with the example of Kirkland's own early troubles that Flexner sharpened his message: that thrift, self-help, family unity, hard work, and clear thinking were assets as valuable to the nation in the 1930s as they had been to Kirkland's South in the lean years after the Civil War. Flexner praised the South for rejecting federal aid to public education as proposed by the Blair Bill in the 1880s, arguing that it was better that southern schools be built on the sounder rock of local resources and better that the southern people, instead of becoming dependent on federal patronage, might know the "satisfaction of looking upon the results which they have achieved through self-sacrifice and effort."[8] Suffering, as Kirkland the nineteenth-century liberal knew, built character. The blessing of poor beginnings, Flexner knew, was that they spurred youth to move beyond them and in the process to leave some mark of its passing. So, at least, his own life seemed to testify.

Flexner's first large step beyond his beginnings he owed to his eldest brother Jacob, druggist, later a physician, and, after father Moritz, the family patriarch. It was on Jacob's insistence and on Jacob's money that young Abraham entered Johns Hopkins University in 1884. In the two years that it took him to earn his degree he acquired there not so much a body of knowledge on a particular subject but an exposure to learning, a first under-standing of what real scholarship was (something that he would refine con-siderably over the years), and an enormous admiration for the people devoted to it and for the institution that made such devotion possible. It was the Johns Hopkins that Daniel Coit Gilman (whose biographer Flexner became) had built and that he still ran according to a few simple principles: unswervingly high academic standards; sound and clear teaching of those sound and clear subjects that could in fact be taught; the advancement of knowledge through sound and clear scholarly research. Research on the German model was the building wave of the future and Hopkins proudly blazed the way. To provide outlet for it in the day before university presses, Gilman established and subsidized there the *American Journal of Philology* (Kirkland was an early subscriber), the *American Journal of Mathematics, Studies in Political Science,* and later the *Journal of Experimental Medicine.* But it was outlet only for the best. Gilman impressed on his early faculties the distinction between important research and idle publication: *Viel arbeiten, wenig publizieren.* It was the Hopkins of Basil Gildersleeve, Franklin Spieker, Herbert Baxter Adams, J. Franklin Jameson, and Richard T. Ely, men of the first American generation of professional academic scholars, and it was understandably an exciting place for an exceptionally bright student from Louisville.

Flexner read classics under Charles D'Urban Morris. It might well have been something else, for he did not become a classicist, though he continued to read Greek for many years. Indeed he did not become a scholar or an academic at all. As he remembered it after more than fifty years, his time at Johns Hopkins was an uninterrupted spate of hard work, serious thinking, and patient sitting at the knees of learned masters, something unlikely even there and even for Flexner. How much his assessment of undergraduate days at that very young institution was colored by its later great successes and his own continuing and very happy connections with it can only be guessed. But this is certain: a young Abraham Flexner spent two years at a young Johns Hopkins. Flexner got two years of solid education and a A.B. degree. Hopkins got the lasting gratitude of a man who, as it turned out, would exercise great power and influence for seeing to the institution's growth and replication.

Flexner left Baltimore in 1886 (the year that Kirkland left Leipzig for Vanderbilt), seven years before the opening of the medical school he later lionized in his report on medical education. But before he went he crossed paths only briefly and at some considerable distance with a figure newly arrived at Hopkins and for purposes rather different from those of young Flexner, not yet twenty years old. The figure of which he knew so little then was the round and portly one of William Henry Welch, German-trained pathologist and newly designated leader of the still unbuilt Johns Hopkins University Hospital and Medical School. Flexner recalled President Gilman's announcement in 1885 of Welch's appointment and got his first view of the man, whom he later would know so well, one day as Welch emerged from Gilman's office. Welch was Gilman's answer to founder Johns Hopkins's wish,

Surgeon General John Shaw Billings's advice, and the trustees' commission to commence planning for a great university hospital and later a medical school. He received from Gilman a free hand, and he began by bringing to Baltimore the galaxy of physicians and medical scientists that would at a leap establish Hopkins's authority and reputation. From Philadelphia he brought William Osler and Howard A. Kelly, from New York William S. Halsted, from Michigan John J. Abel, and from Chicago Franklin P. Mall, all like himself German-trained. Their names and deeds belong especially to Hopkins, though to the extent (a very large extent) that they were mentor and model for young missionaries to such faraway places as Missouri, Iowa, Tennessee, and China, they belong to a larger story as well.

But as much as the substance of what they and Welch did, it was the technique that mattered: a president or a chancellor moved by a broad charge, conviction of great need, and the presence of funds; his selection of a scientist-leader who knew the subject and how best to staff and build for it; his selection in turn of people highly trained, eager, ambitious, and committed, who themselves enjoyed great freedom to follow inner scientific imperatives wherever they might lead. Later when Flexner's own prestige and power for shaping medical education became as great as Gilman's, he approvingly saw that pattern repeated many times. The time would come, after World War I, when not all of the bright young scholars would be German-trained, but their intellectual ancestry, often traced through Johns Hopkins, remained nonetheless unmistakable. So it was at the new Vanderbilt Medical School that Flexner had done much to begin and to shape and where he was joined that October 1925 by his old Hopkins friend and ally, the great Welch himself.

After his two-year stay in Baltimore, Flexner returned to Louisville, where he spent the next nineteen years as a secondary schoolteacher and principal, something that made him an educator of sorts though hardly the sort he was later to become. By 1905, in his own estimation he was ready to move on, and fortune nicely turned his way. He went to Harvard in the autumn of that year, with his wife and young daughter. There, in preparation for some new endeavor as yet unknown, he began a deliberate process of filling his mind with, as he admitted, the ideas and materials others had thought of first. He viewed, as did many of his time, the American national genius as a practical one, and he gauged himself and his abilities to fit within that mainstream. He did not want to be remembered as a great thinker or a producer of knowledge but rather more humbly as an opportunist guided by large and unselfish notions of how good could best be done. Humility never became him, but his excursion to Harvard and then to Berlin, to study with the great and to gather to himself some of their knowledge, differs in one important respect from the similar trips taken by so many bright young Americans before 1914. He did not go as a scholar, nor did he return as one. No one single field of study ever engaged him with the tenacity that it must engage true scholars, like those he had known at Johns Hopkins. He went and he returned as Flexner, the educator.

At Harvard he studied physiological psychology but was sadly disappointed in teacher and subject. He read philosophy under Josiah Royce, a more successful encounter, and brushed shoulders briefly with William James. In the summer of 1906, a new master's degree in hand, he sailed with his family for Europe. After short stops at Oxford and Cambridge they made their way, "hearts throbbing," he later remembered, to Berlin. Though dismayed by the kaiser's bluster, the ever-present uniforms, and the generally martial air of public Berlin, Flexner reveled in those corners of German life not yet Prussianized. At the ministry of culture he met Max Reinhardt and was allowed an extensive tour of Prussian gymnasiums, and at the University of Berlin he found teachers who reminded him of his Hopkins days two decades before. Of Carl Stumpf, a leading psychologist, Flexner wrote that "he travels through the complexities of a dry subject on a straight line, cutting however, a broad swath, and turning it into a garden as he goes."[9] Friedrich Paulsen, author of *German Universities,* held obvious attractions for the young American educator whose near future held his own books with similar titles and substance.

He traveled to Florence, talked there with philosopher and psychologist Franz Brentano about secondary school reform, and in Heidelberg that summer he wrote his first book, *The American College.* It drew on his recent experience at Harvard and roundly criticized much that he had seen there: the elective system, the lecture system, assistantships, all things that to him explained why so many students entered college with greater enthusiasm for scholarship than when they left it. The book, which Flexner concluded was ahead of its time, failed in the sense that no deluge of reform followed its publication in 1908. But for Flexner it opened the door to the next step in his own education and in his educator's career—the step that turned him, by 1910, into the reigning authority on a subject that two years before he had known virtually nothing about.

One of his book's early readers was Henry S. Pritchett, president of the then recently established Carnegie Foundation for the Advancement of Teaching, and it was through him that Flexner entered the twin worlds of medical education and the great foundations where he would spend the next two decades of his life and become famous. Through Pritchett and the circumstance of a profession ripe for reform and already en route there, Flexner seized the opportunity to become a different sort of educator.

His report on American medical education appeared in 1910. Another, on medical education in Great Britain and Europe (undertaken for the same purposes as his American report: to reform American, not European, medical schools) followed in 1912. That year he joined the staff of the General Education Board, the forum that he and his colleagues Frederick T. Gates, John D. Rockefeller, Jr., and Wallace Buttrick turned into the greatest external influence on and financier of medical education in the United States until the federal government entered those troubled lists after World War II. Through the GEB, the fortune of John D. Rockefeller, Sr., was applied to the selective rebuilding of medical schools in this country. It was an example Flexner hoped would spur others to imitate and to improve. Vanderbilt was one of those singled out, and over the years it received more General Education Board money than any other medical institution, no small part of which can be charged up to the close friendship that grew between Flexner and Kirkland. Flexner left the General Education Board in 1928 but continued his own education elsewhere: as Rhodes Lecturer at Oxford, as author of *Universities: American, English, and German* (1930), as planner and first director of the Institute for Advanced Study at Princeton. He lived productively in retirement and died in 1959 at age ninety-three.

Flexner's career was unusual. He was an unusual man. Not himself a scholar, he spent much of his life a layman in the sense that itinerant intellectual interests never permitted him the luxury and perhaps the ease of long years spent on a single specialty. Yet he knew and admired many men who were dedicated to specialties of one sort or another, and from their lives it is fair to suppose he took something for his own. Among the scholars he counted as his friends appeared the great and near-great of his times, and to them he left the front-line work of seeing to the growth and transmission of knowledge, which was to him the purpose of learning and what schools and universities rightly were about. For himself he chose to stand on the outside, and from there he wove his way in and out of the lives of the individuals and institutions in whose promise he had reason to believe.

The self-image offered in his autobiography and the records of his life among the mighty are not perfectly congruent. He claimed, for example, never to have meddled in the internal affairs of the institutions he helped, which simply was not true. He relied on those whose fortunes a half a century ago seemed begging to do good works; he worked as their employee. But he did not regard the rich as master, a role more subtly that he kept for himself. Between the givers and the getters, Flexner posed as the educator and played the broker. He was a powerful man in the solid ways that the world measures power. When Flexner spoke, people of means and action listened. In the closed corridors of the foundations, the universities, and in medicine, Flexner, who was not rich, not an academic, and not a doctor, spent his days and learned all the turnings. There is every reason to believe that he enjoyed it; certainly he was very good at it.

But that is Flexner only by half. He was also a serious intellectual to whom knowledge and thought mattered. About such things he was probably more serious than most professed intellectuals; he was certainly more serious than most of the foundation, academic, and medical people who filled his life and who, though often highly educated, were not intellectuals at all. Power was both pleasant and a problem.[10] With it he did good works; he helped to bring the old nineteenth-century gospel of wealth to full expression. Comfortable with both the getting and the giving, he approved of how America worked and happily played his part up to a point. When he first came into the world of the foundations, the fortunes of the General Education Board were dispensed through a small office with a staff of six (which included one bookkeeper and a messenger). During his tenure things changed as the institutions that dispensed great wealth took on some of the features of the enterprises that had produced it, only they ran in reverse. Flexner was fascinated. But he cared about understanding, about seeing things clearly, while in power and out. Eventually power waned, and he later felt betrayed by the Rockefeller philanthropies where he once had studied and enjoyed it. Understanding, which once he had used in the service of power, seemed not always to yield it.

As a philosophical problem, Flexner's difficulty is analogue for another implicit in the union of science and medicine that he did so much to promote. Medicine, he said, must be based on science. Medical personnel must by definition be scientists. Science was something that was learned and worked at; through it, slowly, came understanding. People trained in medicine also cared by habit and instinct about utility; through service to the sick came power. The difficulty was that greater understanding did not always yield greater power, while power itself sometimes beclouded understanding. Flexner the intellectual and the power broker never finally sorted it out, but, more than many doctors, he tried.

Abraham Flexner stood out even among the distinguished guests invited to Vanderbilt's fiftieth birthday party, punctuated so nicely by the opening of the new medical school. He viewed there another monument to progress at a time blessed with plenty and success. He viewed it through an atmosphere in which much seemed within reach. He feted the present accomplishment (which in part was his) of his academic hosts and responded with them to the invitation implicit in such occasions to regard the future bursting with promise and the search for new meanings.

He and Kirkland shared much, including the shores of a Canadian lake where both summered for twenty years. Laymen whose minds moved in similar broad channels, they suffered from the distraction that comes with multiple loyalties. Both men had done things other than build medical schools, and they would do still other things in the future. Kirkland, now that he had realized the promise of building one, would spend much of the ten years that remained in his career less glamorously contending with the problems of running one. Flexner, who left the General Education Board in 1928, subsequently turned much of his attention away from medical education.

Not so with the third man—the physician—whose position as dean of the new Vanderbilt Medical School and professor of medicine stood for accomplishment of a different sort. G. Canby Robinson was dean for eight years and lived in Nashville only four, a tenure and a stay not unusual in a fairly itinerant career.[11] But wherever he went, he carried a single-minded understanding of what it was he should be about. It was an understanding that set him apart from Kirkland and Flexner. He knew them perhaps less well than he imagined, and likewise they him. It was an ignorance that stemmed, ironically, from an education at Johns Hopkins and from a career that conformed in fact in so many ways to the intellectual models that both Kirkland and Flexner claimed so to admire but never managed to practice.

Robinson was the youngest of the three, forty-six years old in October 1925, a native, aptly enough, of Baltimore. There, as a young man, he passed through the portals of a still young Johns Hopkins, where he received his undergraduate degree in 1899 and, on schedule, his M.D. four years later. He later recalled that, more than anything else, his years as a medical student there shaped his future intellectual outlook. They were exciting times. The Johns Hopkins Medical School in 1899 was just six years old and was still staffed by the galaxy of great names, which Daniel Coit Gilman and William Welch had assembled there, plus numerous soon-to-be distinguished assistants. As a beginner, Robinson studied anatomy under Franklin P. Mall and physiology under William H. Howell, George P. Dryer, and Joseph Erlanger. Welch himself reigned in pathology, assisted by Eugene L. Opie. John J. Abel, the first professor of pharmacology in the United States, taught that newly imported German science to Robinson and his classmates, whose first taste of clinical work also came in the second year in a course on physical diagnosis supervised by William S. Thayer. Like virtually all medical students then and later, he chafed to apply all that he had learned in the lecture hall and laboratory. To do so under the tutelage of William Osler in medicine, William

S. Halsted and Harvey Cushing in surgery, Howard A. Kelly in gynecology, and J. Whitridge Williams in obstetrics, as Robinson did during his clinical years, meant to be stamped with the spirit of a select group of the world's greatest scientist-teachers. To observe them and to be judged by them was to be initiated into a new medical age, to be convinced utterly of its efficacy, and to be recruited forever into the cause of its advancement.

At the end of a career that ultimately returned him to Johns Hopkins, Robinson judged that place as the best of all possible worlds for young students training to be doctors. Abraham Flexner's own assessment comes to mind. As he remembered them later in life, his Baltimore years were the beginning of his real education, his first contact with real scholars and scholarship. There was a difference though, less in the general sort of experience they shared there (Flexner of course did not go to medical school) than in the sort of lives they later came to lead and on which the Hopkins experience would come to bear. Robinson did at Johns Hopkins essentially what he did for the rest of his life: he worked at medical education. Flexner read classics but never became a classicist. At Hopkins, Robinson got his first view of a new world, which, though changing in the shape and amount of its knowledge, was intellectually complete almost at birth. For Flexner, Hopkins began an education that led in many different directions. For Robinson, Hopkins was the anchor for a medical career that, however wide it swung, held firm to the canons learned in youth.

Robinson graduated in 1903 near the middle of his class and not quite high enough to secure one of the coveted Hopkins internships under Osler in medicine or Halsted in surgery. After some searching, he took a position as assistant in pathology at the Ayer Laboratory at the Pennsylvania Hospital in Philadelphia, then directed by Warfield Longcope, a Hopkins friend who had just replaced Simon Flexner (Abraham's brother), who himself had left for New York to head the new Rockefeller Institute for Medical Research. In 1906, Robinson became resident physician at Pennsylvania and two years later, completing his formal education, left for nine months in Germany at the Munich clinic of Friedrich Muller. He returned in 1909 and, after a brief sojourn in private practice and service as clinical pathologist at the Presbyterian Hospital of Philadelphia, he accepted in 1910 an offer to become the first resident physician at the hospital of the Rockefeller Institute.

From there, Robinson's career took off on the series of excursions ("adventures" he later chose to call them) in academic medicine and administration for which he would be chiefly remembered. In 1913, he moved as associate professor of medicine to Washington University in St. Louis, which one year later received a grant from the General Education Board to establish the departments of medicine, surgery, and pediatrics on a full-time or "university" basis, a movement in which Robinson participated and was then a staunch believer. Ultimately he became dean and found in that role, at Washington University and elsewhere, the proper forum for his considerable evangelical and administrative talents.

His performance at Washington University accounted in large part for his selection in 1919 by Kirkland as the man to steer the reorganization of the Vanderbilt Medical School in Nashville. That project (which to Kirkland's chagrin got larger after Robinson got involved) entailed the recruitment of a new young faculty and eventually the construction from the ground up of a completely new physical plant that integrated medical school and teaching hospital after a plan close to Robinson's own heart. It also took longer than in 1919 Kirkland had expected: five full years, in fact, until the happy autumn opening. Robinson did not even move to Nashville until 1924, filling the interim with, in addition to planning and designing Vanderbilt, a term as acting head of the department of medicine at Johns Hopkins and a trip to England and the Continent to talk with medical leaders, visit hospitals and laboratories, and buy books for the Vanderbilt library. From Denmark, his first stop, he went to Berlin, Leipzig, Marburg, Frankfurt, and Munich, where he met with his old teacher and friend from years before, Friedrich Muller. In Holland he visited Willem Einthoven, inventor of the electrocardiograph, and then in the fall of 1922 finally settled for six weeks in London, where previous acquaintances and introductions opened the doors of some of Britain's most renowned medical scientists. Francis R. Fraser, professor of medicine at St. Bartholomew's Hospital, had been a friend at the Rockefeller Institute. He toured Edinburgh and spent time at St. Andrews with Sir James Mackenzie. At Oxford he visited the widow of his old Hopkins teacher and idol, Sir William Osler, and spent an evening in talk about medical education with J. B. S. Haldane. Finally, A. E. Clark-Kennedy, Joseph Barcroft, and Sir Clifford Allbutt, Regius professor of medicine, hosted him at Cambridge.

Robinson stayed at the new Vanderbilt Medical School only three years, until 1928, when opportunity elsewhere made another move seem attractive. This time he returned to New York as director of the New York Hospital–Cornell Medical College, a huge enterprise to be built on land adjacent to the Rockefeller Institute. As it turned out, however, the choice or at least the timing was bad. Planned on a gargantuan scale in the late twenties, the new institution, which did not finally open its doors until the fall of 1932, ran afoul of the depression. The number of beds was drastically reduced and large areas of the handsome new building were left unfurnished. Economies extended to staff and programs too, and as the tensions and administrative confusion mounted, Robinson left under a cloud of acrimony in October 1934.

Officially, he was "retired" (and in fact drew a pension of $5,000 a year from Cornell for the rest of his life) but in name only. He was shortly off to China as visiting professor of medicine at the Peking Union Medical College, another monument to Rockefeller benefaction. Returning nine months later, he settled down to work on what he called "the social aspects of medicine" again at Johns Hopkins, where he produced in 1939 his book *The Patient As a Person: A Study of the Social Aspects of Illness.* During World War II he headed the blood donor service of the American Red Cross and in 1946 retired a second time to become executive director of the Maryland Tuberculosis Association. He retired a third and final time in 1955, wrote his memoirs, and died five years later at his Long Island home, at age eighty-one.

Unlike James Kirkland and Abraham Flexner, G. Canby Robinson belonged to a profession. Academic medicine was a profession being born just as he was coming of age, and into its advance he had the good fortune to fit his own career. It was a profession newly invested with the authority of inductive science, whose methods and habit of mind its practitioners applied with ever-growing success to unraveling the mysteries of disease. Its doctrine of full-time academic teaching, serious scientific research, and organic ties between medical schools and universities called forth a new caste of functional high priests—Canby Robinson among them—dedicated to promoting its progress. Their success could be read in faculties across the country and their influence in the practicing profession for more than half a century to come.

Robinson helped push and shove his generation into that newly built, light, and lofty chapel that housed the grail of modern medicine. There, he and his academic-scientific fellows fought the good fight according to rules set out in their German-Baltimore catechism. Demanding much of themselves and others, they did good works and so earned the esteem of those they served. But with every discovery that moved them closer to understanding there arose, confounding their success, the suspicion that understanding moved in response to the growth of their own knowledge. Truth changed. Beyond that light and lofty chapel, in modern medicine's dimmer sanctuaries, even their evangelism faltered. Method might remain absolute, but attitudes changed. Canby Robinson personified the new profession of academic medicine, and in it his faith was wholehearted. His and his profession's expectations were high, their accomplishments many. But the very intensity of that faith also made it vulnerable, not to other competing beliefs that it had even then all but banished and still largely holds at bay, but vulnerable to internal dangers less easily combated, if only because they were less easily recognized.

Weakness, internal or otherwise, was not what Vanderbilt's celebrants had come to hear about in the fall of 1925. But those who gathered on Thursday, October 15, in the new Neely Auditorium for an after-luncheon speech boringly entitled "Purpose in the American University" learned, probably to their surprise, that much of American secondary and higher education had no purpose. They heard not uplift but a catalog of evils and providential stupidities. Salvation, they were told, lay in reconciling increasing pressures for intellectual specialism with the need for broad culture, a commonplace more now than then. It could be done. The example of Sir William Osler, a medical man, proved it, as did that of Thomas Huxley, Louis Pasteur, and Matthew Arnold, all people who "had mastered large, though different fields of human thought and endeavor—had mastered them so thoroughly that, aside from their special intellectual interests, they saw life broadly and saw it whole." How exactly those worthies had managed it—or how they would counsel future educators to manage it—the audience waited in vain to hear. It was a speech, and therefore more assertion than argument. But the speaker, who was Abraham Flexner, was clear at least on this: that the "extension of human interest resulting from the development of the inductive and experimental sciences has deprived culture of its singleness of meaning."[12]

Those were strange words to mark the opening of a medical school that was itself a monument to "the inductive and experimental sciences." Reaction to them is not recorded: not Kirkland's, not Robinson's, not anyone else's (beyond a newspaper reporter's happy account of the great Mr. Flexner's speech at Vanderbilt). But the new medical school and hospital whose beginning was celebrated in October 1925 represented much that medical reformers since the turn of the century believed such a place should be. In that, Abraham Flexner, James Kirkland, and G. Canby Robinson, the two laymen and one physician who were its chief architects, found ample satisfaction. Their new school was built, staffed, and its course clearly set. Their accomplishment was secure; they had done the best they could. The history of that new school beginning in 1925 would become a study in the durability and the erosion of their original design for university medical education and research. Other places would come to share that design and the high expectations that it spawned among both the servants and the served. Other places too would bear the burden of Flexner's warning.

PART ONE

Question of Possibility

The True Measure   **2**

Behind that happy opening of the new Vanderbilt Medical School lay at least half a century of medical education in Nashville. More than most cities, in fact, this one prided itself on a long and distinguished medical past. Typically recounted, it was a past where perseverance in the face of long odds made eventually for triumph over adversity and the establishment of values and institutions judged worthy by the community. Too, it was past as foundation: on it others later built good things. It was an early chapter of a history whose design was linear and cumulative. Just as the after-dinner speeches commonly said, the great individuals of yesteryear, sung and unsung, made possible what we, a later generation, brought finally to fruition. Simultaneously, they are memorialized and we reassured. Affirming the ties that bind us with our history, we perform an age-old rite of community solidarity. We embrace our ancestors, and presumably they us.

Most nineteenth-century histories of American communities render their tales in a fairly heroic spirit. Today local history has moved on to other presumably more sophisticated and objective styles. Still, the old histories tell something useful about the authors if not always about their subjects. Boldness, real or imagined, mattered mightily to those who took upon themselves the job of recording a community's history, if the heroic characters who fill their pages are any measure. To talented and enterprising individuals acting either alone or in voluntary covenant with like-minded fellows, such historians attributed much progress and many good works. So defined, change was welcomed and the future filled with promise. The future, however, sometimes represented more than the sum of the hard work and good intentions that had come before. So the history of medicine in Nashville suggests. The new Vanderbilt Medical School that opened in 1925 was not the product of the city's long and revered medical past. Not that the discontinuities were absolute: some people, some ideas, and some problems bridged the old times to the new, but against the weight of others theirs bore ever more lightly. The individuals and the money that built it were new, the idea and the model that inspired it likewise were imported. It was a true carpetbag enterprise. But like other older and more notorious carpetbag enterprises, the agents (like Flexner and Robinson) of this one were as much invited as they were invaders. Nor could their quick and easy success be accounted for without the involvement of an enthusiastic local scalawag (like Kirkland), whose zeal for uplifting his native region was commensurate with the outside resources available to do the job. The essential contours of this enterprise's history do not fit the linear, cumulative ones usually ascribed to such communities and institutions. Nashville's old medical history included the predecessors but not strictly speaking the ancestors of those who followed, even though those who followed paid ritual respects to the shadow if not the substance of that older generation.

During the years when Kirkland was busy locally establishing himself as chancellor and working out in his own mind what a real medical school ought to be like, Abraham Flexner was approaching the problems of medical education over a different route. By the turn of the century Flexner too had established himself as an educator of a sort. The private school he had founded in Louisville had brought at least local renown and profit enough to send his brother Jacob to medical school and brother Simon to work in William Welch's laboratory at Johns Hopkins. When Flexner himself tired of his work as a schoolmaster and moved first to Harvard in 1905 and then to Europe, his own life too soon turned toward medicine. To his first book, *The American College,* which he wrote in Heidelberg, he later traced his entrance into the field of medical reform, thanks to the fact that it was read by Henry S. Pritchett, president of the Carnegie Foundation for the Advancement of Teaching.

As Flexner recalled in his autobiography, he returned from Europe in 1908 in need of a job. The Carnegie foundation, whose work since its founding in 1905 had focused on raising the standards of American colleges and creating a more uniform system of higher education, seemed a good place to look. With an introduction from Ira Remsen, Daniel Coit Gilman's successor as president of Johns Hopkins, he appeared at Pritchett's New York office happily to discover that Pritchett knew his book and shared many of its ideas. They lost little time in exploring future possibilities. Flexner at first thought Pritchett had mistaken him for his bacteriologist brother Simon, then head

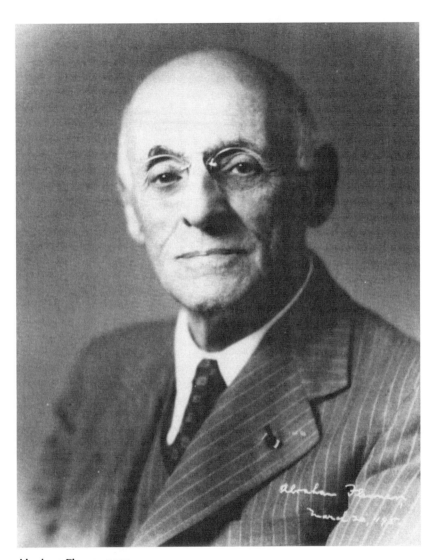

Abraham Flexner, 1953

of the Rockefeller Institute for Medical Research. Pritchett was not mistaken. But he was about to commission a survey of American medical schools, and Flexner the layman and the educator—but not the doctor—was just the person he needed. Pritchett may have been attracted by Flexner's experience at Johns Hopkins, whose medical school would become a measure and model for reform in other places. He was almost certainly moved by Simon Flexner's recommendation of his younger brother. Plus, he had read and liked Flexner's book. Flexner evidently liked what he saw too. He accepted and, with a small salary and a large expense account, shortly set forth on his omnibus tour of the country's 155 medical schools and incidentally on the career that would make him famous.[1]

The full reasons why Abraham Flexner was selected and why he accepted are lost forever in thoughts and conversations never committed to paper, but a few things are clear that surely were clear to Flexner then as well. The game was well afoot by the time he appeared at Pritchett's door in 1908. The study of medical education that Pritchett asked Flexner to conduct was not the brain child of Pritchett alone but stemmed more or less directly from efforts of the American Medical Association's Council on Medical Education to raise standards in the profession and to reduce the number of medical graduates. The council had been established in 1904 as a central regulating agency for medical education and, led by Arthur Dean Bevan of Rush Medical College in Chicago, its five members deftly orchestrated the reform sentiment that ultimately produced Flexner's famous report.[2] For the academic medical scientists, reform promised to secure science in medicine through the agency of palpable institutions: the new kind of medical schools. For the rank-and-file membership of the American Medical Association, reform of medical education held the potential both for raising the prestige of the profession through science and for increasing income through less competition. With the strength of that alliance, the council laid out specific problems and proposed some solutions. At its first conference in 1905 Bevan pinpointed five "especially rotten spots" in medical education, which in addition to Missouri and Kentucky included his own Illinois, fellow member John Witherspoon's Tennessee, and Maryland, where other schools apparently had learned little from Johns Hopkins's example. The council proposed its own high standards for what a modern medical course should eventually look like and suggested some minimum standards that should apply immediately, such as a four-year course and requirement of four-year high school education for admission. In 1906 it began an inspection of the nation's medical schools and ranked them in three groups: eighty-two were acceptable and dubbed Class A; forty-six doubtful, Class B; and thirty-two unacceptable, Class C.

It was with this movement that Pritchett in 1908 at Bevan's bidding allied the Carnegie Foundation for the Advancement of Teaching by agreeing to sponsor a second survey, this one deliberately by a nonmedical man, who turned out to be Abraham Flexner. Not the least of the consequences of that alliance was that it provided the occasion for Flexner's introduction to the world of foundation philanthropy and medical education. There the school-master found his place. He made much of his opportunity. It took him far from his poor southern upbringing, and over the years, as he mediated between the mighty whose wealth he dispensed and countless supplicants, he likely wondered that he should have come so far. If of his foundation benefactors' great wealth he had any moral doubts, they were surely assuaged by the good works they chose through him to do. Their world became his and he moved comfortably in it. His arrival there was one more small monument to the American promise of mobility and fulfillment for the talented individual: Flexner was a success. Like many successful people, his timing was good and his confidence supreme.

The record would seem to vindicate him. After some preparatory reading and visits to Chicago and Baltimore, he began his tour of American medical schools in January 1909 at Tulane in New Orleans and, in what became the pattern, visited half a dozen or so schools and then returned to New York to compile his notes, summaries of which he then mailed to the schools' deans asking correction of any errors. In a year and a half he had finished his travels and his report, which appeared in 1910 as Bulletin Number Four of the Carnegie Foundation for the Advancement of Teaching.[3] To three generations of doctors since then, it has been conventional wisdom that Flexner's report marked the true watershed dividing the old medicine from the new, and if professions need such watershed from which to date their rebirth, the Flexner Report in medicine is surely better than most. Because it prescribed so much that in fact subsequently happened, it was understandably interpreted as the beginning of a new day in medical education so revered by later generations of doctors.

In a sense it was a watershed; its forceful, fact-filled pages did become catalyst for much change in the medical world. But its general theme was not new, and many important preliminaries had already been accomplished. It could be better described as a masterfully timed and executed capstone to the previous three or four decades of reform effort by educators, medical scientists, and the practitioners represented by a reinvigorated American Medical Association. The report was less innovation than meticulous docu-mentation—but it was documentation and the naming of names, plus careful exposition of a better alternative, and it was an enormously powerful polemic in the hands of reformers. In the preface, Henry Pritchett wrote that the "right education of public opinion is one of the problems of future medical education."[4] Abraham Flexner, Pritchett's employee, fashioned a specialized tool to do that job.[5]

The report came in two parts of roughly equal length. The first contained Flexner's rendition of the history of medical education in the United States, his assessment of what presently ailed it, and his detailed prescription for its reform. He drew plainly on others: on proposals for change that had been in the air for several decades (tightened admission standards, a graded four-year curriculum, full-time faculty in the basic sciences, upgraded clinical teaching), on books like Theodor Billroth's *Medical Sciences in the German Universities,* and especially on the model of the medical school and hospital at Johns Hopkins. Not a medical man himself, he counseled with the best who were, learning from Welch, Halsted, Mall, Abel, Howell, and others what the measure for modern medical education ought to be. The second section reported, one by one, how poorly against that measure most schools stood. If ever embarrassment was summoned to the service of reform this was it. Only Hopkins, Syracuse, and Western Reserve thoroughly passed muster. For most of the 152 other schools, Flexner strained for pejoratives.

Sniffing (mistakenly in most cases) Mr. Carnegie's gold behind Mr. Flexner's visits, even the sorriest places opened their doors and account books. There was brought home to Flexner the apparent impossibility of serving at once two gods: profit and education. There the spectacle of local practitioners trying, valiantly in some cases, not so valiantly in many others, to do jobs that required full-time teachers and trained scientists confirmed his suspicion that rebuilding, not repair, was in order. It was not gentle work, but in the atmosphere of righteous battle then settling over the world of medical education, Flexner found it invigorating. Disciplined, documented, and ostensibly objective, his report quickly achieved the results its sponsors intended, and in the process it raised reforming sensationalism to the status of a minor art form.

Flexner's report was not just a compendium of facts gathered to expose and discredit shoddy medical schools, though it was that too. It was an argument, and to understand the medical schools (of whom Vanderbilt was one) and doctors whose magna charta it became, it needs to be examined with some care. An educated man, Flexner knew some history, and it was surely not by accident that he set his argument for medical reform in a historical context. He began on a note of good beginnings betrayed. During the mid- and late-eighteenth century, ambitious young Americans fortunate enough to have gone to Europe to learn medicine in the hospitals and lecture halls of Leyden, Paris, London, and Edinburgh returned home, and through them, Flexner claimed, "the voices of the great masters of that day thus reechoed in the recent western wilderness. High scientific and professional ideals impelled the youthful enthusiasts, who bore their lighted torches back across the waters."[6] With one such fortunate, John Morgan, the organized medical course that was distinct from mere detached lectures and demonstrations—the proverbial anatomy lessons—came to the United States. It began in 1765 at the College of Philadelphia, whose trustees at Morgan's urging created a chair in the theory and practice of medicine. William Shippen, Morgan's friend, soon joined him as professor of anatomy and surgery, as did Linnaeus-trained Adam Kuhn as professor of materia medica and twenty-four-year-old Benjamin Rush as professor of chemistry.

To their example Flexner added the counsel of Thomas Bond, who with Benjamin Franklin thirteen years before had established the Pennsylvania Hospital. In 1766 Bond wrote *The Utility of Clinical Lectures,* and there Flexner spied the historical mandate. The student " 'must Join Examples with Study, before he can be sufficiently qualified to prescribe for the sick, for Language and Books alone can never give him Adequate Ideals of Diseases and the best methods of treating them.' " That meant bedside teaching where, in words that Flexner said held particular relevance for his own time, " 'the Clinical professor comes to the Aid of Speculation and demonstrates the Truth of Theory by Facts.' " There the professor " 'meets his pupils at stated times in the Hospital, and when a case presents adapted to his purpose, he asks all those Questions which lead to a certain knowledge of the Disease and parts Affected; and if the Disease baffles the power of the Art and the patient falls a sacrifice to it, he then brings his Knowledge to the Test, and fixes honour or discredit on his Reputation by exposing all the Morbid parts to View, and Demonstrates by what means it produced Death, and if perchance he finds something unexpected, which Betrays an Error in Judgment, he like a great and good man immediately acknowledges the mistake, and, for the benefit of survivors, points out other methods by which it might have been more happily treated.' "[7]

Thus, nearly a century and a half before were set forth two of Flexner's own requirements for reformed medical schools: that they be organic parts of colleges or universities and that the teaching be practical, something that required close connections with a large public hospital. A final year's study was offered to students who already had "a competent knowledge of Latin, mathematics, natural and experimental philosophy [and] a sufficient apprenticeship to some reputable practitioner in physic." Consisting of lectures and "attendance upon the practice of the Pennsylvania Hospital for one year,"

Flexner thought it "well calculated to round off the young doctor's preparation, reviewing and systematizing his theoretical acquisitions, while considerably extending his practical experience."[8]

To Flexner it mattered little that much of the substance of what was then taught was wrong. Science left to its own advance would have repaired that. More important, right method and sensible institutional arrangement had been achieved: clinical training, preceptorship, and university ties. On such a base subsequent generations might have built wisely, adding to it new knowledge born of their own more scientifically enlightened times. Although Pennsylvania was joined by other admirable medical schools at Kings College in New York (1768), Harvard (1783), Dartmouth (1798), Yale (1810), and Transylvania (1817), their good beginnings were soon forsaken as the proprietary system, which seemed better to suit American tastes in the nineteenth century, flourished. But for that curse, American medical education might have evolved more sanely and in keeping, said Flexner, "with the general increase in our educational resources. The number of schools would have been well within the number of actual universities, in whose development as respects endowments, laboratories, and libraries they would have partaken." The university connection "guaranteed certain standards and ideals, modest enough at that time but destined to a development which medical education could, as experience proved, ill afford to forego."[9] Proprietary arrangements guaranteed other standards and hardly any ideals at all.

Flexner made the explosive growth of the proprietary schools in the nineteenth century the centerpiece in his ensuing tale of woe. Since their appearance, "medical colleges have multiplied without restraint, now by fission, now by sheer spontaneous generation." He calculated that the United States and Canada together had produced an astounding 457 medical schools and, even though many died young or were even stillborn, a hefty 155 still survived in 1910. Among the worst offenders, "Illinois, prolific mother of thirty-nine medical colleges, still harbors in the city of Chicago fourteen; forty-two sprang from the fertile soil of Missouri, twelve of them still 'going' concerns; the Empire State produced forty-three, with eleven survivors; Indiana, twenty-seven, with two survivors; Pennsylvania, twenty, with eight survivors; Tennessee, eighteen, with nine survivors."[10] It was just too easy. Thomas Bond's admonitions about clinical training were long since forgotten. Science had not made clear to enough Americans the need for expensive laboratories and better-trained teachers. The nation was growing. West went the huddled masses yearning for land and apparently for doctors too. William Osler had said that human beings had distinguished themselves from the other animals by their desire to take medicine, thereby inviting their own abuse. Moreover, the large number of providers and the primitive state of the art kept the price people paid invitingly low. Half a dozen or so practitioners sufficed to form a "faculty," and payment of their fee was all a student usually needed both for admission and for graduation. Predictably the bad drove out the good. As proprietary schools expanded, the medical schools even at Harvard, Yale, and Pennsylvania dissolved all but formal ties with their parent institutions. The age-old honored tradition of preceptorship withered and with it contact between teacher, student, and patient. As students listened increasingly to lectures and studied prepared "quiz compends," they no longer read their master's books, submitted to the master's examination, or rode the countryside with the master "in the enjoyment of valuable bedside opportunities." The few good doctors that the country had managed to produce did not weaken Flexner's point. They had succeeded despite a system geared to mediocrity.[11]

By the misbegotten alliance of growth and profit medical education in the United States had gone in one direction while slowly but surely the practice and theory of medicine had moved in another. Some doctors knew that, and with reports of their efforts to do better Flexner lightened his gloomy account. A trend toward a graded course, its extension to four years and lengthening of the term to nine months, the supplementing of didactic lectures with more demonstration and clinical teaching, all by 1910 were apparent. Admission standards in some schools were rising, and better teaching compelled by creation of state boards also raised hopes. Clinical and experimental laboratories were becoming less rare. The Chicago school that eventually became the medical school of Northwestern University introduced a three-year graded course as early as 1859. Harvard decisively reclaimed its medical department in the 1870s, and, favored of all with Flexner, in 1893 the Johns Hopkins Medical School opened its doors, not for business but for education: "the first medical school in America of genuine university type, with something approaching adequate endowment, well equipped laboratories conducted by modern teachers, devoting themselves unreservedly to medical investigation and instruction, and with its own hospital, to which the training of physicians and the healing of the sick harmoniously combine to the infinite advantage of both."[12]

Much remained to be done, so severe was the damage of the proprietary period. The early improvements Flexner credited typically to the "genuine professional and scientific conviction" of a few right-thinking, not easily discouraged men. He believed ultimately in the efficacy of individual action and in the potency of ideals allied with intelligence. In laymen like Charles Eliot at Harvard and physicians like William Henry Welch at Johns Hopkins he saw what that alliance meant and he took strength from what it had produced even in bad times. Future reform surely would depend on others who were similarly secure in their own convictions and confident of their action's beneficent outcome. But in the future, Flexner was also convinced, even giants would need help. Their faith and hard work had indeed made progress possible and had accomplished not a little, but the largely uncoordinated reforms that had first pointed the way now demanded deliberate strategy and another argument to buttress them. Flexner and his report provided the argument, the foundations a strategy.

Flexner argued from the question of society's needs. Reform of medical schools, he reasoned, might conceivably always be driven in part by farsighted and inspired individuals, but the force of their convictions would in future be supplemented by a social mandate as well. That mandate, in fact, had always been part of the old equation that related medicine's product to people's needs. Into it Flexner now factored the "ideals of medical science," which he said better served the very popular needs whereby the proprietary schools had long justified their existence. "The question is, then, not merely to define the ideal training of the physician"; "it is just as much, at this particular juncture, to strike the solution that, economic and social factors being what they are, will distribute as widely as possible the best type of physician so distributable."[13] His ideals were exotics that flourished only under very special controlled conditions. He wanted hothouses and to get them he struck at the very heart of the proprietary system. What the country needed was fewer but better medical schools producing fewer but better doctors. He was no equalitarian: only the few were fit vessels for ideals, but they could be trusted to serve the needs of the many.

He appealed to recent American history. There was once a time when the undeveloped condition of the country helped explain even if it did not excuse the chaotic state of American medical education. But with the spread of technology ("widely ramifying railroad and trolley service, improving roads, automobiles, and rural telephones") the United States had "measurably attained some of the practical consequences of homogeneity." He meant that the nation was settled and was settling in. Although it still invited thousands of hardly homogeneous immigrants yearly to its shores, its comfortable middle-class character seemed assured. It sought coexistence between stable values and institutions and its ever-worshiped dream of mobility. Though its central government was still relatively small, a bureaucratic style and organization was coming to characterize business, industry, and the professions. Technology, which allowed development of national markets and quick communications, helped integrate the diverse cultural values of a polyglot continental nation to resemble at least a kind of homogeneity. If imperfect, the resemblance was enough to serve as Flexner's bridge to the subject that really interested him and that he had to finesse if he was persuasively to argue for scientific medical education from the premise of social need. He had to make a strong case for the reduced members and the different kinds of doctors he believed a modern, supposedly homogeneous nation required.

Again Germany was the example. It was an older and obviously more homogeneous country where conditions might, said Flexner, mirror for Americans something of their own future.[14] Germany had far better and for its population far fewer doctors than the United States: 1 for every 2,000 people in the country at large and in the large cities 1 for every 1,000. In the appalling contrast with the United States, which then had 1 doctor for every 568 people in the country at large and in the cities 1 for every 400, Flexner read the simple lesson of overproduction. Although some had argued for years that large numbers of doctors meant better medical service, still in 1910 at those ratios there were many American small towns without a physician at all, good or bad. Two conclusions might be drawn. Either there were not yet enough doctors to go around, or no amount of overproduction could compel perfect distribution. Crude sums, Flexner said, were poor measure of how much society actually reaped "of the advantage which current knowledge has the power to confer."[15]

So, towns like Wellington, Texas, with 5 doctors for 87 people, or Killbrook, Ohio, with 3 doctors for 307 people, probably had at best 1 good doctor each and an excess of underworked poor ones. "So enormous an overcrowding with low-grade material both relatively and absolutely decreases the number of well trained men who can count on the profession for a livelihood" and "does not effectually overcome the social and economic obstacles to spontaneous dispersion." Areas that naturally failed to attract doctors would be better served by the more widely extended services of one very well-trained doctor (Flexner believed that a physician's "range" increased with competency), who might even be a salaried district physician, rather than by hoping to attract to every hamlet more numerous less-qualified people. To remote but promising areas, on the other hand, Flexner believed good ambitious doctors would not hesitate to go. That they had not he blamed the bloated medical schools: "We may safely conclude that our methods of carrying on medical education have resulted in enormous overproduction at a low level, and that, whatever the justification in the past, the present situation in town and country alike can be more effectively met by a reduced output of well trained men than by further inflation with an inferior product."[16]

The large cost of educating young people in the new scientific ways tended naturally to limit their numbers. Even the resources that the philanthropic foundations soon made available were finite. But Flexner sought to justify in terms of service what science in medicine demanded and would receive anyway. Thus he opened up the problem of what would happen if the knowledge produced by science through observation, experiment, and induction did not relate to the perceived needs of people growing ever more expectant of science's service. If it did not relate, then pressure from outside science and medicine might compel the scientists to attack problems from which the limited state of their knowledge should have disqualified them. Science might suffer or even be changed altogether. That one day the demand for service might outstrip the supply of useful knowledge derived from science was not, however, Flexner's immediate problem, and in 1910 it did not vex him greatly. For the moment reform was the thing. Through it science and service seemed perfectly joined: "The modern point of view may be restated as follows: medicine is a discipline, in which the effort is made to use knowledge procured in various scientific ways in order to effect certain practical ends."[17]

Flexner's sponsors and Flexner himself were committed to reducing the number of poorly qualified doctors and low-grade medical schools because they believed that only then could science be advanced and the medical needs of the country be better served. That advancing the cause of science should claim high social priority was not quite yet the orthodoxy it later became, but it was an appealing idea and Flexner helped it along. Trickier even then were pronouncements about the needs of the country for medical care; there, Flexner turned to the trusted model. His system for determining what the country needed took as reasonable figures the German ones: 1 doctor for every 1,000 people in the cities, and 1 for every 2,000 people in the country, or, averaged, a ratio of 1:1,500 nationwide. In the United States, those thousands of poorly trained physicians already in practice and who accounted for the present overcrowding would soon be history.[18] Henceforth by limiting the production to 1 new doctor for every increase of 1,500 in the general population, Flexner proposed over the next generation to establish the proper ratio without causing a shortage. Thus he calculated that the increase in population of 975,008 outside the South for the year 1908 required production of 650 new doctors. Death, in the meantime, had removed 1,730 from practice and, if only one out of every two such vacancies were filled, another 865 new doctors would be added, for a total of 1,515 (though he believed that many vacancies should remain unfilled for a decade to come and that therefore a figure of 1,000 adequately represented true needs). In fact, 3,497 doctors were actually produced outside the South in 1908, or two or three times as many as the country needed. Nor was the South, whose relative material and educational poverty justified, some felt, continuance of commercial schools with low standards, any exception. There, the states of the old Confederacy plus Kentucky gained 358,837 people in 1908 and lost through death 500 physicians. At a ratio of 1:1,500, 240 new recruits could serve the population increase while 250 would fill half the vacancies and make for a total of 490 for the year. Instead, 1,144 actually were produced by southern medical schools (plus 78 southerners trained in Baltimore and Philadelphia). Whereas barely a third that many could hope to earn a decent living, the poor South had "no cause to be apprehensive in consequence of a reduced output of higher quality." Its requirements, "in the matter of fresh supply are not," Flexner concluded, "such as to make it necessary to pitch their training excessively low."[19] On this effort as on so much else the South must now rejoin the union.

Fewer and better doctors gotten simply enough by *producing* fewer and better doctors summarized Flexner's plan. Endowed, discriminating, and standardized, the new type of medical school would accomplish that as directly as the old type of medical school—commercial, democratic, and idiosyncratic—had caused the problem. His specific proposals for what that new type of school should look like along with abundant ridicule for the old type made up the balance of the first part of his report. Familiar enough today, they became then a handy general blueprint for much rebuilding. Small wonder that so many schools looked so much alike and found in their alikeness such cause for pride.

He began at the beginning with standards for admission. The first subjects studied in the medical curriculum—anatomy, physiology, and (as biochemistry was then known) physiological chemistry—assumed real preparation and manipulative skill. Basic knowledge and skills in biology, physics, and chemistry, for which an already crowded medical curriculum allowed no time, had to be taken for granted. No self-taught person or even a high school graduate likely had them. Only a college course of at least two years provided these things. With luck it provided much more. Modern doctors needed not only instruments and instrumental knowledge to take the accurate measure of disease but also other even scarcer "apparatus" (Flexner's word) to take the measure of the sick people in their charge. He wrote:

Specific preparation is in this direction much more difficult; one must rely for the requisite insight and sympathy on a varied and enlarging cultural experience. Such enlargement of the physician's horizon is otherwise important, for scientific progress has greatly modified his ethical responsibility. His relation was formerly to his patient—at most to his patient's family; and it was almost altogether remedial. The patient had something the matter with him; the doctor was called in to cure it. Payment of a fee ended the transaction. But the physician's function is fast becoming social and preventive, rather than individual and curative. Upon him society relies to ascertain, and through measures essentially educational to enforce, the conditions that prevent disease and make positively for physical and moral well being. It goes without saying that this type of doctor is first of all an educated man.[20]

Flexner believed that that kind of education was had at college or not had at all, least of all in medical school whether old or new. College then was the place for future doctors to begin.

Too few did. As Flexner summarized them, the entrance requirements of American medical schools divided them into three groups, two of which merited attention. Out of 155 medical schools, 22 demanded for admission at least two years of college work; approximately 50 more asked something like a high school education. The balance (the worst of the commercial establishments) touted an array of usually unenforced standards that seemed to bottom on basic literacy. Schools in the first group were presumably already on the road to reform and it was from the second that other good schools must be culled (Vanderbilt belonged to this group). Their chief problem with admissions was the notorious matter of "equivalents." Flexner learned here never to take catalog statements at face value but to compare them with the actual credentials of students admitted. The often-wide discrepancy told him that if a school advertised any form of sliding scale in its admission policy, then "the real standard is perilously close to the 'equivalent' that creeps in modestly at the bottom." In the actual conduct of the subsequent medical course such permissiveness meant that the real standard of work was set up by the bottom, not the top. The teaching of elementary, premedical subjects actively discouraged enrollment by the smaller number of well-prepared college students whom the schools should instead be courting. The "equivalent" in the phrase "a high school diploma or its equivalent" was no more than "a device that concedes the necessity of a standard which it forthwith proceeds to evade." The results, as confessed to Flexner by medical faculty with small reason to exaggerate, could be read in the quality of the student body: " 'The facilities are better than the student'; 'the boys are imbued with the idea of being doctors; they want to cut and prescribe; all else is theoretical'; 'Men get in, not because the country needs the doctors, but because the schools need the money.' "[21] Undemanding as the actual course was in many schools, their still-high student attrition rates—20 to 50 percent in the first year—confirmed their laxness (at Hopkins less than 5 percent dropped out).

It was a social as much as an educational issue. Proper doctors could not even in the best medical schools be cut from other than proper students to begin with. To Flexner and his fellow reformers a better class of students needed to be coaxed into medicine, and means meant frankly to accomplish that required no apology. Their critics' protest that a "poor boy" would by high standards be eliminated from pursuit of a medical career they answered thus: to no social estate, rich or poor, was attached any right to the practice of medicine. The needs of society best dictated the kinds of individuals to whom that privilege should be accorded. The schools that typically justified low standards by claiming service to the poor, themselves poorly served society's needs, which were paramount to any individual's ambitions. Such schools were not, moreover, even "cheap." "Equivalents" enabled admission of more students, presumably some poor ones among them. But depending as they did exclusively on fees, they never waived tuition or offered scholarships to students of meager means, who did not necessarily get what they had paid for. At least, for about the same price elsewhere they could have gotten something much better. Four years at "equivalent" schools in Baltimore, Philadelphia, and Chicago then cost about $1,420, while for $1,466 at the University of Michigan the "poor boy" for the same sacrifice might have had two years of college work in preclinical science and fours years of medicine. "Low entrance requirements flourish, then, for the benefit of the poor school, not of the poor boy."[22]

To be figured accurately in the long run, however, medical education's social as well as its individual costs had to be rung up. In tuition fees alone, Flexner figured that about three million dollars was being invested annually in medical schools. For less than that, he claimed, the country could better educate the smaller number of students it really needed to supply a more efficient medical service. Counting the waste caused by the incompetence of poorly trained doctors, the savings became even greater. Those who had once planned to enter medicine but who were barred by higher standards society could employ elsewhere more usefully anyway. To serve society's medical needs, the "poor boy" had as good a chance as the rich one, if he began for the right reason: simply, because he liked it. If he could demonstrate competence at it then his course was set, happily for him regardless of reward and rightly for the society that would be well served by him. In the context of arguing that well-trained doctors did not necessarily shun small towns that promised smaller incomes, Flexner said that it was a matter of taste, not income, that led people to the scholarly and professional life of which he thought medicine a part. That taste and intelligence knew no class bounds was not to say that those who shared such tastes when educated in the new kind of scientific medical schools would not themselves one day constitute a class of their own whose proprietary pretensions in their profession might have appalled Flexner.

That not-so-distant future was beyond his control, but it did seem to Flexner that if proper people could be gotten into the medical schools, a reformed and highly standardized curriculum would there transform them into the scientific doctors the country needed. That curriculum became over the years something of an article of faith in American medical education, and though it was tinkered with here and expanded there, it remains today fundamentally intact. It was not original with Flexner. It consisted of a four-year course (to which two years of college was prerequisite) divided sequentially into preclinical and clinical subjects. Anatomy, physiology, biochemistry, pathology, and pharmacology (plus introduction to physical diagnosis) took up the first two years. Medicine, surgery, pediatrics, obstetrics and gynecology followed in the last two. The preclinical subjects the student learned less in lecture hall than in laboratory; the clinical subjects less in amphitheaters than in hospital wards and clinics. Wherever, students learned by doing much in the spirit of the old preceptorial tradition. But now they learned "facts" sanctioned by science and, in addition, learned a way of thinking that enabled them through clinical or experimental research to arrive for themselves at new facts. No mere pupils but rather physicians-in-training, talented young people moved by high scientific ideals passed an active apprenticeship.

The facilities where they might do so were still in 1910 sadly lacking, a fact that in part occasioned Flexner's polemic. By his tally roughly thirty schools were then equipped and staffed to teach the preclinical sciences to a truly modern standard, though many more claimed to and did not. Flexner took that number as evidence that the laboratory movement, though inadequate, was firmly rooted and its future assured. With it, however, the reform of clinical instruction had not kept pace, for the fundamental reason that the practicing profession itself had still "in large measure to be educated." Not until the professional and pecuniary interests of local practitioners in the university teaching hospitals were overridden would the quality of clinical instruction equal the quality of students' preclinical preparation for it. Only by constant exposure to abundant and varied "clinical material"—sick people whose illnesses demonstrated the pathological principles of disease—could students learn to relate the knowledge acquired in the preclinical training to tangible manifestations of disease. It was imperative that hospitals be controlled solely by university administrations through full-time teaching staffs. The first purpose of such hospitals should be patient welfare, which would be promoted by the teaching and learning that occurred there. No longer present on sufferance but on the contrary "part of the hospital machine," medical students learned by watching and by doing under the careful super-vision of wise and able doctors who were their partners as well as their mentors. Like other university professors, these clinicians needed to be sala-ried—and content to take less than they might on the outside for the privilege of teaching and doing research. All "academic salaries paid to the right men are [too low]," said Flexner, the professional student of academe. "But there is no inherent reason why a professor of medicine should not make something of the financial sacrifice that a professor of physics makes."[23] They could not have it both ways: science and a consulting practice developed for merely professional or commercial reasons did not mix.

Flexner's requirements for university hospitals thus were high: sufficient size, integration and coordination of teaching facilities with the laboratories of the medical school, a teaching staff that was also the faculty of the medical school, control of teaching and treatment exclusively by that staff. Any of several arrangements might accomplish this standard: a cooperative endow-ment as at Johns Hopkins, state support and connection with a state university as at Michigan and Iowa, or through genuinely effective mutual affiliation as between Lakeside Hospital of Cleveland and Western Reserve University or between Barnes Hospital and Washington University in St. Louis. No form would be easy to establish. Building new laboratories from the foundation up was easier, strangely, than renovating a hospital system that had evolved independently and had long served other gods than science and teaching. Historically, hospitals and medical schools in the United States had not grown up together. When the schools became convinced first of the financial and later of the scientific importance of some sort of clinical instruction and sought access for their students to these "temporary homes for sick people," the restrictive terms they got were far from what they needed. Excessive competition assured "that privileges be divided and restrictive," something not helped by the typical inferiority of the students that was "an insuperable obstacle to any teaching method which sought to use them in the wards in any responsible way whatsoever."[24] Whole new hospitals were often required to make this part of reform work, and they were expensive, extraordinarily so as it turned out. No form of architecture and building cost more than hospitals. Operated as university teaching hospitals had to be (as essentially public service institutions even though they might technically be private), little else seemed to demand such large and steady subsidy.

All of this Flexner knew and candidly documented in his report. If ever there were a dauntless salesman, he proved himself here and with expensive goods at that. Perhaps he suspected that given such long opening odds, any subsequent large accomplishments (in which he would play a large part, though he did not in 1908–1909 know that) would be lauded even more fulsomely. Or, perhaps simply as a zealous reformer, he would redeem the future from utter squalor. Either way, his success would seem to have been large indeed. As his sponsors wished, he fashioned a powerful educational tool. And his layman's prescription for the reconstruction of American medical education persuaded countless doctors who with much talent and energy gave their careers over to its realization. If not in all its detail then clearly in its essential substance, the report read the future for the next thirty years remarkably well. Even though, thanks to the large role Flexner personally played in that future, the report became a self-fulfilling prophecy, it certainly need not have been.

Had Flexner gone back to his work as a schoolmaster in Louisville—instead of to work as a foundation master in New York—things may well have turned out the same. Medical schools became firmly attached to the universities, most of them in medium- and large-sized cities. Their admission requirements and their curricula were reformed and uplifted as he said they must be. Their faculties and their hospitals truly became dedicated to teaching, not practice. The weak and commercial schools closed; the survivors sought and found, outside the profession either with the philanthropic foundations or state governments and sometimes with both, the gold required by reform. To Flexner's 1910 maps rendering his proposal for the reduction and geographical distribution of medical schools, history conformed reasonably well, certainly to his own satisfaction. Medical sects, though withering incompletely, were pushed by scientific medicine further beyond the pale of respectability and safely out of competition. The coercive power of state regulatory bodies and boards of medical examiners compelled ever higher and more exclusive professional standards. Postgraduate work was transformed from its original role in medicine as an "undergraduate repair shop" to an intensive, elective, specialized activity largely within the university system, all as Flexner foresaw.

Also as he predicted, medical schools exclusively for women would disappear and, though not formally barred, women would not flock to the coeducational (but in fact largely male) schools. "Now that women are freely admitted to the medical profession, it is clear that they show a decreasing inclination to enter it. More schools in all sections are open to them; fewer attend and fewer graduate. True enough, medical schools generally have shrunk; but as the opportunities of women have increased, not decreased, and within a period during which entrance requirements have, so far as they are concerned, not materially altered, their enrollment should have augmented, if there is any strong demand for women physicians or any strong ungratified desire on the part of women to enter the profession. One or the other of these conditions is lacking—perhaps both."[25] Flexner rested his argument on statistics for the years 1904–1909. Apparently it did not occur to him to suspect that official declarations of equal coeducational opportunity might have been less than sincere, at least not in the way he had suspected the sincerity of official pronouncements about general admission requirements that were in fact honored largely in the breach. Like many men—and women—Flexner was not always perfectly consistent.

Medical education for Negroes, he said, should be concentrated in only two of the seven black schools then in existence; the two were Howard University in Washington, D.C., and Meharry Medical College in Nashville. He presumed that black education would be separate from but equal to that of whites, granted that, as a poor and backward people, blacks' needs were somewhat different from whites'. Hygiene, not surgery, best fitted them, and it was the missionary role of the only two schools with any promise to train young black doctors so to serve their own people, in the towns but still largely in the rural South. On this matter, whites, on whose benefaction the success of Howard and Meharry depended, should be especially moved. Said Flexner: "self-interest seconds philanthropy." Ten million blacks lived in close contact with sixty million whites, and hookworm and tuberculosis were no respecters of the color line: "The Negro must be educated not only for his sake but for ours." Although Flexner was later accused of supporting the campaign to cut all medical education for blacks, his views on the matter in 1910 were for that time neither particularly ill-advised nor ignoble.[26]

Thus Abraham Flexner's report summoned purpose and a plan for the future. Its argument for the acceptance of great possibilities carried for a time all before it and gave its author, not theretofore a man who conspicuously sought limelight, celebrity for a lifetime. Of another book far distant in subject though not dissimilar in spirit (Alfred Milner's *England in Egypt*), Flexner's contemporary Winston Churchill said, more than a mere book it was "a trumpet-call which rallies the soldiers after the parapets are stormed, and summons them to complete the victory."[27] So did Flexner's report. With it began in earnest the campaign to establish, consolidate, and secure. Not original, it became a seminal catechism for reform whose origins, as time passed, would wrongly be ascribed largely to Flexner alone. Wherever reform's origins, its results numbered among others the new medical school and hospital that Flexner helped christen at Vanderbilt in 1925. At such places younger people answered his "summons" to "complete the victory," and theirs was a story of a great success. It was also a story of grand designs trimmed to fit other fates.

To Flexner, the report was a systematic whole that unfortunately did not suit all those who in years since have posed as its disciples. The highest purpose of modern medicine, it said, was the practical application to people's needs of scientific knowledge discovered at bedside and bench. In medicine, science and service were joined. It was a broad faith that welcomed many comers less catholic than Flexner himself, whose narrower interests later stirred dissension. In time the faithful divided particularly into two groups that read back into the report their own law and made of Flexner their own exclusive prophet. To many academic doctors and probably to most doctors in private practice in the United States, the report was the fountainhead for the doctrine of scientific excellence. They pointed to its repeated emphasis on sound training in the basic sciences and mastery of the scientific method. They approved of clinical training in teaching hospitals where apprentices carefully learned by doing under the eye of watchful masters.[28] To some other academic doctors and fewer though often vocal doctors in private practice, Flexner's other message was long and wrongly drowned out by that chorus of scientific excellence. Flexner, they said, did not really place the highest worth on medicine as science as such but on medicine's "social function." They cared most—and said he did too—about matters of prevention, public health, and most broadly, public service.[29]

Selective quotation was easy enough; the great man seemed to provide abundantly for all partisans. He provided in fact for none at all. He did not segregate medicine as the pursuit of scientific excellence in the abstract from medicine as a humanitarian social service. One indeed was prerequisite for the other. Until the art of medicine became "scientific" (according to standards Flexner enumerated but did not originate) and thus acquired the means actually to do something useful, it made little sense to talk nobly about the medical profession as "an organ differentiated by society for its own highest purposes."[30] Until they became properly scientific, it was positively dangerous to regard physicians as a "social instrument" at all. And unless maintained in that status by new knowledge sprung from scientific research, their power would dwindle relative to the expectations it generated. To seek the truth through science and to do good by applying that truth through service to humankind described the natural history of essentially one idea, if not always one person. And no more than any writer did Flexner have the power to control how his words eventually might be interpreted. As the framers of the United States Constitution demonstrated that words and phrases capable of broad interpretation last the longest, so it may have been with Flexner's report. But its longevity owes at least as much to luck as to design, and Flexner was not just then building a monument to self. He hoped that his work would be put to immediate practical use, in the large work of reform. He tried therefore to be clear and not to mislead.

It is not the smallest or least remarked irony that the Flexner Report helped achieve the standardization of general medical education just as, thanks to science, the practice of medicine privately and in university teaching settings was becoming less general and more specialized.[31] As that happened the powerful alliance of interest between the practitioners and the academic doctors that had united them behind reform in the early twentieth century broke down. Although Flexner claimed that he had called for no undue standardization and rightly pointed to allowances made to account for local conditions (as in the South), the drive to ensure the creation of essentially one kind of doctor for many different needs eventually ran afoul of critics who said that practice demanded something else. Finally, Flexner also had put the case for scientific medical education in utilitarian terms, something that certainly made much tactical and historical sense. Medicine had always been understood as a service; that was its justification. To advertise its newly enhanced ability to perform that service seemed a sure way to convince a practical people of its worth (and the price was high). Scientifically trained doctors served better. With new knowledge they eased suffering and saved life as no doctor had ever done before.

But medicine had not always been science, as science came to be understood in Europe in the late nineteenth century. As science, medicine's new knowledge came over an inductive route different from the one followed by earlier empirical doctors. Thus understood, science was a new means to an old end, and its method could indeed be applied and directed to ends deemed desirable by other than strictly scientific values. "Science declares war on hookworm, on tuberculosis, on cancer," pundits ever since proclaimed, fairly reflecting both the large hopes encouraged by science in medicine and the scientists' willingness to try to satisfy them. But the true mandate of science in medicine or in anything else was internal; its knowledge was developed by observation and was verified by experiment. By its own rules and procedures was it found right or not right. Medicine, however, proved a peculiar and especially troublesome kind of science. Verification of its knowledge was never enough; justification through utility was needed as well. The historic art of medicine whose purpose was to serve thus complicated the evolving science of medicine whose purpose, in addition, was to know. Ever since, they have been all mixed up in the happy but very helpful phrase "the art and science of medicine."

To argue for science from utility, as Flexner did, was to invite conflict with its method, which sometimes ran to nonutilitarian ends. Perhaps the method was wrong, perhaps the understanding of utility too narrow. What to do if science did not serve in the ways imagined for it was the question implicit in Flexner's argument and in the history of the schools modeled on it.

Gathering Substance 3

Most loyalties are multiple, usually comfortably so until by some shift of sentiment or interest a choice is forced. That happened most memorably in American history in 1860 and 1861 when southern Americans felt compelled to pick between the jealous gods of liberty and union. It happened first in American medicine around the turn of the century when a profession newly anxious to raise its status and self-esteem perceived that the means to that end—expensive scientific medical education—mixed poorly if at all with profit. On that Flexner did not equivocate, and high mortality among proprietary schools immediately before and after his report appeared to prove him right. Munificent subsidy from foundation philanthropy shortly replaced the stingy support of local investors and solved the problem. New medical schools and hospitals institutionalized the union of science and medicine. It worked wonderfully but not all at once. The actual mobilizing of resources required to make it work at Vanderbilt in the 1910s affords a pertinent illustration.

By the standards that Flexner proposed for American medical schools, Vanderbilt in 1910 was not much to look at. After a decade and a half of operation as part of the university, it remained a place where old proprietary forms and habits coexisted unsatisfactorily with younger "university" ambitions. James Kirkland, for the price of a new building, had enticed allegiance from the medical faculty on whose good will and hard work alone the enterprise turned—for the chancellor, with his slim exchequer, had nothing more to offer but good words and wringing hands. He knew already what Flexner discovered on his whirlwind whistlestop inspection of Nashville's medical schools in January 1909.[1]

53

The main body of Flexner's report mentioned Vanderbilt specifically nine times, six to hold it up as a bad example of general problems, three to praise it, if only for worthy efforts under trying circumstances. On admissions he was critical. First-year students, for example, were found already to be studying in the medical school for two months without having submitted any preliminary credentials to an examiner.[2] The high drop-out rate attested to the inadequacy of admission standards. Out of the first-year class of seventy in the 1908–1909 school year, those dropped, passed conditionally, and failed totaled 44 percent. Nor did Flexner care much for anatomy lessons: "Elsewhere, dissecting-rooms are indeed found, but the conditions in them defy description. The smell is intolerable; the cadavers now putrid, as at Temple University (Philadelphia), the Philadelphia College of Osteopathy, the Halifax Medical School, and in many of the southern schools, including Vanderbilt."[3] The school's financial arrangements meanwhile were hopeless.

Flexner claimed never to have used a questionnaire, though it is doubtful if all his information was gathered during his short visits alone.[4] Indeed, after his visit to Vanderbilt in January 1909, he corresponded with the medical school authorities there at least three times, seeking the kinds of information that went into the final report. The first inquiry was nothing if not a "questionnaire" asking seventeen questions, the answers to which reveal more about the state of medical education at Vanderbilt than either Flexner's few references to it in the report or any of the university's own public announcements.[5] Given the incentives that the medical schools in general had to cooperate with Flexner's investigations (fear of the onus of noncooperation and hopes for possible subsidy suggested by Flexner's connection with Andrew Carnegie's foundation) and the character of the two men (William Dudley and Lucius Burch) he dealt with at Vanderbilt, there is good reason to trust those answers.

However he gathered his information—whether during his personal visits or later through questionnaires—Flexner found at Vanderbilt and elsewhere what he set out to look for: lax enforcement of low standards, poor facilities, part-time faculties, and meager or nonexistent endowments. Flexner's was not then an especially difficult job. Even had they wanted more to hide from this itinerant minion of medical uplifters, the schools like Vanderbilt likely could not have done so, at least not for long. Flexner's stated belief that medical schools whether public or private were in fact public service institutions[6] became steadily more persuasive as the curve of popular expectation for the good they could do trended steadily upward. Vanderbilt, which was certainly not among the worst schools he judged, was hardly among the best either, and it had much about which to be embarrassed. But like the vast majority, it welcomed exposure—as part of what it rightly perceived to be a larger campaign to build up what Flexner's report ruthlessly tore down. "If I can be of further assistance to you," wrote faculty secretary and professor of gynecology Lucius Burch, closing his reply to one of Flexner's queries, "in the noble work that you are undertaking, elevating medical education, it will be my pleasure to serve you at any time."[7] Even granting the quite real incentives, such willingness took stout hearts and thick skins.

Kirkland's were among the stoutest and the thickest, and it was with characteristic deliberateness and patient faith that he set Vanderbilt to the task Flexner had assigned it. Throughout his long reign as chancellor, Kirkland was nothing if not possessive about his university, and the lead he now took in rebuilding its medical school was only the premier of numerous episodes in which he both proposed and disposed and in general had his way. The opening moves were already afoot in advance of Flexner's report and confirmed the wisdom of Flexner's first prerequisite for reform: consolidation. Nashville early in 1909 still had three medical schools for whites: Vanderbilt, the University of Nashville, and the University of Tennessee. Seeming excessive even to their interested practitioner-faculties, the local profession that year arranged a merger between the University of Nashville and the medical department of the state university that, though it was to run initially until 1912, proved so unsatisfactory that within a few months numerous faculty from the University of Nashville contingent had resigned and offered their services to Vanderbilt. Students too deserted and as a consequence Vanderbilt became with the 1909–1910 school year a larger if not a better operation. After 1910 and after both Pritchett's and Flexner's outside recommendation, consolidation gathered steam. In mid-June 1911 Kirkland reported with pleasure that negotiations had led to an agreement whereby the University of Nashville medical department had agreed to quit the field altogether, and the University of Tennessee medical department had agreed to remove itself from Nashville (first to Knoxville, eventually to Memphis). To accommodate displaced professors, Vanderbilt reorganized its faculty, made some new appointments, and began its new role as Nashville's one white medical school with a roster typically (for then) top-heavy with senior people: twenty-five professors, seven associate professors, plus various lecturers and assistants. What mattered most, though, was that Vanderbilt now stood alone: practically, it was the only remaining institutional object for local professional pride and efforts at reform. So reduced to a single local factor, an equation was now at least imaginable in which that one institution could be deliberately matched with outside talent and resources in the objective of radically changing its nature.

Kirkland meanwhile was not unaware of the large substantive shortcomings of his medical school with or without local competition. A litany of complaint and warning he kept constantly before his board and thus, permanently minuted, before history as well. He understood the direction of the Council on Medical Education's national campaign to upgrade medical schools first by rooting out the most inferior of them.[8] And he understood that while strenuous efforts of devoted teachers thus far had kept Vanderbilt apace of the council's requirements, it could never by itself be expected to meet the anticipated new challenges of a rapidly upgrading profession. New knowledge demanding new education was rendering obsolete old institutional arrangements; science, unlike practitioners, could not survive on fees. Without large endowment (the medical school then had none at all) he found it impossible to conceive how Vanderbilt could provide the expanded hospital facilities and pay the salaries of the full-time scientist-teachers by which the credibility of all schools would shortly be judged. Although he knew its tactical value and himself had engaged in it for fifteen years since taking the medical school into the university, the technique of muddling through would do no longer: "It is clear that the time is coming, perhaps in all our professional work—certainly very speedily in medicine—that this work must be abandoned or liberally supported."[9]

Short of a threat but clearly a warning, Kirkland's preaching on the matter deftly apportioned praise and blame on those whom he would badger and cajole into better ways of thinking and doing: "Our department is therefore recognized as one of the best and perhaps the very best school of medicine in all the South. We have prestige, our graduates have made a splendid showing before state Boards, our faculty have been loyal to the highest interests of the University and their department." He added: "We have invested a great deal of labor in the work of this department. We have a long and honored list of alumni. Our medical faculty has worked and is working faithfully with very small remuneration." It was curious, then, that into the Elm Street building (which the university had erected but whose maintenance and equipping were the responsibility of the medical faculty) during a full fifteen years had been put practically no new equipment beyond a few hospital beds. To outside eyes good intentions mattered even less, Kirkland wrote: "The work of our Medical School has been severely criticized by the offices of the American Medical Association and of the Carnegie Foundation. It has been with difficulty that some of these criticisms have been kept out of the public prints."[10] What was more, within two years Vanderbilt would be compelled under the American Medical Association's classification system to increase significantly its hospital facilities and to enforce more rigidly its admission requirements.

The shortcomings were not really the faculty's fault. Hospital wards and new laboratories for chemistry, physiology, and anatomy cost a great deal, more than even the most devoted and wealthy practitioner-teachers on their own could or would ever provide. Nor were they the ultimate object of Kirkland's persuasion. He would do his best to keep them on his side (something that in the next decade would not always be easy) and to enlist their support for the changes that he knew they alone could not bring to pass. As he lectured, his true aim became apparent: "The pressure of public sentiment and the influence of Medical Association will soon drive from the field all ill equipped institutions and leave medical education in the hands of the great universities that are able and willing to make large expenditures in this cause."[11] Wanting above all to build at Vanderbilt a "great university," Kirkland the layman first had to have a modern endowed medical school, which partly defined it. The effect for him of cementing medical school to university was quite the same as it had been with Flexner, though the logic ran in reverse. Flexner's concerns seemed narrower: to infuse the medical school with the spirit of research, attach it to a university. Kirkland's seemed broader: build a great medical school as partial means to the end of building a great university.

Medical education and medical science already served by enthusiastic new converts and soon to be fueled from the nation's greatest fortunes had taken on new velocity, intolerant of old habits and old institutional arrangements. Vanderbilt might very easily be left by the wayside with the many other schools that Flexner said should be. Of that Kirkland, who was no believer in a charmed history for his beloved school, was sure. He was also sure that salvation, if it came, must come from the outside.

This acknowledgment of the need for outside help was fitting, for Vanderbilt owed its very existence to northern philanthropy, though of a more personal sort than it would later become accustomed to. The old Commodore (so-called because before building the New York Central he sailed a fleet of ocean liners and Hudson River steamboats) gave his namesake university a total of $1,003,600—$1 million for land, buildings, and endowment, and $3,600 to endow the Founder's Medals, given annually to first honors graduates in each school of the university.[12] His descendants carried on, some more munificently than others. In the lean beginning years William H. Vanderbilt, the Commodore's only son, donated $150,000 for the construction of Wesley and Science halls and the gymnasium, and by his death in 1885 had added $300,000 in bonds to the school's endowment.[13] Two of his sons gave more than their grandfather: Frederick W. Vanderbilt, whose approximately $5 million came largely through testamentary bequest,[14] and William K. Vanderbilt, part of whose smaller total of about $1.5 million (most given during his lifetime) touched directly on Kirkland's efforts to upgrade the medical school in 1910 and on the foundation support he secured to do it.[15]

An exchange of real estate negotiated between Vanderbilt and George Peabody College for Teachers in 1910, whereby Kirkland planned to acquire a spacious new setting for his medical school, was contingent on cash payment by Vanderbilt of the difference in value between the two pieces of property, an amount initially estimated at $25,000 (it eventually figured out at $33,820). Because general endowment funds were not to be encroached upon, the arrangement depended on some outside benefaction, something that Kirkland none too modestly claimed to have anticipated and neatly to have seen to. Here reentered the old family patron and Kirkland's other carpetbag allies whose names figured henceforth ever more prominently in the evolution of American medical education at Vanderbilt and elsewhere. Of the funds required to finance the exchange, Kirkland had secured from William K. Vanderbilt in the summer of 1909 a promise of $150,000, a sum that became fifteen months later the match for a like amount from a newer foundation patron, the General Education Board. Together, they constituted the largest sum to come to the university at one time since the original donations of the Commodore, and it was with understandable excitement that Kirkland so reported on October 25, 1910: "No hour in our history since its foundation was ever so filled with the prospect of advancement and educational improvement as the present one. Matters to be decided by the Board at this meeting [final approval of the exchange of property with Peabody and the affiliation that implied] are not casual incidents, but are the result of years of forethought and hard labor, and many are the workers who have contributed to make possible the present issue."[16] As the issue related to the Rockefeller philanthropy in particular it was hardly casual indeed.

Donations from a member of the Vanderbilt family were always welcome but hardly new. But the grant from the Rockefeller philanthropy was new, and it represented the beginning of a long and lucrative relationship of another sort between Vanderbilt and institutionalized philanthropy. Over the next three decades the General Education Board would become the largest single supporter of medical education in the United States, and of the more than $60 million it had dispensed by 1928, Vanderbilt's medical school received more than any other institution. Given both the munificence of that subsidy and the expectations attached to it, something of the General Education Board's origins and personnel bear directly on Vanderbilt's subsequent story.[17] The board's beginning filled another page of the same chapter in the stormy history of North–South relations that accounted for the beginnings of Vanderbilt itself. It began not with the Rockefellers but with others of means and talent whose good will after the Civil War and Reconstruction found in the educationally impoverished South ample field for good works. As genuinely missionary as the Baptist, Methodist, and Congregational churches that practiced uplift through establishment of sectarian schools, northerners like Boston banker George F. Peabody and Connecticut textile magnate John F. Slater pursued educational renewal along more secular and ecumenical channels. With the suffering South as his target, Peabody gave $2 million in 1869 to endow the Peabody Fund; Slater gave $1 million to his own fund and dedicated it specifically to the education of southern Negroes, long the favorite object for northern reformers. From within the region a cadre of progressive southern educators made willing and vital partners in reform: Jabez L. M. Curry, distinguished Confederate veteran and long a supporter of public schools; Walter Hines Page of North Carolina, editor, later diplomat, and conjurer of the South's "forgotten man"; Charles W. Dabney, president of the University of Tennessee; Edwin A. Alderman, president of Tulane and later of the University of Virginia; Hollis B. Frissell, principal of the Hampton Institute; and, of course, Kirkland himself.

It was to Robert C. Ogden, a northerner, however, that credit usually goes for inspiring what would become the General Education Board and for interesting the Rockefellers in it. In addition to being partner in John Wanamaker's department store business, Ogden was a self-styled evangelist for and supporter of southern schools, particularly for Negroes. He had helped found Hampton Institute in Virginia, the first industrial school for blacks, had served on its board for twenty-seven years, and had become its president in 1894. In 1898 he became key organizer of a series of annual conferences that brought together educational leaders from both sections to discuss problems and the strategies for their solution. Three years later, in 1901, with a wonderful show of ostentation in the service of uplift, he chartered what would become over the next few years the first of several private trains on which prominent like-minded and wealthy people toured first-hand some examples of what educational philanthropy could accomplish in the South: Hampton Institute, North Carolina College for Women at Greensboro, and Booker T. Washington's Tuskegee Institute in Alabama. Among the guests on that first excursion was young John D. Rockefeller, Jr., the oil magnate's son and heir, then just four years out of Brown but with a keen interest in shaping the family's educational philanthropies.

Some of those philanthropies were already large. Such giving as the senior Rockefeller's liberal endowment of Vassar College and Brown University and even his building from the ground up of the University of Chicago had been essentially personal in nature (much like the Vanderbilt family's support of their namesake institution in Nashville) or if not personal then mediated through the services of faithful retainers like Frederick T. Gates. But by the turn of the century Rockefeller's fortune (like Carnegie's) had grown so enormous and the demands for its philanthropic use so heavy and so varied that a specialized institution for giving was called into existence: the foundation. For the promotion of general educational reform first in the South and then nationwide (the bright idea that Rockefeller, Jr., brought back from his trip) the foundation, staffed by experts in giving, seemed the ideal institutional form. It would, so the elder Rockefeller hoped, regularize and make more efficient the wise distribution of his wealth, a job that neither he himself nor his family alone could possibly continue to oversee. At the same time, it would demonstrate anew the beneficence that a capitalist's fortune could make possible.[18]

Due first in part to Ogden's own interests, it appeared that the new foundation would confine its activities to education for southern blacks, but on other advice (from, among others, Wallace Buttrick, secretary of the Baptist Home Mission Society and frequent Rockefeller counselor on southern educational matters, and from Washington and Lee president Henry St. George Tucker, who argued that it was futile to try to uplift southern blacks while neglecting southern poor whites—Page's "forgotten men") it was decided not to limit the project to the needs of any single race but to conceive it in the broadest possible terms. So in January 1902 Ogden, Peabody, William H. Baldwin, Morris Jesup, Curry, Buttrick, and Rockefeller, Jr., decided on the substance of the new philanthropy (taking, as Curry noted, "broad, farseeing views, contemplating a series of years, much money, and wide action").[19] A month later, having added Albert Shaw, Page, Hopkins president Daniel Coit Gilman, and attorney Edward Shepard, the group finalized a broad charter for what they named the "General Education Board," its purpose "the promotion of education within the United States without distinction of race, sex, or creed."[20] Baldwin became the first chairman, Gates was added as a trustee, Buttrick was tapped as executive secretary, and, on behalf of his father, Rockefeller, Jr., pledged $1 million to the new enterprise. The trustees originally had hoped that the board would not be a Rockefeller philanthropy alone, but rather that it would act as a clearinghouse for donations from other wealthy people for the cause of southern education; thus the name: *General* Education Board. Although that hope came to nothing when such capitalists as J. P. Morgan and Andrew Carnegie failed to climb aboard Rockefeller's bandwagon, the name stuck. For the balance of its fifty-eight-year lifetime, the board was backed by none but Rockefeller money. But as a monument (which many foundations in a sense are) it always lacked what so many others had: the name of its founder as part of its own.[21]

The prosaic name bespoke large intentions. The GEB was incorporated by Congress on January 12, 1903, but it had already opened for business the previous April with Buttrick at the helm. In the early years it concentrated, true to its origins, on southern primary and secondary education and farm demonstration work.[22] In 1905, however, Rockefeller, Sr., at the bidding of trusted manager Gates, enlarged the purpose of the board "to promote a comprehensive system of higher education in the United States" and provided an endowment of $10 million to finance it. It was in this new role that the Rockefeller philanthropy first touched the history of Vanderbilt with its grant in 1909 for $150,000, which was the money Kirkland needed to consummate his treasured Peabody arrangement. Gates had counseled Rockefeller, Sr., that in essence his fortune was accumulating faster than he was giving it away and that if he wished a say in its ultimate disposition only two courses of action were possible: "One is that you and your children while living should make final disposition of this great fortune in the form of permanent corporate philanthropies for the good of mankind . . . or [the second,] at the close of a few lives now in being it must simply pass into the unknown, like some other great fortunes with unmeasured and perhaps sinister possibilities."[23] The specter of state confiscation through income taxes and death duties and forced redistribution for uncertain but certainly pernicious purposes—"sinister possibilities" for sure—was not a little in the air just then. Gates's alternative thus amounted to an ultimatum, which the Rockefellers proceeded to accept. Rockefeller wanted to keep at least some general control over the disposition of his property; Gates showed him how to do it.

Comparing aims to accomplishments in its support for colleges and universities, in the field of higher education the board was less successful than later it would be in medical education. Rockefeller aid, declared Gates, must not be scattershot but deliberately administered "to contribute, as far as may be, toward reducing our higher education to something like an orderly and comprehensive system, to discourage unnecessary duplication and waste, and to encourage economy and efficiency." Specifically, board funds should be distributed so that there will "gradually emerge a series of institutions of higher learning which shall be for the United States territorially comprehensive, harmoniously related, individually complete, and so solidly founded that it will, as a whole and in all its parts, survive the vicissitudes of time."[24] It was a large order that was never filled, but the strategy it proposed—of coercing comprehensive reform through giving—proved eminently serviceable. On higher education generally the board learned techniques it would employ again in medical schools, which proved more amenable to systematizing than colleges and universities. The procedure became familiar. Exposure through investigation was followed by selective support for the most promising places, with that support usually conditioned on local contributions.

Here then was the perfect field for the beneficent dispensing of Rockefeller's millions, through the offices of experts whose business it became to know all there was to know about higher education in the United States. Convinced there were already too many schools, the board never founded a single college but gave its aid to existing strong or at least highly promising places sensibly situated in centers of population where a local constituency could be expected to supply students and some money. "A few of our colleges are so located as to assure influence, permanence, and power," Gates wrote. "Many are so located that they must perish and ought to do so."[25] In the board's New York offices a series of maps plotted this principle of optimum strategic location with clusters of colored pins depicting where colleges in fact were and where, based on the prospects of enrollment and patronage, the "law of college growth" dictated they should remain. Gates calculated that roughly a quarter of the existing schools would meet the country's needs and that that number could in fact realistically be formed into a system of higher education and be adequately financed.

The nation's general growth and birth rate in the twentieth century confounded that calculation, while local pride continued to frustrate Gates's ideal of territorial distribution. Still, the board's policy of selective support did provide the solid financial footing that made many schools for the first time relatively secure institutions. It gave almost exclusively for permanent endowment, demanding almost always that its gifts be matched within a certain time period by a specified sum from other sources, and many were the institutions surprised by their own success at raising the funds required to receive the board's grants. The results at least in funds generated if not in a system built were gratifying. Between 1902 and 1925 the board dispensed for general endowment about $60 million to 291 schools (Rockefeller having greatly increased his original contribution). To get it the schools themselves raised $140 million.[26] The board's view of its role as stimulator of other public and private support for higher education seemed thus vindicated, likewise its policy of buttressing only those in whose promise it already had good reason to believe.

That notion of "promise" remained always somewhat fuzzy, and never was the board in its support of higher education in general able to articulate the explicit criteria for support quite as convincingly as it did with medical education.[27] But evidently there was promise at Vanderbilt, enough at least to attract the $150,000 of Rockefeller money that Kirkland with such satis-faction reported to his trustees in the fall of 1910. Ever awake to new sources of support, he had watched the movements of the Rockefeller board since its beginnings and specifically those of its first secretary, Wallace Buttrick, the man he would court most diligently until Buttrick was joined at the board in 1913 by Abraham Flexner. Once a Baptist minister and secretary of the American Baptist Home Mission Society (which ran schools for southern Negroes), Buttrick as a Rockefeller employee made it his business to know well the fund-raising college presidents, appointments with whom so regu-larly filled his calendar. Compared with the imperious Frederick T. Gates, who was his close friend, Buttrick was warm and genial indeed, an artful cajoler and subtle master of many board and committee meetings. Of what he wanted in the end though, he was as certain as his more autocratic colleague with whom for twenty years he guided the work of the board. What he wanted—the uplift of higher education across the country and especially in the South—required, beyond Rockefeller dollars and matching dollars alone, partnership with like-minded individuals well tutored in the uses of such money. With Kirkland as much as with any of his supplicants he found such partnership, indeed almost fraternity. Their correspondence goes back to the early days of the new foundation, Kirkland gently probing the possibilities, Buttrick praising in happy generalities the good work the young chancellor was doing at Vanderbilt and the promising future for his school.

The first fruits, $150,000 conditioned on Vanderbilt's securing an equal sum from other sources, came in 1909 under the board's campaign to bolster the endowments of selected promising colleges and universities. It is impor-tant to remember that Kirkland made the request in the context of his by then long-running campaign to associate the new George Peabody College for Teachers with Vanderbilt and to obtain for Vanderbilt's failing medical and dental departments Peabody's old south Nashville campus where at least there would be room to grow. Two sorts of expenses were thus entailed. First, there was the cost in the exchange of property as worked out between the two schools: what Vanderbilt got was deemed to be worth approximately $33,000 more than what it gave. Kirkland also believed that there would be other yet unknown obligations rising from the affiliation with Peabody and the growth he anticipated would stem from it. To meet those costs Kirkland had to go outside, and his choices resulted in a happy combination of the older personal philanthropy of the Vanderbilt family and the new foundation giving of the General Education Board. The use to which the board's funds could be put, however, was restricted to permanent general endowment for the university, which was fine. Kirkland needed that too. But with his faltering medical department he sensed a more critical or at least a more immediate need. In an attempt to answer it, he asked his new foundation patrons to bend the rules.

He had received word in 1909 that the grant had been approved by the General Education Board. Early the next year he wrote to Buttrick to plead the special case of the medical school, whose fate, he explained, was tied to the whole Peabody arrangement. He asked permission to apply the funds to the as yet nonexistent endowment of the medical school. The answer came quickly and unequivocally from Buttrick, who had conferred about it with Gates. First he offered the good words: "Our Executive Committee made their contribution to Vanderbilt University largely because of our high appreciation of the place and work of that institution in the educational leadership of the South." Next he restated the policy: "It is our wish that the major portion of the sum, if not all of it, shall be added to the free, unrestricted endowment of Vanderbilt University. Mr. Gates joins me in expressing the hope that you may find it practicable to take this course, and to make other adjustments of the matters [the medical school] discussed in your letter." He gave the formal reasons: "Our board believes that institutions of higher learning should have adequate free and unrestricted endowment. We do not make contributions until we have confidence in the management and education policy of a given institution of learning. When such a basis of confidence has been established, then our gifts are placed absolutely at the disposal of the management of the institution. . . . The General Education Board is anxious that its funds shall be used for such free endowment of institutions of higher learning, rather than for the erection of buildings, or even the endowment of specific departments." More to the immediate point, Buttrick explained that at its last meeting the board had specifically considered the whole question of making contributions for the endowment of technological, medical, and other professional education and had reached the unanimous decision "that it was not wise for us to depart from the general policy of promoting the endowment of colleges of the arts and sciences." In keeping with that decision, the board had recently refused to support "one of the best medical schools in the country. You can see, therefore, that any announcement of a considerable gift to the medical college of Vanderbilt University [hardly one of the best in the country] would put us in an embarrassing position." Therefore, Buttrick concluded, the board's offer stood unchanged with the "understanding that you should secure $150,000 with which to purchase for your medical department the campus of the old Peabody College for Teachers" and that its subscription of $150,000 for general permanent endowment of the university would be "payable when the further sum of $150,000 has been paid to the University in cash."[28]

Buttrick knew that Kirkland already had from William K. Vanderbilt promise of the matching funds, and thus to him all seemed ready for a happy consummation.[29] So it seemed to Kirkland too, despite the rebuff on the issue of General Education Board support for the medical school itself. He was by then seasoned in judging the limits of his own supplications; he knew when to wait. Besides, he probably guessed that the ways of the still-young Rockefeller philanthropy were not yet fixed and that last year's refusal might well become next year's enthusiasm. Rules might not bend to his special pleading, but policy might change to meet his and others' larger needs. If that was his guess, it was a good one, for over the next decade, under the guiding hand of Abraham Flexner, the board made medical education a target for large subsidy—medical education at Kirkland's Vanderbilt largest of all.

Patronage by an individual or even by a family like the Vanderbilts was one thing. Frequently casual or sentimental, rarely entailing deliberate philanthropic strategy, it built monuments to an individual's generosity. Patronage by foundations and later by the state was something else. Institutions that patronized other institutions had as their business policy making, not monument building. Artfully fashioning philanthropy into a specialized tool for reform, the Carnegie Foundation for the Advancement of Teaching early in the century thus had effected enormous change in the quality of American colleges, and later the General Education Board did the same for the medical schools. The bounty was greater than the old type of patron had offered, and so were the risks. Some of those risks stayed submerged as long as the purposes of the patrons and the patronized were reasonably congruent, as they generally were in medical education at least for the period when private patronage predominated.[30] But when they more and more diverged as they tended to under public patronage, trimmers naturally appeared who, when the call came for a division, tended that master who paid.

At Vanderbilt the preliminaries in which that new pattern first emerged began with the General Education Board's 1909 grant, which had not been for medical education at all, and with Kirkland's discovery that to deflect a foundation from a fixed policy was beyond even his powers of persuasion. The setting was complete for a scenario of expansion and improvement, but more space answered only one of the school's immediate needs. Higher admission standards—another part of the reformers' campaign to winnow out weak students and weak schools—posed even more fundamental problems. Following the consolidation of Nashville's white medical schools, Vanderbilt enjoyed larger than ever enrollment, 396 in 1911–12, and larger receipts, up from $33,000 to $50,000. Those fees alone supported the school, and even after the move to the south campus, where it was no longer obliged to pay rent to the university as it had since 1895, receipts still did not keep pace with expenditures. But if it was to retain its standing as a Class A medical school, Vanderbilt was obliged by the fall of 1914 to implement admission standards calling for at least one year of college. The result was to reduce drastically both the number of entering students and the receipts from fees. What had been entering freshman classes of one hundred fell in September 1914 to nineteen, and some of them "could not meet the requirements of the department without some indulgence." As the old larger classes graduated and new smaller ones entered, it was estimated that by 1916 or 1917 a low point of one hundred students in all four classes would be reached, after which gradual but slow growth could be expected.[31] By the simple arithmetic of shrunken fees and the rising costs of well-equipped laboratory and hospital facilities, to say nothing of full-time teachers, generous endowment had become the absolute precondition for modern medical education.

To Kirkland, whose business it had been for nearly twenty years to nurse his university's precious general endowment, that was no surprise. To beg, coax, and cajole money for endowment was, he knew, to appeal less to a patron's interest or vanity than to altruism. Gifts for endowment had the power to reproduce themselves far beyond the giver's own lifetime and thus to confer immortality of a sort. What they did not offer potential benefactors was the relatively quick gratification of brick and mortar monuments, and they were therefore very hard to get. To make it easier was the aim of the General Education Board's policy of requiring the colleges and universities it helped to raise equal or greater matching funds from other sources. But Kirkland, a man now desperate for endowment to save his medical school, was beyond self-help. He knew only one other place to turn.

In the first years of the century, the millions of Andrew Carnegie probably had greater luster in the world of philanthropy than even the Rockefellers'.[32] It was his gospel of wealth that had invested giving with a moral mandate, and (most important now for Kirkland) it was his name that was associated with the Flexner Report, which had appeared in 1910 as Bulletin Number Four of the Carnegie Foundation for the Advancement of Teaching. Of the useful fields for philanthropy that Carnegie had listed in descending order of importance in his original gospel, "the founding of hospitals and other institutions connected with the alleviation of human suffering" ranked third, just after free libraries and just before parks. Although quite early (1885) he had given $50,000 to establish at Bellevue Hospital in New York the country's first laboratory for medical research (William Henry Welch would be its head) and once had sent four children to Paris to receive Louis Pasteur's treatment for rabies, he never became famous for medical philanthropy. "That is Mr. Rockefeller's specialty," he told supplicants from countless hospitals and medical schools. "Go see him."[33] And, as was poorly understood by the medical deans who thought they scented in Flexner the promise of Carnegie's money, the Carnegie Foundation for the Advancement of Teaching, which sponsored the report, had for its purpose only the creation of pensions for college teachers, not the support of medical education.

In Flexner's report, Vanderbilt had been singled out not for high praise but merely as the best of what there was in the South. It fit into Flexner's vision of geographic distribution, and in his judgment it held out promise of a great future if it could be invested with new spirit and substance. Contrary to that conventional wisdom about the history of poor but aspiring institutions that says spirit precedes substance, sustaining a school in lean times and thus inspiring later benefaction, Flexner had in mind not the general spirit of institutional pride but rather "university spirit," which truly developed only after large substance had been bestowed. University spirit in medical education meant well-trained faculty who gave their full time to teaching and to science; it meant modern, well-equipped laboratories, and large teaching hospitals where masters and apprentices taught and learned. Good will, dedication, and hard work alone had never yet provided such things, but once substance was found the rest would follow. For Vanderbilt it was first found in 1913; its source was Andrew Carnegie.

Kirkland understood clearly that the university's 1911 investment in the new grounds and plant on the south campus did not alter or in any way ease the fundamental dilemma caused by decreased enrollment and the increased work demanded by higher standards, and in 1912 he predicted that proper medical work could not be conducted for long without investment of $200,000 in laboratories and without an endowment of at least $500,000. Like many a university administrator with ambitions for a medical school, Kirkland naturally turned to Andrew Carnegie, patron of the great report. Unlike most such people, however, Kirkland actually got what he was looking for. Since shortly after publication of Bulletin Number Four of Carnegie's foundation, Kirkland had sought ways to interest the foundation in Vanderbilt's medical school. Because the foundation's report had placed on Vanderbilt much of the burden for the future of medical education in the South, it was not unreasonable, he believed, for Carnegie money to support what Carnegie minds had prescribed. One of those minds was Abraham Flexner's, himself in 1910 off on other projects. The other was his immediate superior and president of the foundation, Henry S. Pritchett. With Pritchett, Kirkland carried on his campaign for Carnegie support, though the foundation itself, limited in purpose as it was, could do nothing. Pritchett's sympathy, deftly encouraged by Kirkland with reminders of the efforts that Vanderbilt had made on its own to implement Flexner's suggestions, paid off in the end.[34] The establishment in November 1911 of the Carnegie Corporation, with its superbly vague charge "to promote the advancement and diffusion of knowledge among the people of the United States by aiding technical schools, institutions of higher learning, libraries, scientific research, hero funds, useful publications, and by such other agencies and means as shall from time to time be found appropriate therefore,"[35] raised his hopes, and ultimately the corporation became a major Vanderbilt benefactor. But so pressing were Kirkland's needs in 1911, 1912, and 1913, that he convinced Pritchett (who would be on the board of the new philanthropy as would Kirkland himself a few years later) to attempt to secure the interest and aid of Carnegie himself.

That raised a problem, even beyond the usual ones entailed in begging for $1 million. Carnegie, as was well known, had always refused to give money to institutions of higher learning that were controlled by religious denominations, not, as he explained, because he was opposed to religion, but because he believed that the true cause neither of religion nor of education was served by such control. Vanderbilt was then still a Methodist institution and at that moment was embroiled in a legal battle that would end in the state supreme court over the issues of the visitatorial or veto powers of the Methodist bishops over actions of the university board of trust and over the self-perpetuating nature of that board.[36] It had been a long and often bitter struggle, which in 1913 impinged directly on the history of Vanderbilt's medical school and threatened for a moment to wreck it. Despite Vanderbilt's sectarian connections, Pritchett had succeeded in getting Carnegie's support for a plan that satisfied both his scruples and the school's needs.

As worked out by Pritchett and formalized in Kirkland's request to Carnegie of May 1, 1913, the chancellor asked for $1 million "to place the medical school at this time upon a permanent basis"; no more than $200,000 would be spent for laboratories, with the remainder to be used for endowment. With the money went an administrative arrangement designed to insulate the part of Vanderbilt that Carnegie was agreeing to support from the rest of the university's Methodist masters, should the courts decide in favor of the church. It was also an arrangement designed to provide the best possible management for the reorganized school. To run it, the university board of trust was to appoint a seven-member board of governors, of which the chancellor was to be chairman, three members of which were to be "men of recognized standing in medical education or medical science," and all of which were to be chosen solely because of their fitness for service and "without regard to denominational consideration." Faculty of the school were to be chosen "from the best men obtainable," and in a foreshadowing of the General Education Board's later demand for "full-time," "the professorships to be filled as far as practicable by men who are primarily teachers rather than practitioners."[37]

In his reply three weeks later Carnegie agreed on all particulars but hesitated on the matter of denominational control, still clouded by litigation. "I approve thoroughly your suggestion that this gift be conditioned on the appointment of a small board of seven persons to govern the medical school, who shall be chosen," he wrote, here changing a word, *"absolutely* without reference to denominational considerations and purely upon the ground of fitness for their duties" (Carnegie's emphasis). Troubled still by the unsettled lawsuit against Vanderbilt that was testing whether the board of trust was independent and self-perpetuating as it then was or whether its members should be chosen by the Methodist church, Carnegie proposed an interim arrangement while the courts decided. He would furnish $200,000 immediately and in cash for the needed laboratories, but custody of the remaining $800,000 would remain with the Carnegie Corporation of New York, Vanderbilt to receive interest at 4 percent "until such time as the question of denominational control has been settled by the court of last resort, its final disposition to be then determined."

In all probability Kirkland would not have carried things this far had he not been fairly confident that the outcome of the suit would be favorable to Vanderbilt—for had it not, the implication is clear that Carnegie would have reneged on the principal $800,000 and thus have left Vanderbilt's medical school as before with no endowment at all. Carnegie closed by explaining his objection to denominational control of colleges and universities (perhaps remembering that Kirkland's Vanderbilt, because of its church ties, had been one of the schools originally barred from participation in the Carnegie-financed teachers' pension program). His position was not, the steel master said, "due to lack of sympathy with religion. It lies in fact that such control by a single denomination rarely means religious development, but nearly always means that both religion and education are subordinated to the interests of the particular organization which is in control. I welcome rather all christian sects, believing with Matthew Arnold, whom I am proud to recall as my friend":

"Children of men! the Unseen Power, whose eyes
  For ever doth accompany mankind,
Hath looked on no religion scornfully
  That man did ever find.

Which has not taught weak wills how much they can?
  Which has not fallen on the dry heart like rain?
Which has not cried to sunk, self-weary man:
  Thou must be born again!"[38]

In response to that, Kirkland remarked to his board of trust innocuously enough that "it is not necessary for anyone to accept these views, but we must admit that Mr. Carnegie has the right to hold them."[39] But he had staked his career at Vanderbilt on the board's acceptance of the Carnegie gift, which, he acknowledged, "has largely been of my own seeking."[40] If the board had not accepted, he said that he would have resigned at once, feeling fully justified in leaving.[41] On the other hand, though the gift was in no way explicitly conditioned on his remaining at Vanderbilt, Kirkland evidently felt that if it was accepted with its provision for a medical governing board of which the chancellor of the university was to be chairman, he would feel a "special obligation to remain at Vanderbilt at least for a year or longer, until the Medical Department can be largely reorganized." Five days after it was accepted he was committed: "If I abandon this enterprise just now, the professors and trustees alike would feel that I had almost betrayed a trust." He stayed.[42]

With four dissenting votes, the Vanderbilt board acted on June 17, 1913, to accept Carnegie's gift and the conditions he had set forth. The dissenters filed a written protest of the board's action, and the Methodist bishops, exercising their alleged visitatorial powers, promptly vetoed it. The nine months from then until March 21, 1914, when the state supreme court decided in favor of the university, was one of the more acrimonious times in the history of town-gown relations in Nashville, and it is an episode that belongs more to the history of the Southern Methodist church and the history of Vanderbilt as a whole than to the story of medical education there, except for the manner in which the row forced into sharp relief the terms of this first alliance between a philanthropic foundation and medical education at Vanderbilt.[43] The keystone of that alliance and the major bone in the throat of its church opponents was the provision for a separate governing body for the medical school. To the Methodist bishops and to anyone else with reason to be jealous over control of the university, the proposed seven-member board could easily appear as an attempt by Carnegie and his minions (by implication, Kirkland) to buy control of part of the university. Almost immediately, invective, mostly Methodist, flew hot and heavy.

On May 31, 1913, the day after the Vanderbilt executive committee had tentatively approved the gift, Kirkland announced the gift to the local press as the "most significant benefaction yet made to medical education in the South" and the "first round million ever given Vanderbilt." To his enemies the munificence of the gift made it the more insidious. Bishop W. A. Candler characterized Carnegie's offer as "a shrewd attempt to get control of a part of the property of Vanderbilt University in order to set up a medical school fashioned according to the peculiar ideas of Mr. Carnegie," and he charged that the gift, conditioned as it was, would "denature the medical school of the Methodists" and raise on its ruins "a Carnegieized establishment in his own image and likeness." Bishop E. E. Hoss, one of Kirkland's chief antagonists through the long church dispute, objected that far from getting $1 million, the university as previously constituted got not a dollar. It was actually giving away its medical department to a new governing body without limitations or restrictions. With $800,000 contingent on the elimination of church control, he contended that money was being used to influence the outcome of litigation. "Carnegie's wealth does not prove his right to leadership in matters affecting the intellectual and moral life of the nation," he said.[44]

It was God or mammon, as reflected in newspaper commentary of the day: southern Methodism "will not and cannot consider the question of money when the question of principle is involved." Some have yielded and "filled their coffers with Mr. Carnegie's gold, and are now luxuriating in their way as secular institutions."[45] Never Vanderbilt! "The majority of the Board of Trust have been making a desperate effort to throw off the control of the Church, and Mr. Carnegie is quite willing to help them." "The charm will not work. The lure of gold will not lead the Church to crucify the Lord or to desert her standards in the educational world."[46] Bishop Candler, who earlier had characterized John D. Rockefeller's gift of $1 million to eradicate hookworm in the southern states as a northern slander on the South, called Carnegie's latest attempt at southern philanthropy "an impudent proposal of an agnostic steel monger."[47] (Carnegie, in his letter offering the gift to Vanderbilt, had signed himself "A true friend of the South.") So on it went through the summer. The Methodist College of Bishops acting as the Board of Visitors of Vanderbilt University, and finding the board's action in breach of the trust vested in it at the foundation of the university, declared the action illegal, null, and void,[48] none of which prevented the university from accepting the first installment of $200,000 (Carnegie being satisfied that the money had been accepted by the proper authorities). It is fair to wonder, had the suit gone the other way, if the bishops would have undertaken to give it back.

Kirkland tried to put the best face possible on Carnegie's demand for a separate board, declaring that by the letter of agreement its actions were subject to the approval of the university board of trust, by whom it was appointed and at least four of whose own members served on it. The university surrendered nothing but merely conceded the immediate direction of the medical department to "a group of gentlemen selected in accordance with Mr. Carnegie's wishes."[49] Carnegie certainly did want independence from church connections in that part of the university he proposed to support, but the governing board that would achieve that independence, constituted as it was by at least three medical "experts," served genuine functional purpose as well. No board, Kirkland explained, could ever be totally independent of the body that created it (in this case the university board of trust), but he took it as an act of confidence and good will that "Mr. Carnegie is willing to accept this arrangement as a pledge of honor on the part of the [university] trustees that the Medical Department will be managed with sole regard to efficient and scientific service."[50] That some Methodists saw in that eminently generous position sinister conspiracy was to Kirkland, a Methodist too, fantastic. "Certainly Nashville and the South," he said with an eye to the future, "can hardly be expected to relish the refusal of a great donation on grounds so puerile."[51] Nashville's newspapers approved of the gift and deplored the controversy it had stirred; the controversy became so fierce that the *Banner* requested a "cessation of hostilities" and finally refused to print any more letters on the issue.[52] How opinion actually divided can never be known for sure, but it was not, strictly speaking, a public matter anyway. Kirkland's fierce championing is probably fair indication that he had much public support behind him.

Even in 1913, with years still to run in his career, he had considerable prestige in Nashville and skillfully nursed its flattering and still fragile self-image as host to educational greatness. It was his self-appointed job so to position his university in the pattern of outside forces newly available for its sustenance that it would become known as a worthy and reliable partner and target for the foundation philanthropists—and thus the greater local showpiece. As showpieces would go, medical schools ranked with the showiest, as Kirkland may well have guessed, whose value, backed by solid substance as they soon would be, few people for years ever doubted. Certainly the local doctors did not, the more progressive of whom saw with Kirkland, though from another angle, the chance for great things. By what right, asked William H. Witt, one prominent local doctor, did the Methodist bishops decline the Carnegie gift? "Whose brain, whose money, whose sleepless nights," he asked, "whose days of labor and evenings of planning does our present medical school represent? Have the bishops or other ministers spent from three to ten hours a week for eight months teaching in the school; have they spent money purely to prepare themselves to do this work; has the church as a church donated money—say $25,000—to see that we did not encounter a discouraging deficit? Not much."[53]

Such possessiveness matched Kirkland's and one day would conflict with it, but at that moment it only buttressed what must have been the widespread conviction in the community that bishops and medical education must part. Would it be that "Your dreams shall not be realized; you shall not teach medicine like you wish to. You shall not have fully equipped and manned laboratories. You shall not investigate the poorly understood diseases of the South. You shall not give your time and skill to the poor . . . for the Bishops and the church offer us no funds with which to do these things?" Witt, whose words these were, was a physician and like Kirkland a Methodist for whom the choice nonetheless entailed little philosophical agony: "You can't run a Medical School like it ought to be served—like it has to be served. Give up your supposed rights—you will have done more good for religion and for the Methodist Church at one stroke than Mr. Carnegie could ever undo were he so disposed."[54]

Mr. Carnegie was not so disposed, and the Methodist bishops, try as they did, could not hold onto their "rights." That which to them symbolized Kirkland's great betrayal and Carnegie's ultimate usurpation—the medical governing board—met for the first time on November 24, 1913, four months before the bishops were finally routed by the court, but it met legally enough to Kirkland and his medical allies. According to the terms by which it served, its architects were concerned at once to bestow on it both the substance of power and the appearance of responsibility to the university. At least four of its seven members were to be Vanderbilt people: the chancellor who served as chairman (Kirkland), and three members of the university board of trust, initially Whitefoord R. Cole, Joseph E. Washington, and John W. Thomas. The term was eight years and all served at the pleasure of the board of trust, which had elected them. Its proceedings and records of all its business transactions were to be always accessible to the board of trust and all actions subject to the board's ratification. Its charge, however, was happily broad: to administer in all respects, financial and academic, medical education at Vanderbilt, only with ultimate authority residing with the university. With it was foreshadowed a kind of autonomy that other parts of the university would never have.[55] Its other three members, who were not connected with the university, made for greater separation. Henry Pritchett, president of the Carnegie Foundation for the Advancement of Teaching and board member of the new Carnegie Corporation, served as stipulated in Carnegie's original gift (ostensibly and partly in truth because of his knowledge of medical education but also surely as personal watchdog for his master). William H. Howell, professor of physiology at Johns Hopkins, and Edwin O. Jordan, professor of bacteriology at the University of Chicago, supplied the scientific expertise also demanded by Carnegie.

At that first meeting they inspected the medical plant (cramped and imperfect), met faculty and students (enthusiastic and hardworking), and were counseled by Kirkland, ever the impresario, on the major problems that confronted them: operation of a university hospital adequate for clinical teaching, provision of laboratory facilities with Carnegie's gift, and procurement of a pathology professor (whom the three outsiders, Pritchett, Howell, and Jordan, were appointed to hire, the four insiders being designated a building committee to plan for the laboratory). Lucius E. Burch, professor of obstetrics and gynecology, was appointed to continue as acting dean, and an advisory council of the medical faculty was set up as a liaison group between the faculty and the governing board.[56]

Although a separate board itself would not always characterize medical administration at Vanderbilt, the idea that the changing nature of medical science and education required increasingly specialized skills for its administration dated from the first Carnegie gift and the conditions the wily Scot had attached to it. The notion certainly seemed a sensible institutional response to the changing state of medical knowledge and the new requirements for its transmission. The gift then marks a double watershed. It was the first large sum of money given exclusively for medical education at Vanderbilt (and among the first given by a philanthropy to any medical school), and thus it marked the beginning of a long and largely happy relationship between medicine at Vanderbilt and the great philanthropic foundations. The grant was unusual in that the decision to make it had come directly from Carnegie the individual much as Vanderbilt family money had come to the university. Since then, Vanderbilt and countless other institutional supplicants would find themselves dealing not with those who actually had made the fortunes but with other institutions created to give those fortunes away. The grant was typical in that it was conditioned, not in this instance on raising matching funds, but on procedural and substantive requirements as specific as the demand for a separate medical governing board and as general as the admonition that the school be conducted according to high university ideals and scientific standards.

As time went on and the relation between the givers and the getters grew more confident, explicit procedural conditions more and more gave way to general substantive ones. Although a board was never again demanded, the later and larger gifts Vanderbilt received from the Carnegie Corporation and the General Education Board came with similar strings, but unlike the Carnegie gift of 1913, in which conditions were explicitly enumerated in the grant (right down to putting Pritchett on the board), understandings in the future were usually worked out quietly ahead of time. The resulting terms of such grants themselves could be left generally broad while the parties remained confident about what was expected of whom. Such conditions, explicit or implied, were not generally then viewed as burdensome or intrusive (controversy over the full-time plan was a major exception, but it was an exception). At Vanderbilt in particular, so at one in spirit was Kirkland with his foundation patrons—Henry Pritchett, Wallace Buttrick, Abraham Flexner—that the letter of their agreements could safely stipulate remarkably little.

The policies of the Carnegie Foundation for the Advancement of Teaching in higher education and those of the General Education Board somewhat later in medical education were excellent early examples of organized philanthropy's power to coerce reform that was in the philanthropists' interests—and in keeping with their ideals. Strange as it may seem from the perspective of more litigious times, those interests and ideals were often held in common by potential beneficiaries and did not merely become so before the tantalizing prospect of foundation millions. If the foundations coerced the advancement of their own interests and ideals, as indeed they did, many there were only too ready to be coerced and who were surely not sycophants. At Vanderbilt the carpetbaggers succeeded so brilliantly because scalawags committed equal energy and skill. Few felt put upon or ill-used, and Kirkland, convinced that he spoke for many, saw nothing in the actions of the foundations at all devious or that was not in essential accord with his own aims for uplifting education in the South. At that moment what a sublime vision it must have seemed: their gold, Vanderbilt's glory.

The Carnegie gift of 1913 heralded darker futures too, not then apparent. With it came acknowledgment that modern scientific medical education was something special. It probably would require special administrative arrangements separating it from the university; it probably would cost far more than other kinds of education; it certainly would call for a dedication to science and to service demanded by no other school in the university. Yet it was Flexner's dictum and the new conventional wisdom that medical schools must henceforth be made organic parts of universities, with whose "spirit" and "ideals" they would be infused thereby forsaking for sure the bad habits of the old, practitioner-dominated times. Through integration the medical schools would get "ideals," a development that was most important to Flexner. The universities would get true institutional completeness, which most of them naturally craved.

But it was always a tenuous union, more asserted than consummated, and contingent always on the continued growth and prosperity of both partners. Besides, convenient as it seemed, the arrangement hid more than it settled. Since the darkest proprietary days, medical education had been nothing if not practical, and though they saw that the basis of its knowledge must be changed and made scientific, Flexner and the reformers insisted that medical education remain practical. To the degree that science, the new source of knowledge, could be bent to service, the old, practical goal of medicine, medical schools would be decidedly more utilitarian than the universities that contained them. The core of those universities was their undergraduate colleges of the liberal arts whose job it was to teach students how to think. In the medical schools attached to the edges of those universities there were some true scientists who harnessed the inductive method of how to think to discrete medical problems and so added to the sum of their knowledge. But for the vast majority of their students destined not to be scientists but practicing medical professionals, the medical schools were places to learn what to think. Learning what to think was not in itself a bad thing inasmuch as more and more of what they learned turned out to be right, but nonetheless it was different to a degree from what universities claimed essentially to be about.

To these problems Flexner ironically had added another never since unraveled. By inviting the medical schools into the universities, he invited veneration there of inductive science whose ultimate wisdom even in 1925 he had come to suspect. What chagrin he felt then is not known, only his warning that the "extension of human interest resulting from the development of the inductive and experimental science has deprived culture of its singleness of meaning."[57] On the bonds of spirit and purpose that supposedly made universities whole, every new million invested in the laboratories, hospitals, and faculties needed for proper medical education was a strong solvent that in time worked a rather different result from that once hoped for. Such difficulties few then might have been expected to foresee. But in the odyssey of Vanderbilt's medical school from 1913 through the 1920s and 1930s there is a fitfulness that accompanies the apparent confidence of these leaders that they were doing the right things. Perhaps it rose from a hunch that for all the wonderful promise of the new medicine, they only held a wolf by the ears. More likely or at least more immediately, it can be ascribed to the discomfitting discovery made by Kirkland and many like him elsewhere that never was there enough.

Medical education (like medical practice then and later) once had operated on essentially a fee-for-service principle. It had also been afflicted with all the shoddiness of the proprietary system, but this at least could be said for it: the relationship between what it offered, the cost of offering it, and the resources available to pay for it was self-regulating in the sense that the market decided. That had worked as long as the substance of what medical schools offered was modest (a little anatomy, a little chemistry, a little surgery) and fixed. It was thus neither expensive nor subject to the rising expectations born of new knowledge. It was in the role of dismantlers of that world that Kirkland, Flexner, and other reformers found themselves. Cost of the replacement world (the world of well-equipped laboratories, large teaching hospitals, and highly trained scientist-teachers), they saw from the start, would be so enormous that only by reaching outside the schools and the profession could those costs be met.

On the resources of the philanthropic foundations first and of the welfare state later, medical education had moral claim alone, though that was a mighty one. But a moral claim unlike a market claim had no built-in governor. It could hardly have been otherwise in face of the transformation in medical knowledge and popular expectation pinned to it that swept over the twentieth century. But that does not alter the fact that medical education seventy and eighty years ago entered on a troubled new time when, though every year richer than ever, it claimed at once and quite reasonably to be every year needier than ever. In 1912 and 1913 when engineering the Carnegie gift and then in lobbying for its acceptance, Kirkland (who was not a man given to hyperbole) warned simply enough that without that million Vanderbilt should soon certainly have to quit training doctors. The gift happily was made and accepted, strings and all, and with it Vanderbilt suddenly had $200,000 in cash to build new laboratories and, more important, $800,000 for permanent endowment—where not a penny had been before. But it was not long before Kirkland, already on the first coils of a long spiral, found the game had only just begun.

The rest of the decade after 1910 followed in that frantic pattern. Acceptance of the Carnegie gift permitted modest reorganization of the medical school in 1913 with the hiring of some full-time faculty in the preclinical sciences and some modest expansion of laboratory facilities. But between even that improved performance and the great future that Flexner had painted for it there was much distance to travel. Kirkland cultivated his growing friendships with Buttrick, Flexner, Gates, and Pritchett throughout the troubled war years, and to them and the philanthropies they represented he pleaded the case for his university. All of its schools badly needed support and it was not for medicine alone that, having successfully thrown off churchly ties, the chancellor had large ambitions. In 1914 and 1915 it was for the undergraduate college, "the heart of the whole institution," that he appealed to the General Education Board.[58] Flexner, who had joined the board in 1913, and Buttrick actually came to Vanderbilt to survey with Kirkland the university's needs. Their recommendation that the college needed $1 million for endowment and $250,000 for a laboratory building set the stage for Kirkland's formal request that the board itself subscribe $300,000, which it did. With even greater than usual difficulty Kirkland labored to get the match from the Vanderbilt family[59] and from alumni, a job that drove him close to despair more than once.[60]

But it was to medicine, still on the periphery of institutions like Vanderbilt, that the foundations were turning with greatest zeal. In 1911 Gates borrowed Flexner from Pritchett at the Carnegie Foundation to explore the possibilities for Rockefeller philanthropy applied deliberately to the reform of medical education. Replying to Gates's question of what he would do if he had $1 million to begin that large work, Flexner said he would give it to Johns Hopkins, whose dean, William Henry Welch, was also president of the board of scientific directors of the Rockefeller Institute for Medical Research, in New York City, itself a Gates creation. Although the proposal to give Hopkins $1 million quickly stirred the first of numerous storms over the General Education Board's absolute insistence on the acceptance of the full-time plan in the clinical as well as the preclinical departments, and although it took two years before Welch felt his faculty was ready to be brought around, the gift to Hopkins (actually $1.5 million) signaled the beginning of support for medical education that by 1960, when the board went out of business, totaled more than $94 million. That sum was divided among just twenty-five schools, of which Vanderbilt received more than any other, $17.5 million.[61]

The early General Education Board gifts for medical education went to Hopkins, Washington University, Yale, and the University of Chicago, and the $4 million that Kirkland finally secured for Vanderbilt in 1919 (which took over two years to negotiate) gives to the history of his relationship with the Rockefeller philanthropy in the 1910s a certain symmetry. In 1909 he successfully had appealed to it for a modest $150,000, which, though for general university endowment, indirectly enabled an early step down the road of medical reform. Carnegie's million notwithstanding, the ensuing decade was a makeshift crippled by a fundamental disproportion between ends and means. In 1919 ministration of several millions more of Rockefeller money repaired for a time that disproportion, but it did more than that. With them were invested in Vanderbilt's medical school and others like it new deliberateness and conviction about the true way doctors should be made. The disposition of those millions and the working out of that conviction in the 1920s and 1930s is the story of new leaders, who to Kirkland's dreams and ideals (which they shared) brought a plan and fresh energy to establish it.

PART TWO

Design for Permanence

An Alliance

4

For many years group photographs of the medical faculty were set on the steps of the school's north entrance, an aptly dignified collegiate Gothic portal inscribed "Vanderbilt University School of Medicine, A.D. 1925." From there, gatherings of usually white-coated, solemn-faced physicians looked out across an open court toward the main part of the university campus.[1] Among the first and probably the most famous of those pictures was the one of G. Canby Robinson and his original new staff.[2] In time, those who stayed at Vanderbilt made their mark on their departments and on their school and so were reverently remembered. But in the beginning it was Robinson's charge alone to translate Kirkland's and Flexner's generous commission into a design of laboratories, wards, clinics, and talented teachers.

Toward its end, Robinson looked back on his life as a series of "adventures" in medical education (as he entitled his autobiography), the Vanderbilt chapter of which was surely the most successful. It fit into his career a little past the midway point; he was forty-seven in 1925, a happy age to reach the top. But unlike Kirkland, who had become a chancellor when even a younger man, it was not Robinson's good fortune to sustain his personal success much beyond his Vanderbilt adventure. When he left in 1928 to head the building of the new Cornell University–New York Hospital, then one of the most prestigious medical jobs in the world, he did not know that the Great Depression would confound his large hopes for that enterprise and that, leaving the position after just six years, he would never again enjoy the untarnished acclaim that once was his at Vanderbilt. The checkered nature of his subsequent itinerant career (he returned to Hopkins in the late 1930s as an instructor) lends poignance to the years when without question things did go his way, and it makes the record of his leadership at Vanderbilt best evidence of the things he truly wanted.

From the time he was hired early in 1920 until tempted away to Manhattan eight years later, Canby Robinson shared the center stage at Vanderbilt with no one, not even with Kirkland. Sly as he was, the chancellor knew that the way good jobs get done was by finding good people and then leaving them alone both to do the work and to reap the glory. Not that his interest in the new medical school ever diminished or that Robinson's ideas and conduct did not on a few occasions give him pause, but in general the chancellor contented himself of necessity with leaving the immediate specialized job of building a modern medical school and hospital to the specialist. Although he peered constantly over Robinson's shoulder and by the early 1920s knew far more about medicine and medical education than most laymen, he knew too that that was not nearly enough. Besides, he had other things to do: the rest of his university required constant tending. It was different for Robinson who, member of a profession as he was and a dean of one school and not chancellor of many, enjoyed the luxury of single-minded devotion to essentially one job. Securing the right new dean had been Kirkland's first order of business (and one on which he worked closely with Abraham Flexner), and key to his agreement with Robinson, then dean at Washington University in St. Louis, was that Robinson would be completely free from any responsibility for running the old Vanderbilt Medical School to concentrate solely on planning and building the new one. For an ambitious and talented physician in his prime, one who had proven his scientific and administrative abilities and who had the good luck to be on the scene just as the foundations were making means available to work the ends he had long believed in, it was an opportunity not to be missed.

Student of Osler, graduate of Hopkins, and veteran already of a deanship, Robinson brought energy and commitment to his Vanderbilt assignment, enlarging it considerably as he went. This he knew would be his main chance to make a mark and do great things, a chance such as fortune afforded few people. He took it with the characteristic alacrity with which he did everything else, from doctoring to sports to travel. At school he had captained baseball, football, and lacrosse teams. He and his fiancée Marian had won the Baltimore city mixed doubles championship in tennis the year they were engaged to be married. He played the banjo, went to the theater, and in 1934, en route to China to serve for a year as visiting professor of medicine of the Peking Union Medical College, he took wife, daughter, and son around the world in the process. A discerning man, he believed in stopping often along

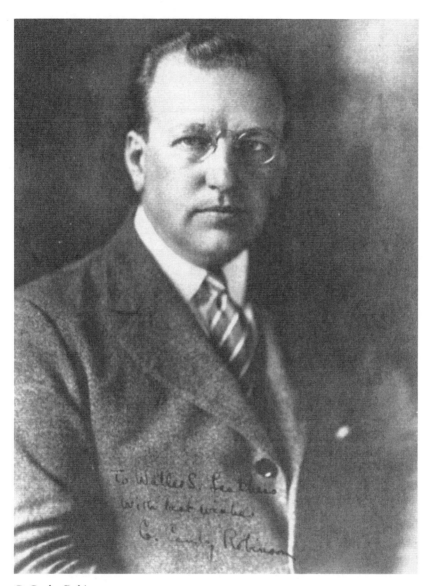

G. Canby Robinson

the way. Across France, Switzerland, and Italy he shepherded his little tribe to all the Michelin sites and recorded faithfully in his diary the glee with which they greeted all those rivers, ruins, and churches. In Naples they boarded a Japanese steamer for the long voyage through Suez, across the Indian Ocean, to Singapore, and finally to Shanghai. All the while he read books on China diligently gathered together back in New York.[3] His public and his private lives, though apart enough to ensure a good marriage and a happy family, exhibited similar buoyant enthusiasm, hardiness, and good will and were in the end much of a piece. For a man who had reached the pinnacle of his profession and had then tumbled so calamitously on bad times, he coped well enough, and for the long years that remained to him (he died in 1960), he kept his self-esteem and generally put his still considerable talents to good use. In the end he managed his life better than his career. Controlling what he could, keeping a sense of proportion on what he could not, finding satisfaction first in worldly success and later in other things, Canby Robinson was a happy man.

Never probably was he happier than at Vanderbilt. He and Marian (Baltimoreans, which made them southerners enough) fit easily into Nashville society. Children Margaret and Boise prospered at private school and made friends easily. Although Quakers by heritage, the whole family attended Christ Episcopal Church, where Robinson and the two children were baptized. During the summers they vacationed on Long Island, driving all the way from Nashville in two Model Ts.[4] If later he would take refuge in such private things, that time in the 1920s had not yet come, so exciting still was the public life and so filled with promise.

It had been ten years from Flexner's report on what was wrong with American medical education and how to fix it, to Robinson's appearance at Vanderbilt, ten years in which Flexner's ideas for reform embodied as policy of the General Education Board had begun to bear fruit. As was their habit, the philanthropists and their foundation masters invested where they caught the scent of previous promise. Thus to Hopkins, Yale, Chicago, and a few others went the first subsidies for full-time faculties and improved facilities.[5] Fine new medical schools resulted, though these nonetheless bore the marks of a gradual evolution. There was no better example than Johns Hopkins, with its curiously eclectic physical plant, located far from the main university campus. Robinson saw to something else at Vanderbilt, where the investment of the GEB (its largest up to then) was made on slimmer collateral (virtually on Kirkland's character alone) yet with more comprehensive design. How comprehensive, Kirkland did not in the beginning suspect. But under Robinson's guiding hand the Vanderbilt project was the first example of how the reformer's ideas about medical education might be comprehended in a single unified blueprint. No piecemeal additions for him: from the ground up rose at a single stroke laboratories, school, and hospital. Architecturally and intellectually complete when it finally opened in the autumn of 1925, the Vanderbilt Medical School was a small but nearly perfect glimpse of medicine's large future. No ordinary job, then, was Robinson asked to undertake five years before. With scope enough for any true believer, it was a job to bring out the vanity of the most humble; if ever someone wanted a monument, here was the chance to build one.

In addition to his own clear-cut ideas of what it all in the end should look like, this particular medical school/monument builder had at first $4 million with which to work. Because it was that and not just Kirkland's charm and his dreams of a great medical school that had enticed Robinson to Nashville, the expectations attached to that gift by the givers and by the getter (Kirkland) bear directly on what Robinson the medical man later managed to do with it. It marked the single greatest fund-raising coup of Kirkland's long and distinguished fund-raising career and seemed confirming proof of what many around him surely had come to suspect: that the chancellor had the key to Mr. Rockefeller's account. Of course he did not, but he did have and was able constantly to draw upon the next best thing: a large store of mutual respect and good will that over more than a decade had grown between him and the professional keepers of Mr. Rockefeller's account. Together they made the deal; Robinson was hired to implement it.

From the time Kirkland first appealed to Flexner for aid for his medical school in 1917 (only temporarily propped up by the Carnegie gift), it took two years to make the arrangements. That was not inordinately long, given the slow-moving nature of the foundation world and the large sums in question, but it was long enough for the harried chancellor who, as he had done before the 1913 Carnegie gift, foresaw how without new money the end was very near. Most important to him was the fundamental question of whether the General Education Board was yet ready to support schools other than those that had already made significant tangible progress toward the modern ideal laid out in Bulletin Number Four. If so, the board would be departing from the policy that had governed its first four grants to Hopkins, Yale, Chicago, and Washington University, when it had put its money where the risks were not inordinately high and where the need for perpetual subsidy seemed remote. By those standards Kirkland's Vanderbilt hardly qualified. Its sole claim to distinction and its only evidence that someone other than Kirkland himself had faith in its future was Carnegie's $1 million, and that had kept the wolf at bay barely four years. Moreover, Carnegie's grant had anticipated no sweeping reorganization along modern lines but had only provided the beginnings of a general endowment and funds for a new laboratory. In fairness, Carnegie was not in the medical reform business; his gift to Vanderbilt was exceptional and part of no large strategic plan such as Gates, Buttrick, and Flexner were then concocting on Rockefeller's behalf. But Kirkland was by then as much in the market for a plan as for the dollars to finance it, and typically he got what he wanted. In April 1917 he laid his sad story before the sympathetic Flexner. For even a hundred students he calculated that Vanderbilt needed at least $90,000 annually. With currently reduced wartime income that meant an additional $500,000 for endowment. With that it could likely only tread water. Improvement, which was needed everywhere, demanded for endowment alone another full $1 million.[6]

Kirkland appended a bill of particulars to his plea and then settled down to wait. Flexner for his part had not forgotten what just a few years before he had written about Vanderbilt, and he did not now turn a deaf ear on its chancellor and his friend. Vanderbilt, he had concluded in his report after cataloging its manifold deficiencies, was the best there was in the southern desert. To it eventually should fall the burden and the glory of leading the South to better ways of thinking and doing. The General Education Board had heard and had answered Kirkland's pleas before—in 1909 and 1915, though not then on medical matters—and Kirkland knew that in the intervening few years the board's resources had grown. When in 1917 he put forth his case for medicine at Vanderbilt, he must have been fairly certain of the answer he would get. What passed informally between him and his foundation friends in the months that followed is not a matter of record, though likely there were anxious but restrained queries from one side and soothing reassurances from the other that all in time would be well. It took more than a year for Flexner to have so ordered his own house to be confident enough to reply for the record that he and Buttrick at least had put Vanderbilt at the top of their southern agenda. "We have not yet, of course," he addressed Kirkland, as supplicant and as friend, "canvassed it with our Board so we cannot predict as to what reception a suggestion of the kind we contemplate may have, but we are very hopeful."[7]

But they wanted to be sure. Early in 1919 they enticed Kirkland to Baltimore to see and to be seen by the complement of Hopkins doctors whose likes would before long be a part of his daily routine. With a cloak-and-dagger touch, Flexner (who then happened to be a patient at Johns Hopkins with a leg injury) and Buttrick (who had come to visit him) conspired with Hopkins gynecologist Thomas H. Cullen (also a summer neighbor of Kirkland's at Lake Ahmic in Ontario) peremptorily to summon the chancellor to Baltimore, at first, Kirkland thought, on account of his troublesome stomach but, as a second telegram explained, actually on account of his ailing medical school. It is a pity that there is no minute-by-minute account of what went on at that little conclave and that only the reminiscences of a few participants document it. But it must have been a set piece of good words, knowing glances, and mutual admiration. For certain it was masterfully orchestrated around two gentlemen-only dinners at the Maryland Club, one featuring Hopkins president Ira Remsen and the other featuring medical dean William Henry Welch, himself recipient back in 1913 of the first Rockefeller medical gift. Kirkland also was featured at both. For the first meeting several members of the General Education Board had come from New York personally to look over their probable new investment, and the heads of Hopkins medical departments were on hand presumably to show the visitor what, after hours, real academic doctors were like. They were good company evidently, so at least Kirkland reported to his wife Mary, and after dinner (likely over good cigars, of which Kirkland was something of a fancier) the talk turned to medical education, what needed to be done about it, and where. By his own account Kirkland guessed that it was his place to listen more than to talk, and what he heard from those distinguished doctors and interested laymen buoyed his hopes that such a get-acquainted session was sure to be followed by real substance.

In a white-coat rather than white-tie setting, Welch arranged for Kirkland to meet with each of the medical school's department heads and to tour under their guidance Hopkins's numerous clinics and laboratories. In addition he was given a thorough physical examination (he was then fifty-nine years old), something he interpreted as the insurance required by his patrons-to-be that their collaborator could see the job through. He was uplifted by all he saw and disgusted by what he knew he must go home to, which was just what Flexner probably intended. If he had not been convinced before that the Hopkins way was the only way, he surely was by the end of the week. The message was clear that if medical education was to continue at Vanderbilt there could be no more shoring up a ship poorly designed to begin with, no more casual million here, casual million there. And before he left, it was the rotund and genial Buttrick who asked, teasingly, if Kirkland could get his present medical faculty to resign to make way for full-time teachers, were the money to become available for real reform at Vanderbilt. Gambling, Kirkland said he could.[8]

The trip also apparently whisked away any hesitation there might have been on the General Education Board, for by the end of February 1919 the board was ready, informally at least, to give Buttrick and Flexner authority to begin working out details. With their resolution that "the officers of the Board are authorized to submit to the Board a definite proposition looking to cooperation with the authorities of Vanderbilt University in the reorganization of the Medical Department of Vanderbilt University," Buttrick and Flexner set out for Nashville in mid-March "for the purpose of conferring with the Chancellor of Vanderbilt University and surveying the local possibilities."[9] They stayed at the grand Hermitage Hotel and, after three days of meetings with Kirkland and local doctors and of inspecting Vanderbilt's motley array of facilities, they offered the diagnosis and the prescription. Of the need and of the opportunity in the Vanderbilt situation they agreed there was little doubt; in correcting it they saw another progressive step in the process of medical reform for which Flexner's report had been the keynote.

In this effort as in so much else that northerners would do for it, the South would be uplifted. Nationwide the worst of the old commercial schools had rapidly been dying out, while those of a better grade were being improved, particularly with regard to higher entrance requirements and better equipment and teaching in the laboratory subjects. Beyond Hopkins, three other institutions in the 1910s had been so reorganized and financed as to place them in the small but growing ranks of "medical schools of modern type": Yale, the University of Chicago, and Washington University in St. Louis. They were the pacesetters for the East and the Midwest, "which other schools will bestir themselves to imitate. Their influence should therefore extend beyond their own immediate achievements, they should train superior physicians and surgeons, increase medical and surgical knowledge, and, over and above all this, stimulate other schools to emulate their example."[10] Not as far as the South, however, was "their influence" apparently expected to reach. There another exemplary beacon was called for. In that vast backward and benighted hinterland, Flexner (perhaps recalling his Louisville boyhood) believed, loomed by far the widest field for the modern science of medicine to prove its worth in useful service. In the South was the test tube to try the much-labored justification for the new science that Flexner had worked out ten years before in composing Bulletin Number Four. The worth of the abstract principles of reform had already been proven at those first, non-southern schools to be subsidized: excellent physicians and surgeons were produced and research was generating new knowledge. But now in the South, so especially afflicted, came opportunity to make doubly plain the practical utility of medicine as science.

It had taken a decade for all the pieces to come into place, but at last they had. Having successfully tried its policy of philanthropy in return for reform, the GEB now had the confidence it needed to risk more nearer the margin, and it would shortly have vastly more money to do so. Its officers had in Vanderbilt and Kirkland hit upon the ideal object for a new regional experiment: "Here is a vast region which, in addition to problems common to the entire country, such as tuberculosis, venereal disease, and typhoid fever, has its own peculiar problems in malaria, pellagra, and hookworm disease. To deal with these, medical training, medical research and organized hygiene of the highest order are required." Starts had been made at Augusta, Charlottesville, and elsewhere, but still "not a single medical school in the entire South possesses the facilities or the personnel needed to train men to meet existing conditions or to carry on the research by means of which unsolved health problems may ultimately be mastered." The consequent lack of proper standards left the South prey to a host of ill-trained physicians and patent medicines glaringly huckstered in the press and on the billboard, and for its backwardness the South paid dearly in public health and economic efficiency. What countless advantages awaited if only "it possessed a medical profession trained on numerous lines, and medical investigators competent to attack the difficulties with which the southern sanitarian is confronted. It is our judgment that this can best be accomplished by creating in the South a modern medical school which will set up higher ideals and from which better trained men will pass into medical practice and medical teaching throughout the section."[11]

Centrally located and growing bigger and richer in best New South fashion, Nashville could plausibly be touted as a strategic point accessible to all in the region. It also boasted Vanderbilt, "an institution which has played a leading part in creating and maintaining scholarly standards in the South," and a fit place clearly for radiating future enlightenment as well; the presence of Kirkland guaranteed that. Wrote Flexner the flatterer: With "vision, energy, and leadership," the chancellor had perceived at once what aid from the General Education Board could mean.[12] Kirkland concurred completely that only radical reorganization could work the anticipated wonders and that to that end the present faculty would surely make way for change, particularly for the recruitment of academic doctors from the country at large. So Vanderbilt met Flexner's key condition: the promise of the full-time plan.

Flexner then mustered the facts. Once a typical southern school, too poor and too large, Vanderbilt had raised standards and suffered the resulting fall in enrollment and income from fees. At the time of Flexner's and Buttrick's visit it enrolled about 125 medical students. Its teaching staff included a few instructors with modern training in the basic laboratory sciences, but on the clinical side few teachers, despite clinical experience, possessed anything like modern qualifications. Likewise, the physical facilities for all departments were, in Flexner's judgment, for future purposes negligible. To the good, the university's medical department did have a fifteen-acre site in south Nashville, an endowment of $1 million ($800,000 if the money designated for the Carnegie laboratory was not counted), and use of the hospital being built by the Methodists.

The endowment yielded $40,000 a year and student fees about $20,000, which together was far short of the $150,000 that Flexner and Buttrick estimated as the annual maintenance cost of the type of small modern school they hoped to build there.[13] For maintenance they said another $1.8 million was needed. In addition, a properly equipped laboratory building would cost $400,000, a hospital building $750,000, and a hospital endowment the same amount again. The total came to $3.7 million. Flexner anticipated a student body eventually of about 200 students, which with some increase in fees would without additional endowment generate about $25,000 for annual maintenance and bring total income to $175,000, a sum he believed adequate to operate the departments of medicine, surgery, pediatrics, and perhaps obstetrics on the full-time, university plan. The salaries that could be paid from such an income even for the head posts obviously could not be large (the highest, Robinson's as both dean and professor of medicine, was $9,000) and certainly not as munificent as the incomes then enjoyed by some of the school's practitioner-professors. But the money would be sufficient, Flexner was convinced, to attract from junior full-time positions elsewhere a talented and promising young faculty. Although prominent consultants and clinicians had their place on the part-time "clinical" faculties of university medical schools, they were not as a rule fitted by the kind of special training in the basic sciences that was required for the research and teaching responsibilities of modern full-time departments. And Flexner had no interest in them for university chairs in medicine and surgery; Vanderbilt initially had no interest in them either. This was the course followed by the Rockefeller Institute (which Simon Flexner headed) in forming the staff of its hospital (where Robinson served as first resident physician from 1910 to 1913), by the China Medical Board in recruiting the staff of the Peking Union Medical College (another Rockefeller project), and by Washington University (where Robinson himself had been involved).[14] The need to get young people early and for the most productive stages of their careers governed. Robinson, whose actual job it was at Vanderbilt to fill Flexner's prescription with the names of real people, succeeded in that remarkably well.

After three days in Nashville, Flexner and Buttrick bade farewell to the chancellor and returned to New York with the ammunition they needed, though for Kirkland at the other end there were still several anxious months of uncertainty. During June he wrote to Buttrick, ostensibly about the bothersome future of the Vanderbilt dental school (which eventually closed in 1926), but in truth for bucking up on medical matters in general. "Please don't mind a bit sharing your troubles with us," Flexner soothed his friend. "We understand their genesis and urgency. We should feel more worried about the future of things medical in Nashville if you weren't worried. Your worrying worries me less than some other people's complacency."[15] Soothing dollars soon followed: four million of them. The GEB voted the gift in July, citing reasons that were culled directly from Flexner's memorandum: strategic location, the need to study diseases endemic to the South, the lack of a first-rate school in the region, and the presence of Kirkland.

But little of the world beyond the GEB board room and Kirkland's office would know of their deed officially until the end of November, for Kirkland needed time to iron out two local matters. First he had to secure the resignations of the present medical faculty, the implied condition of the grant and something he had previously assured Buttrick and Flexner he could do. As well they might have, the old medical faculty greeted Kirkland's news of a great Rockefeller gift with something less than glee. The chancellor pointed out that the gift was to them the ultimate compliment because it came at least in part on the strength of noble efforts made by them under less than ideal conditions. That was a half-truth at best, and for many of those practitioner-teachers, who had truly given much for little, it probably made no happier the prospect of a future at Vanderbilt (if they were to have a future there at all) served under new, young, and outside masters. Still, with many of those Nashville doctors Kirkland's stock was high and their loyalty to him enough that all in the end signed the paper that left them serving solely at his pleasure. In the large and urgent task of reorganization that lay ahead, read the carefully worded (the words were in fact Kirkland's) final resolution, "we are ready to render assistance, but realize that the initiative must fall to others."[16] He also had to settle the status of the Galloway Memorial Hospital, which had been in various stages of planning and construction since 1916, and there too he worked things out well enough for the time being. Short of money, the Methodists agreed to relinquish control to Vanderbilt with the understanding that the hospital would be completed and equipped by the university and would become the teaching hospital for the soon-to-be reorganized Vanderbilt Medical School. It never did.[17]

With those two matters resolved, Kirkland and the GEB were ready to proceed with the formalities of applying for the now committed money and then to announce it with suitable public fanfare. In September Kirkland submitted to the GEB, for Buttrick's and Flexner's editing, drafts of the three documents that were needed from Vanderbilt in order to make the request official and to satisfy the conditions of the grant: the faculty resolution containing their resignations, the resolution of the executive committee of the Vanderbilt board of trust accepting those resignations and authorizing the chancellor to seek aid for the planned medical school reorganization, and the letter that Kirkland on behalf of his board would send to Buttrick as president of the GEB requesting aid in the amount of $4 million. Kirkland had drafted them all and confidently told Buttrick that "I assume that there will be no difficulty in having them executed according to my views."[18]

He was right, but first the Rockefeller men made in each document small but significant changes. The most urgent of the three was the faculty resolution (the faculty being scheduled to meet shortly) that referred to the need to build up at Vanderbilt a "worthy school of medicine." The very day Kirkland's letter arrived in New York a telegram shot back suggesting instead that the phrase "worthy school of medicine" be changed to "school of medicine modern in type, facilities, equipment, personnel, and ideals." The wire was signed "Buttrick Flexner," but the wording (which was adopted) was almost certainly Flexner's.[19] Three days later came a letter from Flexner about the other two documents. The second paragraph of Kirkland's draft of the executive committee resolution read: "The Chancellor of the University is hereby authorized to present the needs of the School of Medicine to the General Education Board and to such other philanthropic societies and individuals as may be disposed to help, making such requests for assistance as he may deem wise." In the final draft the phrase "educational agencies" had replaced "philanthropic societies." Finally, in the proposed formal letter of request to Buttrick, Kirkland explained that Vanderbilt sought not "small and temporary improvements of a weak organization, but a radical reorganization which would amount to the establishment of a new school." He added (evidently still aglow from his Baltimore visit the previous winter): "We have in mind a duplication in this section of the country of the Johns Hopkins Medical School—not, of course, in its present perfected condition, but as it was in its early years." Hopkins man that he was, Flexner offered instead: "We have in mind to attempt to accomplish in this section of the country the kind of service to education, to medical science and to humanity that can in these days be accomplished by a modern medical school."[20] That covered more bases and hinted more directly at the limitless good expected to come from this enterprise.

None of this editing changed at all the substance of anything Kirkland wanted to say, but it did reveal that to Flexner nuance was important. He preferred to view the General Education Board (and foundation philanthropy generally) less as the mere dispenser of part of the Rockefeller or some other fortune and more as an equal partner with those institutions it helped.

Although the phrase "educational agencies" was patently less accurate than "philanthropic societies" as a definition of the General Education Board, it suited better Flexner's self-image as an educator, and the words were most likely his own. They implied equality between patron and patronized; Vanderbilt too, after all, was an "educational agency." "The new opportunity to invest your life is also an equally new opportunity to invest ours," he wrote to Kirkland late in 1919. "The undertakings are mutual and cooperative. Your effort means our effort, your joy means our joy, and vice versa. Dr. Buttrick and I therefore rejoice in your opportunity and in the opportunity which you and Vanderbilt afford us."[21]

Flexner was an agent of one of the world's largest accumulated bodies of capital designated for charitable disbursement and therefore a very powerful man. Power and wealth—even when not his own—were then still new to him, and being a man of good taste and considerably more than average intelligence, a certain modesty and self-effacement about it all naturally became him. So did some disingenuousness. Well it behooved him and his patrons at least to appear to identify society's broadest interests with their own; in philosophical vagueness was shelter from charges of special pleading. Hopkins clearly enough was to be the basic model for many if not most of the newly built and rebuilt medical schools in the decades after 1910, but people other than Buttrick knew—and resented—that the Hopkins men formed "a sort of mutual admiration association." It was more prudent, if wordier, at least in the public record to have as a goal not Hopkins but "the kind of service to education, to medical science and to humanity that can in these days be accomplished by a modern medical school." What grander themes were there than education, science, and humanity to bestir the talents and energies of right-minded people and to assure maximum public accolade for the agencies whose policies those themes were seen to guide?[22]

Such adjustments safely made, the formal public announcement came on Thanksgiving eve 1919. It was also homecoming weekend at Vanderbilt, which assured an enthusiastic and larger than usual audience for Kirkland when he went before two special assemblies of faculty, students, and friends to tell the good news. Before noon the afternoon papers were out with extra editions and large headlines, and on the street corners newsboys shouted of the great gift to Vanderbilt.[23] To the doctors and apprentices on their separate and, so they thought, soon to be vastly improved campus, Kirkland, in his own words, "told the story simply but eloquently." The faculty of course already knew, but to most of the students this announcement was proof to the rumors, no doubt circulating for some time, that big things were afoot. To Kirkland too it was surely a moment for innocent excitement.

With some understatement he wrote to Flexner a few days later: "In my talk to the medical faculty and students I made fullest acknowledgement of the interest you both [Flexner and Buttrick] have taken in our enterprise, and I let it be understood also that the enterprise was still somewhat in your hands." Although naturally apprehensive he was also feeling very happy and fraternal. He let it show, sharing with these men who were not just his benefactors but his friends, too, homey talk of holiday football and hunting: "I trust you are far from your office environment in thought, and that you will have good weather and great joy. At this end we have a homecoming of alumni, all of whom will come with thankful hearts over the great news. This afternoon we have a football game, and I am planning a quail hunt for tomorrow and Saturday. I wish I could put the results of my efforts on your table and Dr. Buttrick's. Perhaps, after all, this would not be enough for a Thanksgiving dinner."[24]

Local rejoicing climaxed with a public meeting on the night of December 1 in the Ryman Auditorium, orchestrated by James Stahlman, editor of the *Nashville Banner* and lifelong Vanderbilt partisan, but the splash was heard well beyond Nashville.[25] Flexner reported that "a number of the best local men [in New York] have spoken to us on the subject and all of them have without exception endorsed the project as wise and timely in the highest degree," adding, plainly pleased with himself, "I do not believe the Board [GEB] has ever done anything that has received warmer appreciation from the judicious."[26] The General Education Board's clipping service gathered notices of the Vanderbilt gift from forty papers around the country and no doubt there were more. The Nashville boosters may have set the largest headlines, but New Yorkers (whose city was headquarters for the other end of the new partnership and was Rockefeller's town to boot) read the news in seventeen of Gotham's then prolific newspapers, from the *Times* and the *Wall Street Journal* (which devoted to it five precious lines) to long-since vanished dailies like the *Globe,* the *Mail,* and the *Telegram.* Boston, Rochester, Chicago, St. Louis, Muncie, and Madison all got the news, and from Richmond to New Orleans old Confederates and New Southerners alike read of this, the latest and the biggest-yet Yankee doing in Dixie. Among editorial writers was ample encomium for the Rockefeller philanthropy's munificent service to humankind through the promotion of medical progress.[27] (One writer, however, in the *Richmond News-Leader* also worried that in light of its own proximity to Hopkins and of the General Education Board's large gift to Vanderbilt, Richmond might be left out of the board's future plans for the South. It was.)[28]

Most papers, however, simply copied the memorandum that Kirkland had prepared for the occasion with Flexner's advice and consent.[29] A press release better than most, it supplied enough information to sustain the excitement the event was supposed to generate, but of necessity it also left much unsaid. Only the eye-catching $4 million came before the large and quotable general theme of recognition "in accordance with the most exacting demands of modern medical education." Next there was credit to the local faculty who had sacrificed much to gain much for their school and who were from that moment committed publicly to "unconditional cooperation in the establishing of a new school of medicine in Nashville as an integral department of Vanderbilt University." Detailed plans had "not as yet been developed" but it was announced that the Galloway Hospital would be completed and an additional hospital unit and a modern laboratory built in the near future. The public also learned of the planned "appointment of an increased number of professors, giving their entire time to the school and hospital, in both laboratory and clinical branches." It was surely Flexner who took this opportunity to remind the world of the good works the GEB had already done to aid the development of promising medical schools, reciting down to the penny names and numbers that made good copy: "Johns Hopkins Medical School, Baltimore—$2,210,874.11; Medical Department, Washington University, St. Louis—$1,000,000; Medical Department, University of Chicago, Chicago (of which one half was contributed by the Rockefeller Foundation)—$2,000,000; Yale University, New Haven—$582,000." Kirkland certainly had no objection to the addition of this information, for it put his university in some very distinguished company and only highlighted the magnitude of its own good fortune. "The gift to Vanderbilt is the largest that the Board has ever made for this or any other purpose," began the last paragraph, "and it will suggest to the people of Nashville and to the entire South, as well as to the whole country, the importance which the Board attaches to creating in the South at this time a medical school of the most advanced modern type." So Vanderbilt would save itself by its (and the GEB's) exertions and the South and beyond by its example: "It is to be hoped, and indeed believed, that the new school will have, not only in the South but throughout the whole country, a stimulating influence. It is impossible to measure the effect on medicine and public health, which will be exercised by the creation at Nashville of a medical school which may serve as a practical demonstration of what can at this time be accomplished in their field."[30]

It was a good piece of work: enough facts, the right length (two double-spaced pages), the grandest good words saved for the end. It was also, purposeful design aside, a fair measure of the limits of Kirkland's knowledge about what would happen next. What did happen next and for several years to come was much to-ing and fro-ing, as the principles—Buttrick, Flexner, and Kirkland—saw to it that the new partnership really was one. Until the new school was built and opened in 1925, they corresponded constantly and logged many days and nights on the Pullmans between Nashville and New York (it was then a twenty-four-hour trip). That Kirkland leaned so heavily on his foundation friends after he already had their money was sure sign that he one day might want more of it; it was symptom too of his own insecurity when it came actually to implementing the large designs dreamed of for so long. His friends knew of his apprehension and, true friends that they were, did their very best to help. Never in this part of the history of their relationship did anyone overbear; at least no one complained of it. Only later, when the laymen were joined by the physician (Robinson, the new dean) and the relationship became triangular and therefore more complex, did awkwardness arise.

But before anything was started, events occurred that gave to Vanderbilt's progress in the 1920s a dimension larger than may have been guessed locally. The GEB grant to Vanderbilt of $4 million, like its early grants to Hopkins, Yale, Washington University, and the University of Chicago, had come from the general funds given to the board by John D. Rockefeller, Sr. In addition to the initial $1 million with which the board was founded in 1902, there had been seven other gifts totaling close to $32 million, none specifically designated for medical education.[31] Since 1914 and its first medical grant ($1.5 million to Hopkins), the GEB generally had felt its way, knowing that there was obviously much still to be done. Its own resources were not enormous, and in medicine it could hardly have embarked on a costlier field for philanthropy. No one knew all this better than Abraham Flexner, who since coming to the board in 1913 from the Carnegie Foundation for the Advancement of Teaching had become head evangelist for the reforms in medical education proposed in his report and a close figurer of what the bill for those good things was likely to be.

It would be higher by far, he figured in 1918, than the GEB's resources then could bear. Unwilling to give up his plan for building up nationwide a series of strategically located, thoroughly modern medical schools whose example "would point the way," he campaigned naturally for more money. Buttrick sent him to Frederick T. Gates, charter member of the GEB and long the senior Rockefeller's chief confidant in matters of philanthropy. Gates in turn approached Rockefeller, Jr., also a member of the GEB and himself as deeply involved in giving away the family fortune as his father once had been in acquiring it. A memorandum eventually was submitted to Rockefeller, Sr., setting forth the present sad condition of medical education in the United States, pointing out the urgent need for increased resources and improved facilities, and detailing policy proposals should the GEB come into position to direct the large work of upbuilding.[32] Flexner's approach succeeded, and between 1919 and 1921 Rockefeller, Sr., made grants to the board of some $45 million (both principal and income were to be used) restricted to medical education in the United States, thus more than doubling the assets of the foundation and making the cause of medical education (after the raising of faculty salaries in liberal arts colleges, for which Rockefeller had designated $50 million also in 1919) its largest single activity.[33] How best to apply such a sum was a matter of some concern to the GEB and one that occasioned formulation of a deliberate and separate policy to deal with it.

The basis for that policy was set forth in a memorandum prepared by Flexner and submitted to the board for discussion in December 1919.[34] Like most large blueprints, this one over the years it was in effect underwent some tinkering and modification, but in its original form it marks a coda to the Flexner Report a decade before and is fair indicator of how he saw the future. Although cast as a proposal for the board's consideration only, the paper contained a forceful series of "general policy considerations," all of it, if not quite ex cathedra, bearing nonetheless Flexner's own by this time considerable personal authority on the subject. If any members of the board had doubts about the wisdom of Rockefeller's having given so much for the single purpose of medical education, Flexner set out at the beginning to remove them. There was no other field of education, he declared in the memorandum, "in which we are as clear as we are in the field of medical education with respect to what is needed and what can be and should be accomplished." Although the sum of human suffering from disease was still enormous, "the method and the technique by means of which successive diseases may and probably will be ultimately conquered are now clear enough to suggest the proper educational procedure to be followed in the training of physicians who can apply such knowledge as has been won and who can utilize their current experience for the increase of knowledge and skill. Modern medicine is then a definite, logical conception." That settled, it was easy to adduce educational prerequisites for the study of medicine, the kinds of facilities and resources needed to support it, and the objects to be aimed at by the medical schools. "We are therefore justified in saying that we know what a modern medical school should aim to be."[35]

A practical man, Flexner judged that many areas of the United States were still unready (as they had been unready in 1909) to support the ideal type of medical school. Educational, financial, and social conditions were uneven at best and could not summarily be made otherwise. "Until they become fairly homogeneous [a word he had used before], the same type of medical education cannot be everywhere realized." The choices for the GEB, then, were either to wait until conditions in the United States became as happily homogeneous as they allegedly were, for instance, in Germany, or to try a different approach to the problem. Waiting posed a serious difficulty, for in his deed of gift Rockefeller, Sr., had stipulated that all interest and principal should be expended within fifty years—a long time perhaps, but not necessarily long enough for a polyglot nation so completely to change its nature. Rather, Flexner proposed, would it not be much better if the new fund were employed "for the immediate *improvement,* rather than the immediate *standardization* of medical education in the United States"? If such were the policy, "it would seem desirable to vary the form and object of our cooperation, according to local conditions."[36] Conditions in the East, for example, already admitted of nothing but the very best type of school, and though many inferior ones still existed there, none should expect any help from the GEB. In the South, by contrast, secondary schools and colleges were not yet sufficiently advanced to furnish more than a select few medical schools with the kind of student body they required, while local financial resources, again in contrast with the East, were extremely limited. The board had already committed to but one regional flagship, the establishment of which at Nashville "should provide a concrete embodiment of the modern ideal, which will be a constant source of inspiration and stimulus." Existing schools in Virginia, Texas, and Louisiana that held promise for considerable improvement but were not yet first-rate led Flexner to ask "whether in the South it would not be both wise and necessary to assist at the moment something other than the best."[37] In the West there was a mixture of a few superior eastern-style schools, with many more struggling ones in whose promise the board might well invest.

Flexner's memorandum also raised the issue of GEB assistance to other than privately endowed institutions to which up to then it had limited its support. Gates was adamantly opposed to such a change and he fought Flexner bitterly over it, reportedly never forgiving him when Flexner proposed aid to the University of Iowa and won the board over to his viewpoint.[38] How, practically, to do the greatest good over the widest area was for Flexner more important than the ideological purity Gates espoused, and he reasoned that if the board did not so open itself to applications from publicly supported institutions (he counted only eight or ten non–state medical schools in the whole South and West), it would find its work virtually limited to the East where the need was smallest to begin with. Thus, though possessed as ever by certain knowledge of what the ideal medical school should look like, Flexner with a practiced and pragmatic eye for what was really out there claimed to eschew standardization in the real medical schools he sought to uplift. Or at least he proposed that in order for the GEB to get on with its work of applying Rockefeller's new gift, it needed to cast the net broadly enough to cover the entire country, which was not blessed as yet with many incipient Johns Hopkinses. This proposal entailed no backing off from the essential content of the medical school curriculum and the specific institutional arrangements that distinguished a real medical school from a fraud— all defined a decade before in his report and as nonnegotiable as ever. But it did admit that, if in the next two or three decades the job of placing medical education in the United States on a modern basis was to be accomplished, taxation would have to be relied upon, particularly west of the Mississippi and to a degree south of the Ohio. Rather than skimp on the true standards and pare down the colossal $200 million he estimated it all would cost, Flexner and the board were willing, in that sense, to go public.

But whatever the financial arrangements settled on to meet those staggering costs—aid to tax-supported state universities, aid to schools conditioned on the raising of matching funds (an increasingly common demand), or, as had been the case with the first Vanderbilt grant, GEB underwriting of a total project—what mattered most was that by those various means one common end would be served: bringing "medical education throughout the United States to the level made possible by the recent progress of medical science." No guesses, no hunches, no leaps of faith were wanted here: *"We know how to train competent practitioners and investigators in the field of medicine and surgery. We know with sufficient definiteness how many establishments of this kind the present needs of the country require and in most cases where they ought to be located. We know how medical schools and hospitals ought to be organized and how they ought to be related to the general educational system, secondary and higher, of the country."*[39]

Of such knowledge schools like Vanderbilt became the embodiment as the GEB marshaled its resources and the talent of its officers for a final assault on the shoddiness of American medical education. It would be a big push where success well rewarded the conviction and hard work of its planners. But it rested, as do most such campaigns, not on the clarity and soundness of the general orders alone but on the skill and the energy of ambitious captains and lieutenants: the line officers who with still unfinished careers to care for bravely faced the prospect of an extended action in a good cause and hoped distinction would come of it.

The New Man   **5**

On the steps to the north entrance to the new Vanderbilt Medical School the camera captured their likeness. Among them, balding, tending to the portly, and with horn-rimmed spectacles and bow tie, was G. Canby Robinson, dean of the new medical school. He had first become known to Kirkland, not surprisingly, through Flexner. Robinson, Flexner told Kirkland in October 1919, was in charge of an exemplary medical plant and educational operation at Washington University. "Wouldn't it be a good idea," Flexner asked, "for you to run over to St. Louis, confer with Dr. Canby Robinson, and look over their plant?"[1]

Flexner himself and his cohorts were then scouring the still small scientific-medical world for suitable candidates for the new deanship, and it was not specifically with Robinson in mind as a prospect that he wanted the two to meet, or if that was his purpose he did not admit it. Throughout the partnership of the GEB and Vanderbilt—at least as long as Flexner was connected with it—Flexner was ever at great pains to make it appear that the real decisions were made in Nashville and not New York, which in a sense they were (though they were also almost always the same decisions that would have been reached in New York too, so close was their collaboration). In this instance, whether it was to inspect Washington University's physical plant preliminary to meeting with consultant Winfred Smith, or to inspect Canby Robinson, or most likely both, Kirkland did, as his friend and patron counseled, "run over to St. Louis." Flexner knew about Robinson through at least two very reliable channels: his brother Simon, director of the Rockefeller Institute in New York in whose hospital Robinson had been resident physician from 1910 to 1913, and from his own and the GEB's dealings with Washington University where Robinson, first as a member of the department of medicine and then as dean, had participated in the reorganization of that school along modern Flexnerian lines. Flexner liked both Robinson's work as a scientist (he had established a respectable reputation for his studies of the heart) and, even more important for the task at hand, Robinson's budding administrative talents.

Kirkland went to St. Louis in November, before the gift to Vanderbilt was formally announced, anxious both to see the impressive facilities there and to confer with the dean. As Robinson remembered the encounter, Kirkland appeared in his office, announced that Vanderbilt was to receive $4 million from the General Education Board for a complete reorganization, and asked counsel about a suitable new leader. Kirkland listened politely to Robinson's suggestions and then asked what the dean thought of himself for the job. "I replied that I had not thought of him," Robinson wrote, "but would be glad to give him consideration although at that moment I was quite unprepared to make a decision."[2] Whether Robinson remembered it correctly or not (Kirkland left no record of the meeting), he was certainly flattered and intrigued by the prospect, and he took up Kirkland's invitation both to visit Vanderbilt and inspect the local situation and to confer with the officers of the GEB about the project.

He came to Nashville five days before Christmas 1919, and Kirkland gave the entire day to touring the young medical man around Vanderbilt's plant and talking over "a thousand things" concerning its imminent reorganization.[3] Years later Robinson wrote disdainfully about what he saw there: "About five miles from the main campus of the university on the other side of the city . . . a heterogeneous group of five or six buildings dominated by the unfinished Galloway Memorial Hospital on what was known as the South Campus. . . as to the other [other than the Galloway] buildings—one had been built as a college in about 1850, another was occupied by the Vanderbilt Dental School, and a third had been built to house the University of Nashville Medical School which had been taken over by Vanderbilt. The original Vanderbilt Medical School building, about two blocks away, had been converted into a small hospital and dispensary which, with the Nashville City Hospital not far away, provided the facilities for clinical instruction. Viewing this array of buildings, it was natural to wonder why the General Education Board had selected Vanderbilt for its special attention."[4] At the time, however, Robinson the candidate put it rather more diplomatically: "I can see no reason why Vanderbilt University should not take a very important place in medical education," he wrote to Kirkland a few days later. He even added a little banter about Nashville's amenities, which he was surely comparing with those of St. Louis: "I had an opportunity to visit the library and to walk through the shopping section of Nashville after I left you and was much surprised to see what attractive shops and fine buildings you have."[5] He had also, of course, had the opportunity to take measure of Kirkland and his university and to decide that he wanted the job.

That at least was Kirkland's judgment, who had himself decided that he wanted Robinson. "I am of the opinion that Dr. Robinson is willing to come to us [and] accept the deanship," he reported to Flexner even before receiving Robinson's cheery letter about Vanderbilt's bright medical future (brighter presumably for Robinson's hoped-for participation) and Nashville's nice buildings. He would have to have an assistant dean "who will relieve him of routine student work," and the matter of salary had not yet been discussed. From his spy in St. Louis, Eugene Opie, professor of pathology at Washington University, Kirkland learned that Robinson was then receiving about $5,000; as to what he should get if he came to Vanderbilt, Kirkland pleaded advice from Flexner and Buttrick.[6] In the meantime, Robinson arranged to meet Buttrick and Flexner. They talked three times in a thirty-day period, in St. Louis, Nashville, and New York. There are no records of their conversation, though from them Robinson clearly received the assurance that the GEB was committed to development of a genuinely first-rate medical school in the South and that it would commit the financial resources needed to do the job. Buttrick and Flexner were no doubt convinced again that here they had their new dean, so confirming Kirkland's own judgment.[7] Thus assured, Kirkland made the formal offer in mid-January. As professor of medicine and dean of the medical school Robinson would be responsible for reorganizing the faculty and designing and building the new plant. In the meantime he would have no teaching or administrative duties in the old school, which would continue to be run by an acting dean. His salary on a full-time, university basis would be $7,500 per year.

Robinson turned it down. He wanted more money, and his argument for it is a good example of the problem of trying to attach to the perennially underpaid academy the profession of clinical medicine whose members—unlike most professors of English, history, mathematics, or physics—had other attractive places to go. In four closely written longhand pages he explained himself in a way that he hoped would keep the door open. He told Kirkland that when full-time clinical teaching had been adopted in St. Louis, heads of clinical departments had received salaries of $10,000 or more, a sum that had meant more then than later. That was good pay indeed during World War I, but said Robinson, "I considered these large salaries, as did practically all people engaged in medical education, as essential for the success of this plan, and naturally looked forward to obtaining such a place myself." The importance of good pay was really all Flexner's doing, whose authority Robinson now summoned in the calculation that Kirkland listened to him. Full-time had proven very expensive, and Flexner had tried to keep salary scales in hand. It was "partly through his influence" that two appointments to professorships in clinical departments at Washington had been made at lower figures, but both men, neither of whom had before attained professional rank, were quite young and untried, and both were given to understand that their salaries were for a probation period only. But Robinson still felt in 1920, as he did four years before in St. Louis, "that large salaries are essential to the success of the plan which Mr. Flexner had advocated."[8]

In his counterproposal he tried to have it both ways. He would accept the position at $7,500 "with the privilege of accepting for my own personal use two thousand five hundred dollars from fees collected for professional services rendered to patients in the Vanderbilt University Hospital and from unavoidable consultation within the limits of the City of Nashville." What he meant by "unavoidable" was anyone's guess, but he did point out the sacrifice he was thus generously making, inasmuch as his salary would not reach $10,000 until the Vanderbilt Hospital, site of his proposed consultations, had been reorganized and put in satisfactory running order (he apparently did not anticipate earning $2,500 in "unavoidable" extramural consultation). Such consultation, happily, would not "add any additional burden on the university and will not require any more work outside of the purely academic confines than would be necessary under any other condition." Again, what other conditions there might conceivably be were unclear, but it was clear that Robinson interpreted full-time differently than Flexner, if only to help get a better salary. At St. Louis, he told Kirkland hopefully, paying patients brought into each of the clinical departments about $5,000 yearly "in spite of the fact that as much of this work as is compatible with the best interests of the school is directed to the part-time members of the staff."[9]

There was then no way to stretch limited resources. And what better way besides to relieve the financial pressures on the schools supporting the full-time plan of clinical teaching, "without in any way impairing the chances for accomplishing the things for which it has been established?" Robinson was master of the well-placed but vague phrase that alluded to large altruistic purpose for the real purpose of winning a smaller argument. But his confidence in his ability so to win over Kirkland was less than total, for (perhaps believing that Kirkland would consult Flexner anyway and that with him lay the key to the problem) in the same letter he proposed to go to New York to take up his plan with Flexner himself. Kirkland from their first meeting in St. Louis had encouraged Robinson to confer with the officers of the GEB, and Robinson had done so on two occasions already. Robinson was aware that a third meeting might have the appearance of going over Kirkland's head, and he hastened to add that "I hope you do not consider that I am pressuring and doing so, but I believe I am acting as you would advise in this matter." Indeed, Kirkland had no objection. He knew Flexner better than Robinson did, which was perhaps why he was so generous in the face of Robinson's presumption. "I can frankly say I am anxious," Robinson wrote, "to have Mr. Flexner accept this plan and advise you accordingly. I am taking it for granted that you and Dr. Buttrick would be strongly influenced in matters relating to the full-time plan by Mr. Flexner's opinion."[10]

He was presumptuous, but correct too. Kirkland did listen to Flexner. Robinson only overrated his own power of persuasion and thus misjudged what Flexner would tell him. Robinson went to New York at Vanderbilt's expense, and what passed between him and Flexner can only be inferred from later events; likewise what passed between him and Kirkland, whom he also saw there. In Flexner's office he probably laid out his interpretation of full-time, as he had in his counterproposal to Kirkland. Flexner, by this time deft at saying no with a smile, probably allowed that was not what he and the board had in mind at all. Because Flexner held all the cards, beyond the pleasantries there could have been little else to say. That clear, it was in the more opulent setting of the City Club where a compromise of sorts was worked out with Kirkland. It involved less principles than money.[11] Robinson clearly would work for less than $10,000, but he was worried lest he not be paid more than any other member of the faculty, all of whom had yet to be hired and whose salaries could not be known. He did not want to be discriminated against because he was the first appointment. That being the real problem (or the only real one remaining, inasmuch as Flexner was immovable on the other), Kirkland, not raising the offer a penny, proposed that Robinson receive $6,500 as professor of medicine, $1,000 for the extra work of the deanship, and, in the event any professor was appointed at more than $6,500, Robinson's salary would increase by that amount—that is, that his salary would always be at least $1,000 higher than any other salary in the school.

Back in St. Louis Robinson promptly accepted, on the full-time basis as Flexner understood it and without costing Kirkland any more money. Robinson wanted the best he could get but he wanted the job more and, his bluff called, the mood changed. "I can assure you," he wrote Kirkland, accepting the offer, "that I am willing and glad to undertake the new work as we have discussed it, with enthusiasm and with all the energy and care of which I am capable. I am looking forward with happy anticipation to cooperating with you in this splendid enterprise." To Flexner he wrote with more chagrin: "I finally agreed to Dr. Kirkland's second proposition which was not very different than the first and I am as ready to plunge into the work at Nashville with our differences behind us and forgotten."[12] Kirkland meanwhile suggested to Flexner that "we may congratulate ourselves that we are bringing this important matter to a satisfactory conclusion."[13]

Everyone seemed pleased.[14] For the record and for his own board Kirkland wanted only one more thing: that Robinson set forth in writing his understanding of his position at Vanderbilt. "Please try to avoid too many technical details," he counseled his new medical man. "Trustees do not like to be bound by measures that may hereafter prove unwise. There is no question about their readiness to carry out the plans suggested by me; we only want to have matters in as flexible a form as possible."[15] Accordingly, Robinson summarized what he and Kirkland had agreed to. Vanderbilt was in possession of approximately $5 million ($4 million from the GEB, $1 million from the Carnegie grant of 1913) and land and buildings valued at $500,000, all to be devoted exclusively to the expansion of the medical school. It was "the intention of the University to conduct a medical school of the best type, according to the approved methods as now understood in medical education." Further, "the University will make every effort to secure additional funds, whenever the present funds shall prove inadequate for the immediate needs of the school or for future development." The departments would be organized "on the University or so-called whole-time plan as recommended by the General Education Board as far as the funds of the school will permit." Robinson outlined his authority and responsibility as dean and professor of medicine, referred to the resignations of the medical faculty that Kirkland then had in hand, and stipulated that there would be an assistant dean to deal with routine administrative work. Together with the chancellor he would make the decisions regarding construction and equipment for the new buildings and select the architects and other experts needed for the project. The only new thing he suggested was that the term "director" be substituted for "dean" in describing his new post, "dean" being reserved for the officer responsible for daily administration. The switch, he said, was in keeping with "the modern tendencies of medical education" and had recently been adopted by the China Medical Board for the Peking Union Medical College and by the new school of public health at Johns Hopkins.[16]

Kirkland had no objection to any of it (though the dean/director matter seems to have been mislaid, Robinson being called only "dean" while at

Vanderbilt), believing that now "we have a satisfactory working plan."[17] He did ask Flexner's confirming judgment, and Flexner typically tinkered with a few words but also thought Robinson had admirably sketched everyone's intention.[18] Only on the question of how explicit they should be regarding Robinson's responsibilities at Vanderbilt (beyond planning the new school) did they disagree, Flexner wanting clearly to free the new dean from any possible teaching involvement until the new school was in operation, Kirkland reluctant "to elect professors with the proviso that they shall draw salaries and be free from all obligation to the School until such time as new hospitals and laboratories are ready for service," which time no one could predict. It "would be a very great mistake to announce to the public that we had secured Dr. Robinson as Dean but that he would have no definite duties or relation to the school for two or three years." The wording on that point was kept vague for Kirkland, but as Flexner and Robinson wished (and Kirkland having no substantive objection), Robinson was in spirit at least bound only to a school that did not yet exist.[19]

His appointment was to begin on July 1, 1920, but even before he had formally resigned his St. Louis post Kirkland was after him about specific Vanderbilt medical matters. Negotiations were already well advanced with James Jobling at Columbia to head pathology, and Walter Dandy, a young Hopkins man, was high on the list of surgery. As usual the correspondence was three-way, but Kirkland was obviously eager to shift much of the medical burden to Robinson's shoulders. Neither Jobling nor Dandy in the end came to Vanderbilt (Jobling wanted too much money and stayed in New York, and Dandy, though mentioned as a possible successor to Halsted at Hopkins,[20] was also too expensive and not inclined to accept the full-time plan as Flexner understood it).[21] But the occasion of their consideration reveals something of the new dean's approach both to faculty recruitment in particular and to the large job of medical school reorganization generally. Working through a network of predominantly Hopkins friends and colleagues, Robinson as dean-designate only and with still large responsibilities in St. Louis gave what time he could to Vanderbilt. Jobling, he thought, could be persuaded to return to Nashville, where he had been professor of pathology at Vanderbilt from 1914 to 1918, if a small cohesive group of similar medical scientists were also brought in at the outset. While in New York to confer with him about that prospect, both men called on Donald Van Slyke, then at the hospital of the Rockefeller Institute and a man Robinson believed to be one of the best biochemists in the world and likewise someone who would contribute enormously to a good start at Vanderbilt. And at Cornell, Robinson cast an envious recruiter's eye on leading anatomist Charles R. Stockard, a Mississippian by birth to whom he hoped a Vanderbilt appointment would offer an appealing opportunity to get out of New York.[22]

None of these men in the end ever joined Vanderbilt's faculty, but those who eventually did were selected for like reasons. From the outset Robinson was intent on assembling a core faculty of individuals whose scientific attainments and personalities equipped then to attract others to junior posts. As quickly became apparent when Jobling decided he could not come to Vanderbilt for $6,500 (which was less money than he was getting at Columbia, though Kirkland argued it would go further in Nashville), Vanderbilt could not hope to compete with the larger salaries paid for senior posts in the Northeast. It might then have to settle for promising younger talent. That, Robinson was certain, was best decided from the inside by a medical person and not from the outside by a layman. As much as he respected Flexner's ideas about the general course that had to be set for medical education, he was a jealous captain who knew best the sort of crew he would have under him. At Kirkland's bidding, for example, Flexner had made the first investigations of Dandy as a prospect for surgery at Vanderbilt. With Buttrick in tow he had gone to Hopkins and had learned from others there that Dandy was one of the most promising surgeons in the United States. They watched him teach at the bedside, and they came away highly impressed.[23] Robinson took the occasion to make clear to Kirkland that sometimes Flexner overlooked things that were desirable and necessary in someone considered to head a complex department like surgery. Apparently he felt Dandy something of a prima donna lacking in qualities needed to conduct that staple of training in surgery, the surgical clinic. Not content to rely on Flexner, he insisted before making a final judgment on consulting his friend Alphonse Dochez in New York and in inspecting Dandy more closely for himself. That he eventually looked on Dandy more favorably did not change his feeling that "Mr. Flexner must speak as an outsider [who] has never been actually involved in medical education."[24] At least Flexner had not been involved as only a doctor supposedly could be, something that to this particular young medical man made all the difference.

Flexner probably heard all that from his friend Kirkland, but being a man whose outsider's involvement in medical education gave him perspective some doctors did not have, and with a thick skin besides, he continued to insist for the record at least that "we must . . . make it plain to Robinson and all these young fellows that the General Education Board is not the source of authority."[25] Robinson's perception (largely accurate) that it was the source led him sometimes to chafe against it and sometimes to appeal to it over Kirkland's head—but always for the purpose of consolidating his own plans for what he hoped to do at Vanderbilt. Even as Kirkland had him busy at this early stage weighing candidates for key posts, it became apparent that the plans might require both more money and more time to accomplish than the chancellor, already years weary with medical school troubles, probably had in mind. How much more money and time would not become clear for some months yet, but even in those first few weeks there were signs. Thus when Kirkland, refusing to improve on his offer of $6,500, found it necessary to drop Jobling from consideration for the pathology post, Robinson implied that such first-rate men were worth what they cost and to lose one, who was otherwise eager to come, over money matters was foolish: "I do not feel that the spirit of extravagance should be allowed to creep in, although it is necessary to give the impression from the beginning that the school is to be built up by a group of men of the first rank."[26] On the other hand, when Kirkland eagerly pressed the search for a chief surgeon and Robinson was unsure, Robinson urged that while he shared Kirkland's impulse to get started, "still we must make haste slowly."[27]

Events over the next year made clear what exactly that mysterious admonition meant, and Robinson emerged as the dominant force in shaping them. Faculty matters for the moment pushed aside, the new dean had his first meeting on plant design with architects Charles A. Coolidge and Henry R. Shepley and consultant Winfred Smith in Baltimore early in May 1920. In the same month he was introduced formally to the then–Vanderbilt medical community, to the accompaniment of what he recalled as glowing after-dinner speeches by Kirkland, Whitefoord Cole, president of the university board of trust, and Lucius E. Burch, dean of the medical school. The next day, with many of those same doctors, he boarded the train for the New Orleans meeting of the American Medical Association, a comradely time passed with the help of numerous hip flasks and poker games.[28] For the record at least, Robinson was much pleased with these southern doctors: "The profession as a whole is in my opinion greatly superior to that of St. Louis, and altogether I have obtained a very pleasant impression"; and "unless I am a failure as a judge of men, I can assure you [Kirkland] that they will be of the greatest assistance in the future of the school."[29]

It all seemed an auspicious beginning, and had things taken hold at that moment so it might have remained. But it was the end of the academic year, which in those less hurried times meant a lull in university affairs, even medical ones. Kirkland and Flexner retreated to their cottages in Canada; Robinson that June moved his family to Baltimore, there to be closer to the architects and consultant Smith and to get the best vantage (which Hopkins surely was) on possible recruits to fill posts at Vanderbilt. He too sought respite in the country, at Blue Ridge Summit in Pennsylvania. It was there in the summer of 1920 that he conceived the piece of mischief that soured his dealings with Kirkland, placed Flexner and Buttrick in an embarrassingly awkward position, and threatened an early end to his own career at Vanderbilt.

From the beginning Kirkland had encouraged his new dean to visit other medical schools as a help to planning Vanderbilt's. Vanderbilt would pay the fare. In August Robinson embarked with friend and future professor of medicine at Hopkins, Warfield Longcope, for the West Coast to look at medical schools at the University of California and Stanford where there had been innovations in the administration of teaching hospitals.[30] He returned via the Mayo Clinic in Rochester, Minnesota. Back at home he drew up totally new plans for Vanderbilt and prepared to stake everything on them. It was no small thing that he did that autumn and winter—to take on at once both Kirkland, his immediate employer, and the awesome Rockefeller philanthropy that ultimately was his patron. Had he been a man of less brass and more prudence, later history might have remembered him only as one of a number of competent but cautious medical administrators. Whether he had history on his mind when he decided so dramatically to change all the rules is not known, but he surely did have in mind, for whatever reasons, dramatically to extend his reach to touch his ideals. For the last time in his career his reach did not exceed his grasp.

He lacked Kirkland's subtlety and with him there were no trial balloons. He launched his plan full-blown late in September with the clear expectation of a quick answer. Copies of his twenty-two-page proposal for the reorganization of the Vanderbilt Medical School went simultaneously to Kirkland, Flexner, and Buttrick, with letters that warned of big surprises to follow.[31] "I realize that it presents some big problems," he said with some understatement to Flexner, "which we must work out together, and I trust we can arrive at some definite arrangement."[32] To Kirkland, in whom he believed he had a natural ally, went a long handwritten missive in which he tried to shift responsibility for his ambitious proposal from himself, its author, to the General Education Board: "When they contributed the sum of \$4 million to Vanderbilt for the Medical School, they carried out what seems to me a big piece of business on a very superficial knowledge of the matter." Robinson the physician, who naturally had much better knowledge, nobly cast himself not as beggar but as savior: "I shall try to make him [Flexner] feel that I am someone anxious to help him and the Board out of a somewhat delicate situation. Everyone is looking toward Nashville as an enterprise of the General Education Board, and if they do not provide sufficient funds to accomplish a reorganization of a first class order, they will be regarded as making a very poor use of their large resources."[33]

At that Kirkland, though he was a patient man and one who had dealt with deans before, probably boiled. It took him nearly two weeks to reply, and when he did, he politely accused the doctor of prescribing a course of treatment no one could hope to pay for. Progress, for Kirkland the liberal, came inevitably enough with evolution and slow growth. His career had been spent nurturing a lot from a little; small wonder that plans for medical utopia offended his natural sense of moderation. He likewise, he wrote Robinson, could draw up an ideal blueprint for his university that would, alas, require an annual income of $4 or $5 million and thus an increased endowment such as no individual or group could possibly underwrite. Nevertheless he admired boldness when he saw it and admitted Robinson's was a wonderful plan "but unfortunately required a wonderful amount of money. . . . It is unwise to expect any such enlargement of heart in any quarter as your plan calls for. No great institution was ever built that way."[34] Flexner, ever careful to avoid the appearance of meddling (and who had consulted his brother Simon at the Rockefeller Institute), told Robinson that he and Buttrick had found his proposal embarrassing in that it seemed something better taken up first between the dean and his chancellor.[35] Kirkland, meanwhile, hopeless though he thought it was, gave Robinson free rein to get what he could from Rockefeller's agents. No one, he said, would be more pleased if Robinson succeeded—and no one more surprised.[36]

Brash and presumptuous as Robinson's action may have appeared to his seniors, it was well calculated to tempt their vanity and ambition. In his action he guessed Kirkland's mind correctly: he offered to help give to Kirkland's precious Vanderbilt an instrument of enormous power for education, scholarship, and service—things upon which the chancellor had built his life. He also knew where Flexner had much invested. He had read Bulletin Number Four and now read it back to its author. Coordination was his theme. The coordination of clinical and preclinical departments and of medical school with laboratories and hospital must be deliberate from the planning of the building through to the organization of departments and curriculum. And coordination of the entire medical enterprise with the larger university whose name it shared also had to be actual and not nominal. They must be in the same place. If Flexner's dictum were applied, Robinson implied very clearly, Vanderbilt's medical school would have to move across town.

So Robinson elaborated. Much could be said for Flexner's favored German "institute" concept in which each department lived happily on its own, often physically apart from other departments. But much more might be accomplished if a medical school itself were formed into one large institute whose subject would be the study of disease in human beings. No medical school, Robinson claimed, had yet been organized with such a fundamental conception, but the time had now come to try at Vanderbilt. People were available with the proper training and point of view in all the necessary sciences to assure success; they would guarantee the institute's single-minded pursuit of scientific truth while facilitating the application of such discovery to the treatment of disease. The idea of coordination as Robinson advanced it entailed both the physical contiguity of the various departments and a certain degree of interlocking of personnel on the various staffs. No matter where research work might originate, for example, the heads of the laboratory or preclinical departments must assume responsibility for the work done in their respective fields. Obviously, they would have to be chosen with an eye to their relation to the school as a whole as well as with regard to individual attainments and potential. On selection of the initial group of such individuals the success of the whole school depended. They must be enthusiastic and wholly convinced for themselves that university medicine was not a passing fancy or a chapter on the way to something else but a worthy and permanent object for a life's work. They should be young, fresh in their careers, more intent on the future than bound to the past, receptive and ready to share fully in the work of developing the whole school. From the organization of a medical school on the basis of coordination of departments would flow much needed reforms in the medical curriculum. It would invite the mutually beneficial integration of laboratory and clinical studies that in time would mold a new, more competent scientist-practitioner.

The people who would do all this would have to be paid salaries sufficient to provide what was commonly considered a pleasant standard of living, with enough to put something aside for old age. Yet the numbers Robinson proposed were hardly extravagant and, with the exception of the salary of the professors, surely demanded of academic doctors real sacrifice to live the life of the mind. The scale was the same as had recently gone into effect at Robinson's old school, Washington University: professors, $6,500 minimum with an average of $7,500, their appointment permanent; associate professors, $3,500 to $5,000, their appointment for five years to be indefinitely renewable; assistant professors, $2,500 to $3,500, their appointment for three years to be indefinitely renewable; instructors, $1,500 to $2,500, with yearly renewable appointments; fellows, $800 to $1,200, also with yearly renewable appointments. The scale for professors was an absolute minimum and was not equivalent to that of $5,000 set when Washington University reorganized its medical school in 1910. Indeed, it was far below what had been necessary to pay full-time teachers in the clinical subjects even in 1914.

Robinson doubted whether he had recommended sufficient salaries, especially for the heads of clinical departments, and the question of maintaining a uniform scale or of permitting some discrimination raised further practical difficulties. He proposed, though, no difference between the heads of clinical and laboratory departments, on the assumption that no faculty member received more than a "living wage" and that size of salary in no way measured the service each rendered to the school. Even though the greater complexity of the clinical departments and the added responsibility borne by their heads could argue in favor of a certain amount of discrimination, additional returns from private consultations should be permitted only where the facilities and staff were such as to enable the head of a clinical department to cultivate the same university spirit of scientific ideals as would a head of a laboratory. "In other words, intellectual return must be such as to eliminate the desire for private practice, and the salary must be such that family obligations are not constantly urging an increase in financial returns." Part-time or "clinical" personnel would receive small honoraria only: $200 to $500, which in Nashville might make staffing some of the clinical specialties difficult. Ideally such posts should be filled with promising young individuals who for salaries of up to $2,000 could be induced to settle in Nashville as part-time teachers. And while the spirit of the old medical faculty was "a splendid asset to the new school, which we cannot afford to turn into a liability," their professional ability as teachers could not be determined "without a careful study of the individual men."[37]

To assure the success of those ideals and to bring together such a faculty there also would have to be guarantee of adequate physical facilities. This, Robinson knew, was the single weakest part of the original plan to reorganize the Vanderbilt Medical School on the south campus. If built there the medical school would be permanently separated from the main university campus and thus forever forfeit of all the blessings contiguity supposedly promised. So for years Flexner had argued in general; so Robinson now argued in particular. Certain in his own mind that a new start had to be made on the west campus with the rest of the university, Robinson proposed a courtlike design with hospital on the south end and medical school on the north, with laboratory departments arranged in such a way as to place the more closely allied subjects in contact with each other and also in contact with pathology, bacteriology, and the clinical laboratories and services.

His specific plans and budgets for various departments illustrated the theory of coordination that was also to be apparent in the design of the buildings. With the too frequently neglected laboratory departments, the scientific heart of the modern medical school, great care especially must be taken (a familiar Flexnerian theme). "The scarcity of men in the pre–clinical departments of medical schools is the most threatening condition in American medical education today," warned Robinson the clinician. Here science alone must govern. At Vanderbilt these departments "should be so headed, equipped, financed and manned that they will serve to attract medical graduates into anatomy, physiology and the other sciences, and the training of future medical teachers should be considered one of the avowed purposes of the school. The school should serve to draw the best minds of the developing South into intellectual pursuits, and it should stand as an example of what such pursuits may lead to." The world of medical education was watching with expectant interest the scale on which the preclinical departments would be organized at Vanderbilt, and insufficient support for them from the General Education Board would be "a disappointment to an already somewhat discouraged group of workers."[38]

Pharmacology, bacteriology, and biochemistry got special mention in this regard. Although Robinson had placed pharmacology as a subdepartment of physiology, as then befitted its lesser importance as a subject for undergraduate medical students, as a field of research it held large promise and its coordination with clinical medicine was potentially of enormous value. As a developing science whose subject was the relation of the chemical structure of substances to their effects on living tissue, it crystallized the principle of coordination and hinted at its promising future. Correlating chemistry, physiology, and clinical medicine, pharmacology's growth would soon merit establishment as an independent department. Bacteriology, though at many schools incorporated with pathology, at Vanderbilt should be independent from the beginning. It had developed far beyond the study of bacteria as a cause of disease, and immunology and serology had become subjects far too large for the pathologist alone to master. The ties between them and clinical medicine were self-evident, and there was no longer any debate that an expert bacteriologist should be connected with well-organized clinical departments. Such an expert should be provided with a staff sufficient to conduct the extensive work entailed by responsibility for the standards of bacteriological work in the school and the hospital. The same was true with biochemistry, which was coming closer together with clinical medicine. The trained biochemist was an assumed essential part of the modern medical clinic and at the same time was an important investigator, through laboratory research, of the biomechanisms of disease.

Robinson prescribed beyond the laboratory too. He anticipated that one member of the department of public health and preventive medicine should be trained in social service and should teach social medicine to medical students and public health nurses. Such a person would also be an important link between the university and the community by representing the medical school in various public health movements, such as the control of tuberculosis and venereal disease and in infant welfare and public health nursing. So conceived and staffed, public health at Vanderbilt would become an essential factor "in training physicians for general practice in the modern sense"—the front-line doctors whose daily job it was to render esoteric science into mundane service. Pediatrics, which Robinson judged the clinical department in which the full-time plan of development had been most successful elsewhere, also held forth great hope at Vanderbilt, and he called for its early establishment on a university basis. The department could be developed as a subdivision of internal medicine but as a stopgap only, he said, echoing the best German and Hopkins tradition: "The younger men want to work under a master in their specialty, and an experienced man could probably not be obtained as associate professor when there is no outlook toward a professorship." He thought the same for obstetrics and gynecology, which also if at all possible should enjoy full university status rather than rely on the services of the local profession.[39]

In the development of a strong school of nursing, Robinson saw for Vanderbilt an unusual opportunity to perform as great a service to the South as it would in medical education generally. Authorities agreed that the education of nurses should no longer be merely a by-product of the care of hospital patients, and though the establishment of proper facilities and program was beset with considerable difficulty, Vanderbilt should nonetheless strive to take advantage of its wholly fresh start to bring to medical education and hospital administration the unquestioned benefits that would be derived from a strong school of nursing.

Under the heading of administration generally, Robinson proposed to defray the railroad fares of department heads to attend one meeting of a national society each year and to do the same for other members of the faculty who had papers to present at such meetings; this proposal intended, as he put it, "to offset the relative isolation of Nashville."[40] He also asked a fund for lectureships to bring individuals from other cities before the school and the local profession, and he included an item for postgraduate fellowships to meet the living expenses of "especially gifted graduates, in whatever department such men may desire to work, and wherever favorable opportunity for investigations present themselves."[41]

Robinson detailed proposed budgets for each department and summarized a budget for the whole enterprise. For initial annual expenditures (he also calculated "ultimate" needs), internal medicine and surgery, heading the clinical group, demanded most ($37,650 and $35,300 respectively), followed by physiology and pharmacology ($26,350 each), anatomy ($24,350), pathology

($23,900), pediatrics ($22,220), obstetrics and gynecology ($21,300), bio-chemistry ($19,750), public health and hygiene ($18,650), and bacteriology ($18,600). Clinical departments thus would receive $135,120, preclinical departments $139,300. Another $64,450 would be required by X ray, library and record room, medical illustration, mechanical shop, and administrative and general expenses (at $43,050 the largest of any single category). The total anticipated beginning expense came to $338,870 yearly, not including the hospital endowment initially figured at $100,000 but ultimately twice that figure. Robinson figured hospital endowment needs with consultant Winfred Smith at Hopkins, accepting the sum of $1,000 per bed and adding that the amount that could reliably be realized from patient receipts was problematic at best. The initial figure was based on completion of Galloway Hospital with 78 beds and estimated receipts of $28,000, plus ten private self-supporting rooms and payment of $3.00 a day by half of the ward patients. The final figure of $200,000 presumed a new hospital of 330 beds (60 for blacks) and patient revenue of $130,000. Projected initial endowment needs, accounting for revenue from student fees and figuring a return on investment of 5 percent, totaled $6,650,000. Another $5.3 million for building costs and $200,000 for equipment gave Robinson's plan a final price tag of just under $12.2 million—at a time when he had at his disposal Carnegie and Rockefeller funds in less than half that amount.

Money aside, that was how the medical school was built—not in all the particulars, necessarily, but faithful enough to the general lineaments of Robinson's plan. At Vanderbilt the medical school and teaching hospital were deliberately coordinated in form and in function; the faculty was organized on a full-time, university basis, fully in the laboratory branches and as far as funds allowed in the clinical departments; the physical plant adjoined the main university campus; and there was an endowment adequate enough, if not munificent, to underwrite it all. Only a small number of carefully selected students, well-prepared by previous schooling to study medicine, won admission, and a faculty of medical scientists served simultaneously as searchers after the truth, tutors to the apprentices, and servants of the sick. The spirit of objective scientific inquiry reigned simultaneously with the spirit of useful service.

When in the summer of 1920 Robinson wrote it all down, he did not know that on all the essential points he would get his way, but for his new job he plainly had high hopes and was willing to stake everything on them. With Flexner's (whose ideas borrowed from Bulletin Number Four Robinson had made up the core of Robinson's proposal) slow response and evident lack of enthusiasm (which Robinson interpreted as a betrayal of the spirit if not of the letter of the GEB's grant to Vanderbilt to reorganize its medical school on "thoroughly modern lines"), he had little patience, and in an effort to enlist Kirkland in the cause, he offered his doctor's opinion that the great Flexner seemed to suffer "a definite lack . . . of information regarding details of medical education. He has a number of theories, but as he has had no opportunity to put them into actual practice himself [as presumably only a doctor could], he really doesn't know whether they work or not."[42] Kirkland, a layman too and one to whom $5 million seemed ample, took that coolly enough and to protect himself with his foundation patrons distanced himself as much as he decently could if not from the substance of Robinson's proposal (in which he recognized much good) then from its brash presentation. "I do not see any good that can come of a conference over Dr. Robinson's plans," he wrote Flexner. "From the first I discouraged his presenting them to you. My constant reply to him whenever he pressed the matter to my attention was 'wait and work. No great institution was ever built that way. Trust evolution.' "[43]

Between him and Robinson ensued a time of strained relations, Kirkland ever pushing to move ahead with the building program on the south campus for which architects Coolidge and Shepley were then preparing plans, and Robinson ever pushing for an answer from the General Education Board and for Kirkland's support.[44] The breaking point came in January 1921 when Kirkland frankly advised Robinson that it should be clear enough from the General Education Board's unwillingness to discuss Robinson's large plan that "your ideas cannot now be carried out, at least in the way you indicate. They would say doubtless, that assurance of continued interest and support of the Vanderbilt Medical School did not mean that large additional funds would be placed in our hands before the enterprise was ever begun."[45] That to Robinson was precisely the point, and Kirkland seemed to miss it. Robinson had calculated carefully how much a small modern medical school and teaching hospital would cost, and in that calculation he was neither wildly extravagant nor far from what Flexner himself in other circumstances had calculated. But if the enterprise was "ever begun" with other than a comprehensive plan in mind, no amount of money later could salvage what had initially been poorly conceived. Medical education simply was not like that anymore. The blueprint was complete; the future had been foreseen, and a shortsighted man it was who for simple lack of money hesitated to align himself with it.

Robinson's answer was to quit, or very nearly so. He took the high ground, appealing to ideals and modern standards betrayed. He had taken the job, he said, with the impression that the General Education Board would actually stand behind the development of a modern medical school and that he, the board's officers, and Kirkland were of one mind in their understanding of what was meant by "modern standards." But confronted with Kirkland's response to his plan that "we must take the resources provided and make the most of them," and with Flexner's that "the Vanderbilt medical project like similar projects elsewhere—past, present, and future—would have to be an evolution, and, as such, would have to win its way," Robinson concluded that their consensus had dissolved and that he for one would not compromise. "I feel bound to hold to certain ideals of medical education, which are being fostered by some who are earnestly endeavoring to elevate the American standards, and I cannot participate in a project which does not embody these ideals. They have been expressed in my original plan. A large sum of money and a free hand are necessary for their realization in Nashville."[46] The building program should not proceed until the main substantive issues had been settled. Not to settle them now and to Robinson's liking meant negligence: "I am unwilling to assume the responsibility for the care of patients in a hospital in which thorough modern medical practice cannot be carried out, and for the teaching of students in a school that is inadequate in facilities and staff. The present resources are not sufficient to furnish these requisites. I take the attitude that the officers of the General Education Board are under an obligation at least to me if not to Vanderbilt University, to do everything they can to furnish these requisites."[47] Otherwise he was not the man for the job.

Although the threat was forceful and frank enough to make Kirkland angry,[48] he refused to be drawn into a philosophical debate over the meaning of modern standards in medical education, and like the good lawyer he would have made, he kept the argument narrow and well-focused. They differed not on ideals but only on the resources needed to realize them. Kirkland agreed that in the long run more money would be needed, but for the moment he was content to make a beginning with what he had and so prove by his actions the real worth of his ideals. It was a cautious tactic befitting a man well-seasoned in fund raising and unconvinced that modern medical schools should be exempt from the usual laws of institutional evolution. He feared giving offense to his friends and patrons with whom over the years he had nursed much good faith,[49] and while not averse to putting himself across the course of a wandering miracle, he would not become with Robinson a party to demanding one. "We must not seek points of disagreement. These do not exist. The only difference between you and me is the difference of opinion as to the wisdom of projecting certain requests, amounting almost to demands, into the present problem of organizing the new medical school. I have thought it unwise to do this. You have thought it should be done. What is also very important to remember is that you have had your way. If your ideals are accepted by the General Education Board you will have won a victory, and no one will rejoice more than I."[50]

Whether Robinson's claim that the officers of the General Education Board had "virtually agreed, at least to me, to stand behind them and properly support the medical school project"[51] was ever anything more than just his claim is not a matter of record. Whatever did pass in conversations between Robinson and Flexner, Robinson's own anticipation and ambition (to say nothing of his ideals) likely led him to read back into his memory of those conversations promise of whatever resources the job required. So Kirkland may have suspected; at any rate he knew that universities were not built on implied commitments. Confident both that the General Education Board would not enlarge upon its present grant and that Robinson meant what he said, Kirkland did not beg the dean to stay. He had no new suggestion to make and no new terms to offer. If Robinson, dealing directly with the board, could get something better, well and good. If not, Robinson as he himself admitted was the replaceable part.

Kirkland was half right and half wrong. Robinson surely was serious about quitting. He had left himself no convenient retreat, and had his plan been finally rebuffed, care for his self-esteem likely would have impelled him to seek his fortune elsewhere. But Kirkland mistook the hesitancy of the GEB for disfavor, and ever reluctant to overplay his hand, he left the strident begging to Robinson. However much he opposed Robinson's tactics, he was as good as his word when he declared in favor of Robinson's ideals, and he willingly compared the alternatives of moving ahead with the south campus plan or starting afresh in west Nashville. Kirkland's memorandums on that subject are models of conciseness and fairness and reveal a man who was, as he claimed, understanding of ideals but by habit constrained by budgets.[52]

The difference between the two options lay essentially with the financial advantage of delay. By then no one expected that the $4 million of General Education Board money then in hand would build an ideal facility on the south campus. As Robinson's earliest drawings showed, expansion was anticipated so that ultimately the south campus would require as much in plant and endowment as the west campus. (For the west campus he contemplated immediate investment in new construction and medical school and hospital endowment totaling $9 million; for the south campus, $5.8 million, of which the value of the old buildings to be used, the amount paid out on Galloway Hospital, and the additional work to be done on Galloway accounted for $538,429.) In the meantime, the south campus plan could progress slowly with a new spirit and in the hope of larger things to come. The west campus plan, on the contrary, called for a thoroughly modern school of adequate size from the day it opened.

That was the meaning of Robinson's ideal plan, and that was what made it so tempting, not just for Robinson the physician and medical educator, but for Kirkland the layman and university builder. Kirkland had been down that road of haphazard growth and of barely muddling through before, and he knew there was no magic in it. How tempting must have shone the possibility, however remote, that at one stroke at least one school of his university might ideally be provided for. On the merits he convinced himself. "If the expenditure of money for medical education is justifiable," he wrote, "then it also follows that postponement of such expenditures at a sacrifice of [quality of] work is not economy but an educational loss. If such postponement is necessary it can be endured, but if larger resources can be secured and immediately expended the increased outlay is justified by every argument that justifies the original expenditure. The chief advantage of the West Campus location is that it brings the University into one consolidated institution. It helps us to unite Vanderbilt and Peabody. It solidifies all the educational work of the city. It will give the greater satisfaction in the light of ultimate history."[53]

But before "ultimate history" would have a chance to say, four million additional dollars would have to be conjured. By the early spring of 1921 there were signs that they could be. Flexner (who recognized his own prescriptions when he read them) had all along been less opposed to the substance of Robinson's proposal than to its ultimatum-like presentation.[54] And from Charles Cason, former Vanderbilt alumni secretary who then worked for the Rockefeller Foundation, he and Buttrick had learned that their friend Kirkland had no special reasons for wanting to keep the school in south Nashville but was only reluctant to ask for the funds to move it.[55] To enable a thorough study with preliminary plans and estimates showing comparative costs and advantages, the GEB had appropriated $10,000 shortly before Christmas 1920. At the General Education Board internal discussion had begun over a possible change of site, Flexner counseling with financial expert and fellow secretary Trevor Arnett as to what the costs would be and the precise kinds of information that should be asked of the people in Nashville.[56] Flexner and Robinson met in New York in March 1921 to discuss the west campus plan, at which time Flexner's mind was made up, as evidenced by his eagerness to discuss such details as the dimensions of laboratories and whether or not it was necessary to make the nurses' home a fireproof building. They agreed on the large matter of the size of endowment, and Flexner spoke encouragingly about the prospects for obtaining the additional money to make the move.[57]

Flexner and colleagues meanwhile were conferring with their counterparts, James R. Angell and Henry Pritchett at the Carnegie boards, and early in April they summoned Kirkland to New York to finalize a formal application to be submitted at once to both foundations.[58] It was decided that Vanderbilt should ask for the round $4 million that Kirkland's memorandums indicated would be needed. The answers came late in May. The Carnegie Corporation appropriated $1.5 million on the condition that an equal amount come from another source. By arrangement the General Education Board supplied the match.[59] "This gives us $3,000,000 for the new enterprise," Kirkland wrote to Robinson in Baltimore. "I am sorry we did not get $4,000,000 but we shall have to see what we can do with the total sum now at our disposal of $8,000,000."[60]

This time he got no argument. Originally (when Robinson had been hired), there had been available $5 million (the General Education Board's $4 million grant of 1919 plus the still unspent $1 million that had come from Andrew Carnegie in 1913), a sum that Kirkland and the officers of the General Education Board once thought enough to do the job on the south campus. Robinson's ideal plan of 1920, which required starting from scratch on the west campus, stated that no less than a princely $12 million would do. Kirkland in his own evaluation of the proposed move said it could be done for $9 million. As such things go, $8 million was not a bad figure to end up with. With it—and with Robinson's ideas about coordination—they did the job.

Courts and Corridors   6

Seldom are ideas so nicely embodied in brick and mortar as in time they would be at Robinson's new Vanderbilt Medical School. At his Blue Ridge retreat in the summer of 1921 he made a rough sketch of how it all might look; although it took two years to elaborate the plans and another two for construction, the final product was remarkably faithful to his first drawings.[1] The building—which still stands and which with additions still houses much of the medical school, all of the outpatient clinics, and until 1980 housed the hospital as well—is a monument to an era in American medicine when the union between research and teaching and between science and utility for which Flexner and the reformers had long fought was still fresh and expectant. As Robinson the medical man determined, and in more than the common-place sense, its function begat its form. With the help of young Boston architect Henry R. Shepley and associates, Robinson conceived a structure that for the first time in this country would house under one roof all the facilities needed for the laboratory and clinical training of students and for the research that made scientists of their mentors.

The deliberate physical coordination of all those facilities, which was the heart of Robinson's philosophy of medical education, resulted in a sprawling six-story structure (including the basement open on the east or the Twenty-first Avenue side and the top floor, which housed store rooms and kennels), extending 458 feet north to south, 337 feet east to west, and enclosing 3,390,000 cubic feet of space. From the air it looked not unlike a large ticktacktoe board: two center quadrants enclosed grassy courts, and from the center and western corridors extended long wings that made for open courts, one facing Garland Avenue on the south, the other the rest of the university on the north. The courts were by-products only of a grid design that Robinson devised to achieve optimum arrangement of interior space. To the internal ones there was no easy access, which meant that few wandering medical scholars or apprentices ever paused there to think great thoughts or just for a moment to escape the scent of ether and alcohol. As the years passed the courts filled up with blowers and an occasional grazing experimental sheep. The court formed on the west by the 1938 addition to the hospital was filled in entirely in 1964. The open north court (where the pictures were taken) was enclosed in the 1950s by the erection of the A. B. Learned Laboratory and still constitutes (except for the noise of the air conditioners that also inhabit it) a pleasant thoroughfare from the medical school to the university, doors thoughtfully having been included through the laboratory. Even the elms still remain, beneath which freshly minted Vanderbilt M.D.'s once received their diplomas.

Dominating the interior landscape were the mammoth corridors off which were strung, to untutored eyes (that is, the eyes of patients and many a new doctor and nurse too), a bedlam of laboratories, offices, wards, and countless other cubicles. But to Robinson, the proud and knowing father, it was a masterpiece. Expressing his ideas about coordination between the clinical and scientific branches of medicine and his belief learned from the model of Hopkins and the German universities that research was the key to new medical knowledge, the building bespoke an educational philosophy that marked Vanderbilt long after Robinson's original layout succumbed to the endless remodelings entailed by fifty years of hard use. With the courts and corridors he sought to solve the problem of bringing the laboratories into closest possible contact with the clinics and the wards, and in the clean linear pattern that resulted could be read the intellectual presumption of the new medicine as hammered home by Flexner: that from science, service of a high order naturally grew. There would be no separate laboratory buildings at Vanderbilt standing in lonely grandeur aloof from the daily work of a teaching hospital. And there would be no ward or clinic not close enough to a laboratory so as to make the trek from bedside to bench easy and indeed obligatory. Off the court facing north toward the university campus, laboratories and staff offices formed three sides: on the first floor biochemistry and dissecting rooms for anatomy; on the second histology research, tissue culture labs, and preventive medicine; and on the third floor, pharmacology, pathology, bacteriology, and physiology.

The teaching hospital was arranged around its own open court facing south. On the first floor in separate wings were the medical and surgical

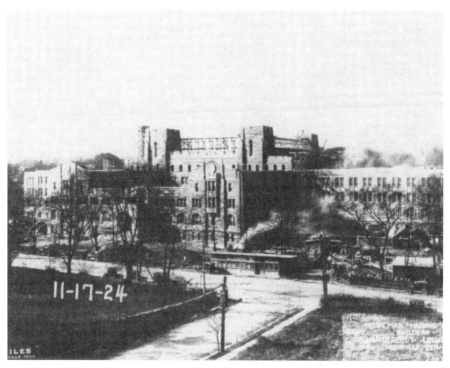

Medical School and Hospital under construction; view across Hillsboro Pike,
November 1924

outpatient clinics. They were connected to the north end by a corridor running
east and west, off of which were housed a plaster room and consultation and
treatment rooms for otolaryngology and ophthalmology. On the second and
third floors above the respective clinics were medical and surgical wards. By
placing the outpatient clinics directly beneath the hospital wards of the same
service Robinson hoped to break down in the minds of both staff and students
the distinction between inpatient and outpatient services. To that end there
was to be a common record room and a unit record system so that each
patient would have but a single record even if treated at times in the hospital
and at other times in the clinic. The south ends of the wards featured open
solariums overlooking Garland Avenue; off the corridor between them was
a covered porch. Key to the whole arrangement was the joining of the clinic
and ward side to the laboratory side through the laboratories of the clinical
departments in such a way as to bring into close proximity the preclinical

laboratories most closely allied to them. Thus on the second floor of the east corridor, clinical chemistry laboratories connected medical wards with the main laboratories of pharmacology; directly above, clinical physiology joined medical wards with physiology. On the west corridor, experimental surgery sat astride the path from anatomy to the surgical wards; above it, clinical bacteriology joined more surgical beds to pathology and bacteriology. Robinson hoped that such arrangement of space would help eliminate the barriers between the laboratory and clinical departments and generally encourage a spirit of cooperation throughout the institution. There would be no "watertight" compartments here. On the contrary, the layout assumed that the influence of the basic sciences would be felt constantly by the clinical staff and by the students throughout their training.[2]

On the first floor in the center of the east corridor in between the medical dispensary and the biochemistry department, the library occupied a position that Robinson hoped would be analogous to the hub of a wheel (there having deliberately been no provisions made for separate departmental libraries). Stack room on one side, reading room on the other, it was a walk-through affair suited less for long bouts of scholarly research than for easy access and convenient reference by busy people. A museum was connected to it and serviced by the same staff. The front or east corridor of the building (of which the library was the back side) housed the variety of other facilities required by a modern teaching hospital. On the first floor the admitting office on the southeast corner of the building adjoined the main entrance hall of the dispensary and, close to Robinson's own heart, space for the social service department. The main lobby of the hospital faced on Twenty-first Avenue, while around the corner to the north the hospital superintendent and other administrators had their offices. One flight up was the domain of the professional staff: quarters for interns and residents who then, Hopkins-style, lived in the hospital, and doctors' and nurses' dining rooms separated by a serving kitchen. The two wings above were given over to private rooms for patients who paid fees and, on the front of the building, to an open roof for patients.

The main hospital ward on the second and third floors of the two wings that pointed south themselves represented a departure from the large open wards then in general use in the United States and they borrowed from the plan of the university hospital in Copenhagen, which Robinson had visited in 1922. The basic ward unit, of which there were four, comprised a still-large 30 beds, but they were so distributed that 4 was the maximum number of beds consigned to any single undivided space. Beds were placed lengthwise so that patients did not have to look out the east- and west-facing windows.

The ward clerk's office plus linen, utility, and bath rooms separated the main portion of the wards from the smaller rooms that together contained 14 beds. And in keeping with the philosophy that the students should be incorporated as far as possible into the work of the hospital, two rooms were provided for them just outside each ward, one a small laboratory, the other a combination study and conference room. A total of approximately 170 beds was planned, including 27 for private patients, 16 for contagious cases, and 23 for blacks, who were segregated on the fourth floor around the corner from the operating suite. It was a slim number of beds for teaching purposes but all that could be maintained with the available endowment. The building was to be so constructed, however, that another story could be added to accommodate pediatrics over the medical wards and obstetrics over the surgical wards (though this addition was never in fact built), and the grid plan was so conceived as to permit further extension of hospital and laboratories toward the west (and that addition was completed in 1938). The small number of beds originally provided for placed on the number of medical students a ceiling of no more than fifty per class, a physical limitation that to Robinson and like-minded medical educators was agreeable enough anyway, because the rigorous new educational standards meant numbers needed to be comparatively small. "Fewer and better doctors," had been Flexner's maxim, and for years, even as Vanderbilt's plant grew, its student body did not. Attrition would be low, and of those few who were called most would be chosen.

Long hallways on three floors then encompassed nearly all of Robinson's ideal coordinated medical school and teaching hospital. In addition to the black wards, the fourth floor accommodated only the operating suite, which contained offices for the chief and assistant surgeons and anesthetists, prep and dressing rooms, and, with large windows facing north, a delivery room and three operating rooms. The animal house had a single fifth-floor wing to itself while in the labyrinthian basement were crowded all the people and equipment that made the large building work. The main kitchen came complete with bakery, butcher shop, and fruit, vegetable, butter, and milk rooms; the separate diet kitchen included the dietitian's office and teaching room. There were locker rooms, restrooms, and dining rooms for the service help, all carefully segregated by sex and by race, and ample space for medical stores and mechanical apparatus. On the front corner directly beneath the main admitting waiting room, space had been allotted to occupational therapy; down the hall was the hospital pharmacy, which connected to the dispensing pharmacy above by a circular steel staircase. Records were stored across from the diet kitchen; close by was future stack room for the library, also with a spiral to the main stacks above. The only thing that really did not fit, curiously, was the ambulance entrance, a circular drive through a porte cochere that faced the corner of Garland and Twenty-first avenues. Inside on the right was one lonely receiving ward and a small operating room but nothing that by any stretch of the imagination could be called an emergency room, something that Vanderbilt would not have for some time to come. This room was a receiving station only, and stretcher patients were dispatched quickly to the clinics or more likely to the wards upstairs. As befit its minor status, it shared a corridor with, among other things, the paint shop and the mattress room.[3]

Built of steel and poured concrete with a red brick exterior and carved limestone decoration about the entrances, the building was a respectable example of the collegiate Gothic style much in vogue in the 1920s and 1930s. Inside, the walls of the medical school and the laboratory sections were unfurred and painted directly on brick or terra-cotta partitions. Only hospital and clinic areas were afforded the luxury of plaster. Ceilings throughout were open to the floor of the next story (twelve and a half feet), except in corridors where the ventilating system ran and in the two entrance lobbies, which also received oak paneling in keeping with the Gothic portals just outside. A formidable though not exactly beautiful building, it would be eclipsed for external loveliness by the more pretentious and withal more handsome medical towers shortly to be raised across the mountains at Duke University. Yet Robinson's appreciation of the architectural niceties was probably as keen as anyone's; keener surely was his sense for how the forms could best be made to serve the functions, which was what his new Vanderbilt was all about. Later recalling the congenial relationship he enjoyed over the years with architect Henry Shepley, Robinson described himself as the figurative physiologist and Shepley as the anatomist, whose first collaboration—Vanderbilt—resulted in such a wonderfully functional organism. The building had few decorative frills, but one at least—the Gothic north court entrance to the medical school—found regular and practical use as the dignified backdrop for photographs.[4]

By the spring of 1921 Robinson had won acceptance for his large plan for a building on the main campus that would embody his educational philosophy of coordination, and that plan was not again seriously debated. He knew where he was going; he had the fare and a good idea of what his destination would look like when he got there. Everyone seemed pleased, and it was a happy Flexner who wrote to Kirkland in December 1921: "Now that the Irish question is settled, disarmament under way, and building prices falling at Vanderbilt, I can see that the millenium is fairly well started."[5]

Because it was thought that design and building of the new school would take two years at least (in the end it took four), Robinson, who had been

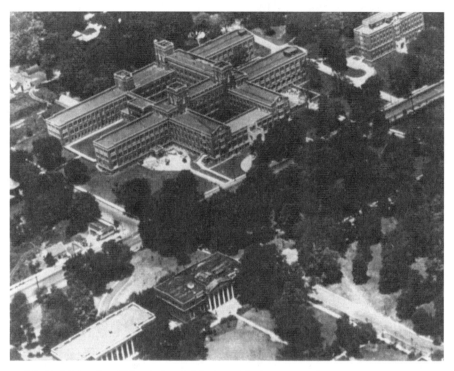

Medical School and Hospital as finished, aerial view, ca. 1928

hired early in 1920 in anticipation of heading a reorganized Vanderbilt within a year or two at the most, found himself temporarily underemployed, a problem solved by an invitation from alma mater Hopkins to serve for one year, beginning July 1, 1921, as acting professor of medicine and head of the department. There he filled an awkward hiatus between the resignation of William S. Thayer and the appointment of Robinson's friend from college and medical school days, Warfield T. Longcope.[6] It was a prestigious if interim post and he took it with Kirkland's and Flexner's blessing. On arrival he found a department whose ranks were badly depleted, and the work of filling them with full-time scientist-teachers was valuable experience for the job of recruitment he would soon face at Vanderbilt. Among those he persuaded to come were Alan M. Chesney, then at Robinson's old school, Washington University, and a graduate of Hopkins whose historian he would become, and C. Sidney Burwell, who as a graduate of Harvard became the first outsider to serve as resident physician at Johns Hopkins. Burwell shortly followed Robinson to Nashville and after Robinson's departure for Cornell in 1928 succeeded him as professor of medicine at Vanderbilt. No one seemed concerned that Robinson himself might be asked to stay on and fill the Hopkins post permanently, and if the matter was ever mooted in Hopkins councils it was done quietly. Hopkins then was looking for bigger fish, and Robinson, having just won his campaign with Kirkland for a splendid new coordinated medical school and hospital in Nashville, no doubt perceived that at that moment he himself had bigger fish to fry—a whole medical school in fact, in addition to his own department of medicine.

Still it is tempting to speculate how different might have been Robinson's biography had it been possible or for him desirable to settle in at Hopkins at that point in his career. So finding himself in the shoes of the man he revered more than any other, William Osler, Hopkins's first professor of medicine (who never, incidentally, became a dean), Robinson in all likelihood would have stayed there, tutoring young Hopkins students in the ways of his own great master and cultivating his own not inconsiderable talents for clinical research.[7] Later in the 1930s, after his fall from grace at Cornell and after a one-year stand at Peking Union Medical College, he again returned to Hopkins. But he returned fifteen years older and as an instructor, not as a professor in Longcope's department. He was not a bitter man in those later years when his career having already peaked seemed stubbornly not to take hold. But he must have wondered once or twice at least how pleasant it might have been simply to have been professor of medicine at Johns Hopkins and to have left to others the glamorous work of building medical schools. Under his Oslerian hand medicine at Hopkins surely would have prospered, and his career might well have been sustained at a high plateau for many happy years. Vanderbilt of course might have ended up a different place for his absence. Although he was not alone among the bright scientist-doctors and administrators of his talented generation, his ambition did find, if briefly, larger outlets than most. Vanderbilt was the first such outlet, and however much fun it was again to walk the wards haunted by so many worthies and however flattering it was to head for a year Osler's own department, in 1922 Robinson's mind was elsewhere.

He finished at Hopkins in June 1922 and spent that summer and fall with his wife and two children on a Vanderbilt-financed excursion to Europe where he visited various hospitals and medical schools and shared with the eminent his ideas about medical education and research—and his plans for the new Vanderbilt.[8] With those plans everyone was duly impressed, none more than Sir James Mackenzie, with whom Robinson spent two happy days in Scotland and who for Christmas 1923 made him a gift of a new style of putter from St. Andrews. "One of the best critical minds in English medicine,"

Robinson proudly wrote of Mackenzie to Kirkland, "said the [Vanderbilt] scheme embodies his ideal which he always hoped to see. He told me his old age would be happier because of our plans. That may sound 'a bit thick' as the English say, from a distance, but I want you to share the pleasure it has given me."[9]

Back in Baltimore in December (the Robinsons did not move to Nashville until the fall of 1924), Robinson took up again the work of planning his medical school from a distance, firming things with the architects in Boston and contemplating future administrative policies and faculty recruitment with Kirkland in Nashville. As the one who was going to be in charge of enticing a new faculty to the as yet unbuilt school, Robinson was eager to pin down guidelines establishing the extent of faculty power over educational and financial matters. He proposed an arrangement (subsequently established at Vanderbilt in the form of the "executive faculty") whereby the heads of the major departments would constitute an advisory board, which in conjunction with the dean and with the chancellor as representative of the university trustees should exercise complete control over educational policy, including appointments and the regulation of interdepartmental relations. How far such control should extend to the apportionment of funds, the fixing of salaries, and the selection of future deans was yet unsettled in his mind, but in that general form of government he was sure lay the new school's best hope of efficient administration.[10] Kirkland generally agreed, though at that still early stage he was reluctant to determine much more than that in any hard and fast way before the school actually began to function in its reorganized form.[11]

Spring and summer lagged by, the architects taking more time with the building plans than promised, and not until September 1923 (just one year before Robinson and Kirkland had hoped to see the new school ready for service) could contracts be awarded, to Hegeman and Harris Company, a New York firm highly recommended by Flexner. As finally agreed to by Vanderbilt and the General Education Board, the building and furnishings were to cost slightly more than the $3 million originally allotted, an overdraft that led Robinson the anxious dean to reiterate to Flexner the badgered patron that the plans (which were to be copied with local modifications by the University of Rochester and which influenced the plans for the new medical school of the University of Colorado) had been drawn with as much economy and simplicity as the requirements of modern medical education would permit, and that further restriction in plant quality or size would seriously jeopardize standards. Even with what was left, Robinson confessed that serious problems could be anticipated in working out a financial program for the proper support of the medical school and hospital.[12]

Ground finally was broken on October 22, 1923, and for the moment the great enterprise was left in the hands of the contractors, which left Robinson to ponder other matters. As he did, he shortly found himself so at odds with Kirkland that, as in 1920, he nearly quit once more. It was a row that neither Robinson in his autobiography nor Kirkland's biographer chose to record, but it bears importantly on the problem in reformed medical education that more than any other subverted at the core both Robinson's ideal of coordination between laboratory and clinical branches of the medical school and, even more so, Flexner's ideal of integration between the medical school and the university. Since it had first been made a condition of the General Education Board's grant to Johns Hopkins in 1913, the university or full-time system for the clinical as well as the preclinical subjects had been the cause of endless hand wringing and considerable philosophical debate in medical schools all across the country, and by the early 1920s both sides had fairly well exhausted their supplies of original argument. Flexner, inspired as ever by the German example, had been full-time's staunchest, most dogmatic advocate, whose insistence on the full-time plan in schools aided by the Rockefeller philanthropy had raised howls from outraged university administrators and from clinicians who saw things differently. As much as anything, full-time drove the wedge between the true academicians and those who professed to be such. As a result faculties self-sorted in response to the General Education Board condition, but only up to a point. Already by the time of the Vanderbilt project, Flexner was under heavy attack for his uncompromising stand, and at Vanderbilt, the GEB's pet, the brief flare-up between the dean and the chancellor in the winter of 1923 illustrated the practical limits of full-time even in the hands of those clearly dedicated to it in theory.

What remained was to hire the new faculty on whose talents the new school, once built, would rest. Prior to the decision to move the entire school to the west campus and make a fresh start, only one new faculty member had been appointed: John P. Peters as associate professor of medicine who, when it became apparent that the new school was still several years away, accepted instead an offer at Yale.[13] By the fall of 1923, with the building program at last settled, Robinson was eager to get on with recruiting. Knowing what he wanted in the way of medical scientists and knowing in general the administrative policies that would govern the new faculty, he needed, before recruiting in earnest, assurance only on the matter of what could and should be paid to get them. The matter became more awkward because the slate was not, strictly speaking, completely clean: there was Robinson, himself the first new man. Back in 1920 he had been hired (with some haggling) at a salary of $7,500, $1,000 of which was supposedly for his work as dean, the rest for duties as professor of medicine and head of the department. Three and a half years later and veteran of several duels with Kirkland, he asked that the question be reopened and stated that unless it could be settled to his satisfaction, he was not the man to attempt to recruit a first-rate, full-time faculty for Vanderbilt. In part, Robinson's present arrangement clearly was embarrassing, because it made his salary contingent on the salaries paid to others whom it was his duty to recommend for appointment. That was something Kirkland understood and agreed should be reconsidered.

But Robinson had also probably sold himself too cheaply to begin with and that opened the whole question not just of his salary but of what clinical full-time at Vanderbilt would really cost. Kirkland found that harder to handle. Between Robinson's own self-interest (he wrote Kirkland that he was at a critical period in his career and that it was not fair to his family to begin his new duties at the new school on so small a salary) and the high ground of principle there was in this instance some congruence. As professor of medicine he wanted $10,000, a sum that he said was commonly agreed upon as early as 1914 as suitable for such a post and that could hardly be considered extravagant in 1923 given that his counterparts elsewhere—namely, professors of medicine at Columbia, Hopkins, and the University of Michigan—were then receiving $12,000 and that Washington University, then trying to fill its chair of medicine, had its offer of $10,000 refused by several qualified applicants. In London (Robinson had done his homework), where the cost of living was considerably lower than in the United States, full-time professors and heads of medicine and surgery could expect about £2,000 a year with various benefits adding another £400. When he added the $1,000 that he still expected to receive as dean, Robinson's proposed new salary would come to $11,000 a year.[14]

Kirkland predictably was appalled, doubly so because he saw the question of Robinson's salary becoming enmeshed (as was clearly Robinson's intention) with the larger one of what numbers would be necessary to attract qualified individuals to all of the other as yet unfilled professorships. At the salaries suggested by Robinson (from $7,000 to $8,000, though whether a competent surgeon would come for that was doubtful), Kirkland figured that the compensation of the six or seven leading professors would come to more than $50,000, "which is twenty-five percent of the total income of the school. I am wondering," he chided "just where we will come out on that basis."[15] In the meantime both men appealed to Flexner, Kirkland confessing reluctantly that unless Robinson could be talked down on his own salary, Vanderbilt (which needed no administrative changes just then) would somehow have to meet it.[16] But that prospect threatened the whole scale and was fundamentally offensive to Kirkland. It ran against his conviction, buttressed by thirty years of experience, that the academic life by nature demanded that certain material sacrifices be endured for noble ends. Never for him had there been any shortage of ideals, whether his own or his deans' and professors', but never had there been enough money either. "I do not see how medical education," he told Flexner, "can be carried on if the extravagant ideas of some of the new leaders are to be followed. At the same time I do not see how we can get the men we need without yielding to their demands. There is a real lack of supply in this field." His position was weak and he knew it. It was also portentous of inflated expectations and troubled times in the larger university: "The extravagant ideas are passing over from medicine to general education. There is bound to be some difficulty if on one and the same campus you pay a medical professor of chemistry $8,000 and a college professor of chemistry $5,000 or less."[17]

But medical education, not the larger university, was Robinson's business, and he staunchly defended his ground. To him the success or failure of the new school for which he had designed such a splendid home would be determined right at the start by the very first faculty. Unlike Kirkland, the layman to whom progress and success in education as in everything else was an evolution prompted by good intentions and hard work, to Robinson the physician it was at that moment at least an act of will—albeit a well-financed one for sure. Others elsewhere, he knew, felt as he did. Thus when he demanded more money for himself and for his colleagues-to-be, it was not primarily to assure them a standard of living befitting the prestige of the rising profession of academic medicine but rather to enable Vanderbilt to attract the best in a fiercely competitive seller's market. Kirkland had argued, unconvincingly to Robinson, that lower living costs in Nashville justified lower salaries and that "every institution must be to some extent a law unto itself in this important matter."[18] But Robinson was by now certain that with a medical school endowment of $3 million, yielding together with fees a yearly income of $200,000, Vanderbilt was badly undercapitalized to do the job that he and (so he thought) Kirkland had in mind. Constantly he badgered both Kirkland to admit the need for more money right away and to ask for it and Flexner to give it. Skillfully Flexner led him on, short of additional commitment. Kirkland told him that it was foolish to anticipate greater subsidy before they had made some showing with what they already had.

Robinson knew that Vanderbilt was small and could not compete with the older schools in the matter of quantity. But it must be able to compete in the matter of quality, even if that meant trimming the sails of the full-time plan. The number of departments fully developed should, he said, be kept to a minimum, their size as small as was compatible with sound teaching, and with the minimum staffs needed to attract high-quality researchers as their heads.[19] While in the preclinical departments of anatomy, physiology, biochemistry, pathology, and pharmacology, full-time was taken for granted and where proposed professional salaries ranged from $6,500 to $8,000 (bacteriology would temporarily be in the charge of an associate professor at $5,000), in the clinical branches he warned that only medicine could be put on a full-time basis and there imperfectly with a full professor at $10,000 and a part-time associate at $4,000. For surgery, where he said it would be impossible to attract a professor at less than market value (which would be at least what was paid the professor of medicine), a part-time local professor at $1,500 and a full-time associate at $3,500 would have to suffice. Pediatrics and obstetrics, meanwhile, would be relegated to subdepartments of medicine and surgery respectively. But he had no doubt that full-time that was not also first-rate was worse than none at all.[20]

The controversy finally came to a head between Thanksgiving and Christmas of 1923, when Robinson (much as he had done in 1920) accused Kirkland of being so preoccupied with financial matters that he had lost sight of the aspirations and ideals that had supposedly given birth to their new enterprise.[21] It was a vexed and testy Kirkland who responded that "I know nothing more discouraging than the study of financial obligation and responsibilities. We could all be intensely happy if we could forget these things. I am not aware that I have ever said a word to you evincing any lack of appreciation in scholarship or in high standards. I have largely made my reputation as a believer in high standards, and for twenty-five years I have worked to promote scholarship at Vanderbilt University. . . . We must remember that the financial burden of the medical school will not be taken off our shoulders by other parties. It will rest entirely on you and on me, and I want you to carry your part of the load." Get the best men possible by all means, he said, but "pardon me if I refuse to forget that every budget must be balanced and every desired improvement must be paid for."[22] It was something that he and Robinson never really got straight and that festered for the remainder of the dean's time at Vanderbilt. To Flexner, Robinson complained that Kirkland feared over-emphasis on research, that he was too fixed to change, and that "he has much the same attitude towards me that a good watch dog has of a stranger in the house." Worse: "He seems to be satisfied with second class men, and I am not willing to be included in that category."[23]

Flexner probably kept that letter to himself and did his best to assure the doctor of Kirkland's and Vanderbilt's fundamental soundness.[24] In the end it all seemed to come down again to money. Kirkland told Robinson that $9,000 was as high as Vanderbilt could go and pleaded that, while in view of the possibilities for future growth his final salary could well go higher, for the moment Vanderbilt's position with the General Education Board would be stronger "if they realize that we are even [now] sacrificing something in order to aid them in carrying through a great enterprise."[25] Robinson came back with a compromise: he would accept $9,000 for the present, provided his acceptance of fees from patients not be restricted by any formal contract, a stipulation made not in the hope of augmenting his income in any way that would interfere with his university duties but, he said, "so that such an augmentation could be relied upon in case my income did not serve to meet my reasonable obligation."[26] That was a fine line, but his fundamental point—that he should be paid more not primarily so he and his family could live more comfortably but because in the national marketplace of medical scientist-teachers he and the others like him on whom the full-time system would depend were worth more—was hard to argue with, though Kirkland tried with his "every university must be a law unto itself" proposition.

There truly was a shortage of supply, and had Vanderbilt been richer Kirkland probably would have paid. But Robinson could not thus have it both ways without running head-on not just into the ever-cautious Kirkland but into Flexner, too, with his purist's interpretation of "full-time." The chancellor was willing to accept Robinson's proposal if his private fees were limited to $2,000 annually. When Flexner heard that, he wired back: "Doctor Robinson's suggestion involves abandonment of full-time plan." In the letter that followed he played well the role of betrayed patron. Responsibility for deciding the matter of Robinson's salary and other conditions of his employment lay entirely with the chancellor and his trustees, "but I think . . . that I ought to point out that Dr. Robinson's suggestion that clinical men be allowed to collect fees, however small at the outset, is the end of the full-time system as it is practiced, and happily practiced [something that was not always true], at Baltimore, St. Louis, and New Haven, and as it is to be instituted at Rochester and Chicago." After the admonitory reminders came the threat: "A moment's reflection will, I am sure, show that no person and no organization would provide millions for the endowment of clinical teaching and research if the clinical teachers and investigators were also free to develop a professional business." Science and fees, Flexner had long said, did not mix. "As a matter of fact the appropriations of the General Education Board—unprecedentedly large appropriations—for the creation of a modern medical school in Nashville were made with the distinct understanding that the full-time plan as practiced in the places above mentioned was to form the basis of the school's organization on the clinical side." With respect to arguments about income, expenses, and standards of living, the clinicians should in Flexner's opinion learn to be like other professors: "clinical men who are unwilling to make some of the sacrifices made by all others occupying academic posts ought not to accept full-time teaching and research posts."[27]

It took a meeting in New York among them all to settle it. What exactly was said is lost with their conversation, but it is a safe conjecture that Kirkland and Flexner brought to bear on the poor doctor their biggest guns, for two days later Robinson accepted the offer of $9,000 on full-time for himself at least, undiluted just to Flexner's liking.[28] His argument had been good but his position was weak. At that moment he did not have any other place to go, and besides he did not truly want to wreck full-time at Vanderbilt. He believed in it as staunchly as anyone (with the exception perhaps of Flexner), and he had built his career largely faithful to it. Nor was he a greedy man ever hungry for larger pay. "I do not look upon money as a measure of what we gain during our lifetime," he wrote Kirkland (who certainly did not either) and meant it.[29] So before the awesome persuasive powers of Flexner and the chancellor he gave in for a gain of $1,500.

The issue that the whole tiff had raised, however, remained as unsettled as ever. How much would it really cost to institute the full-time system and all its accoutrements at Vanderbilt, and was there enough on account to cover it? Robinson continued to believe there was not. Kirkland probably agreed but, having more faith and patience than Robinson, did not admit it publicly. Flexner, whose foundation would indeed invest even more in Vanderbilt, believed nonetheless that more money alone did not itself buy the success of anything, the full-time plan included. As the demand for their service drove up their price, the matter festered as to how well the doctors in the clinical branches could be "coordinated" (Robinson's term) with the laboratory scientists in the other half of the medical school whose skills were less widely serviceable and who enjoyed fewer options to go elsewhere. So too festered the larger question of how well the modern scientific medical school could be coordinated with the university itself.

But Robinson, satisfied for the moment, proceeded with Kirkland's and Flexner's blessing to secure the other new people. Of those he had considered earlier in the midst of other problems, none finally came to Vanderbilt. But by early 1924 others did begin to line up. First came Waller S. Leathers (whose department, preventive medicine and public health, had only just then been provided for by the General Education Board's promise of $10,000 yearly to support it for five years), then dean of the medical school of the University of Mississippi and executive officer of the Mississippi state board of health and a medical graduate of the University of Virginia.[30] As his right-hand men in the department of medicine, Robinson brought with him two bright young internists who in turn would succeed him as professor and physician-in-chief in the Vanderbilt hospital. From Baltimore came C. Sidney Burwell, a Coloradoan and a Harvard M.D., who had trained at the Massachusetts General Hospital and served with the Red Cross in Poland and Russia before Robinson brought him to Hopkins as resident physician in 1921.[31] Hugh Jackson Morgan, a Nashville native and Vanderbilt undergraduate alumnus but a Hopkins M.D., came from the hospital of the Rockefeller Institute where he had been resident physician and protégé of Simon Flexner.[32] For biochemistry Robinson picked Glenn E. Cullen, a Columbia Ph.D. who had been research chemist at the Rockefeller Institute and associate professor of research medicine at the University of Pennsylvania.[33] From the Singer Research Laboratory in Pittsburgh came Ernest W. Goodpasture to head pathology, like Morgan a native Tennessean, Vanderbilt alumnus, and Hopkins M.D.[34] Direct from Hopkins where he had been associate professor of anatomy, came R. Sidney Cunningham, also a Hopkins M.D., to head that department, thanks in part to William Welch on whose advice Cunningham, who had a simultaneous offer from the Rockefeller Institute, came instead to Vanderbilt.[35] In bacteriology Robinson appointed James M. Neill, a Ph.D. and a veteran of the Rockefeller Institute where he had worked with Oswald Avery.[36]

At the rank of associate professor Robinson hired Horton R. Casparis in pediatrics, in the beginning at Vanderbilt a subdepartment of medicine. Like others of his soon-to-be colleagues, Casparis had earned his M.D. at Hopkins and had served there as resident and staff member under master pediatrician John Howland.[37] Robinson chose for physiology Walter E. Garrey, who had been associate professor at Washington University for part of Robinson's tenure there. Alone of Vanderbilt's new staff, Garrey held both the Ph.D. (University of Chicago) and the M.D. (Rush Medical College).[38] In pharmacology the professorship went to Paul D. Lamson, then associate professor at Hopkins and the second Harvard M.D. to grace the new Vanderbilt faculty. He had preceded Burwell at Harvard by a decade, had also trained at the Massachusetts General Hospital, and already had studied abroad in Germany and England.[39] Finally, for surgery, the clinical department that Robinson said could not with present resources be organized on a full-time basis, he managed to get Barney Brooks, a Hopkins M.D. and intern under William Halsted, and whose path first crossed Robinson's at Washington University where Brooks had been since 1913. Brooks came for the same salary as Leathers and Goodpasture ($7,500) but with the provision (which Robinson had asked for and been denied for himself) that he had the privilege of

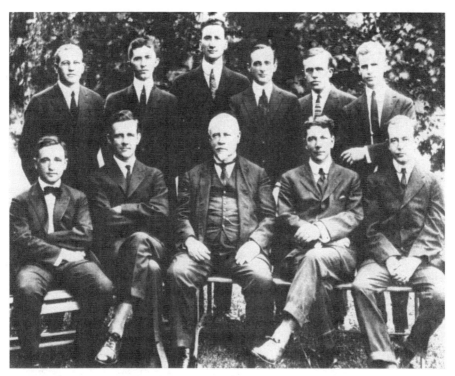

The Hopkins heritage: William Henry Welch (seated, center) and Ernest W. Goodpasture (standing, far right)

accepting fees from private patients occupying the private wards set aside for them in the new hospital. Brooks, who held his post at Vanderbilt longer than any of the other new professionals except Hugh Morgan and Ernest Goodpasture, in fact never pursued a large private practice. But that he was granted the privilege of accepting fees at all meant that the full-time system in the clinical departments, as Flexner defined it, was not then nor ever since securely established at Vanderbilt.[40] Three others appointed at junior ranks by the middle of 1925 should be added to the list: Beverly Douglas became assistant professor of surgery; Alfred Blalock, resident surgeon and instructor; Tinsley R. Harrison, resident physician and instructor. All were Hopkins graduates; Blalock and Harrison had been classmates.[41]

There were then, at full or associate rank, an even dozen new men who posed for that first faculty portrait at the Gothic portal on the north court of Vanderbilt's new medical school.[42] Half of them—Robinson, Brooks, Goodpasture, Cunningham, Casparis, and Morgan—had Hopkins degrees. Only two—Goodpasture and Morgan—had local ties to Nashville or Vanderbilt. Three others—Leathers, Brooks, and Casparis—were southerners, Brooks and Casparis from Texas. All had agreed to come to Vanderbilt for less money than Robinson anticipated. Except for his own, no salary exceeded $7,500, a sum that, while it no doubt appeared princely to many of the university's nonmedical professors, was not enormous, especially not for clinicians even in 1925. Goodpasture even came for less than he had been making in Pittsburgh, which raises the matter of expectations.[43]

Robinson had assembled as talented a group of people as he might have had he had twice the money to offer, and of those he recruited few if any expected or realized large gain. The practice of medicine, responding to the reformers' quarter-century campaign to reduce the number of doctors and improve their quality, was for some doctors (though hardly yet for most) beginning to yield predictably high returns in addition to new prestige. On the other hand, the pursuit of medical knowledge through deliberate research and careful clinical study—which defined the new profession of academic medicine of which these twelve men were vanguard—promised less money and another sort of prestige.

In the decades after 1910 a new figure joined the pantheon of American folk heroes. This new figure was not the medical practitioner, already long ensconced there. The horse-and-buggy doctor who was poorly trained and seldom paid, who knew little of the science of medicine but much of the art, who was immortalized in Samuel Fildef's painting, *The Doctor,* and who later became object for some considerable nostalgia, was secure because of fitting easily into the fondly remembered Currier and Ives image of a once rural and provincial people. Too, the family doctor was secure simply because of the service rendered, which was a sincere purpose. And the doctor was judged as much by the willingness to render this service as by the results. In contrast, the newcomer, whose veneration was then in 1925 only beginning, was seldom pictured attentively waiting by the bedside of a sick child and certainly never in street clothes. This new hero wore nearly always a long white coat and if pictured at the bedside was sure not to be alone with the patient but surrounded by an attentive group of young apprentices in shorter white coats. Or as likely, the popular image revealed the doctor in the laboratory, with the common equipment being a microscope, test tubes, a Bunsen burner. It was in 1925, in fact, the same year that Robinson finished gathering his new medical staff and opening his splendid new medical school, that this new figure of the doctor as scientist achieved a place in popular fiction and thus immortality of a sort, in the character of Sinclair Lewis's driven Dr. Martin Arrowsmith.[44]

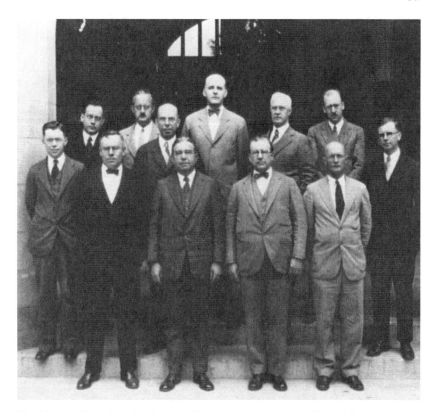

Teaching and learning: the first new faculty, 1925. Front row from left: Glenn Cullen, Waller S. Leathers, G. Canby Robinson, Barney Brooks. Middle: James M. Neill, Paul D. Lamson, Ernest W. Goodpasture. Back: Sydney Cunningham, Horton Casparis, Hugh Morgan, Walter Garrey, Sidney Burwell.

For Arrowsmith, the pursuit of scientific truth led to conflicts with huckstering public health agencies, crooked drug companies, and social-climbing, publicity-conscious heads of New York City research laboratories, to one wife sacrificed to the plague, to a second marriage wrecked, and finally to exile in the Vermont woods. No such melodrama awaited Vanderbilt's new medical staff of 1925, but their own pursuit of new knowledge from which better service might or might not come was faithful in spirit to hero Arrowsmith. And perhaps on occasion it was as fraught with doubt, not about the value of their new calling, but about a culture whose values were practical values and that demanded of them much and left them in the end ironically beleaguered. But their doubts went largely unspoken, and we are left instead to view the recorded ample accomplishments of truly stouthearted men. All the institutional rearrangements that Flexner had said were needed for such individuals to flourish were now more or less complete and, at Vanderbilt, handsomely housed under one expansive new roof. There, they set out after the new knowledge that defined their new profession. To them went a new order of prestige—even awe—bestowed only on healers who as scientist-scholars too could prove themselves.

PART THREE

On Technique

Medicine 7

Canby Robinson was better at building medical schools than he was at running them. Of the two that were his—Vanderbilt and Cornell—he stayed at neither for long: beyond their openings, less than three years at Vanderbilt, less than two at Cornell. His deanship of the new Vanderbilt Medical School saw renewed disputes with Kirkland and less than ideal relations with some of the local doctors, and even as the new school opened its doors others tried to tempt him away. While he did not accept the directorship of the new New York Hospital–Cornell Medical College Association until July 1927 and did not leave Vanderbilt until a year after that, it is fair to say that all the while his eye if not his mind was wandering. At Cornell, a monument to the new medicine more splendid by far than Vanderbilt, he had even less time to make work the wonderful place he had planned. The new hospital and medical school opened in September 1932; by July 1934 Robinson was gone, retired from the center to the edges of the world of academic medicine.[1]

At Vanderbilt as dean of a working medical school, Robinson got along with Kirkland no better than he had as planner of a school not yet built, and it is natural to wonder just how long their uneasy partnership would have lasted had Robinson not received the timely invitation to New York's more prestigious arena. The mere opening of the new school, even though it occasioned some hard-earned sighs of relief and much mutual congratulation, could have been expected to hold no magic for their relationship. Neither man had changed his nature. Although he knew that the running of a modern medical school such as Vanderbilt's now was must be left in large part to the medical staff, Kirkland remained as possessive as ever about his university, of which medicine was supposedly now an integral part, and as nervous as ever over anything that might jeopardize relations with his foundation patrons. Robinson remained as convinced as ever that the standards for modern medical education were nonnegotiable and that, undercapitalized as the Vanderbilt Medical School clearly was, the urgency of its need for larger subsidy overrode Kirkland's belief that it was most prudent first to wait and make a showing with what they had. So they wrangled for the time that Robinson remained. Robinson knew what he was talking about, and indeed by the end of the 1920s the General Education Board did increase the school's endowment by more than $5 million. But those first few deficit-strewn years over which Robinson presided hardly added to his stature in Kirkland's eyes, which saw in medicine no exception to principles of fiscal responsibility and no reason to forsake his old habit of paying as he went.

It was well enough, then, that he and Robinson parted when they did. For his failure to meet his budgets not just in the hospital but in the medical school as well, Robinson on the eve of his departure in the spring of 1928 took the last opportunity he would have to put the case and not, he insisted, merely to make excuses. Departmental budgets had not always allowed, he said, activities on a scale to which some department heads had been accustomed elsewhere. That was Robinson's way of saying that everything at Vanderbilt from the beginning had been too small and too poorly supported to fill properly the mandates of the new medicine, an oft-repeated refrain that Kirkland had been hearing since 1920 and that in eight years had still not shaken his conviction that "every university must to some extent be a law unto itself." But Robinson also pleaded indulgence on the high ground of research, which he said was accelerating now that the organization of the teaching program had largely been accomplished. Whether that was strictly true or whether research accounted for deficits was a moot question. Robinson's successor as dean, Waller S. Leathers, did not expect "to have any real difficulty in keeping the school of medicine within its budget," Kirkland reported smugly later that year. The bookkeeping, though, mattered less than Robinson's certainty that research (like the number of beds needed in a teaching hospital) properly dictated budgets, and not the other way around. Although he himself was by 1928 no longer a prodigious investigator, Robinson gladly championed those of his faculty who were. Rightly or wrongly, he had always suspected the shallowness of Kirkland's commitment to this, the least practical activity of the modern medical school (the last research Kirkland the philologist had done was his dissertation at Leipzig in the 1880s), and in at least one instance he approved an overdraft for research work not with Kirkland's but with Flexner's assurance.[2] The time was still in the future when research alone would swell budgets far beyond the internal means of any school to support, but the proposition that its claims when they came would prove irresistible, and that to them would be attached commensurate expectations for useful application, was fairly hinted at as the departing Robinson sought justification for the record of his deanship.

His resignation from Vanderbilt and his departure in 1928 for, so he thought, greater glories at Cornell occasioned the usual spate of congratulatory good wishes from colleagues and hearty thanks for a job well done.[3] Kirkland too, not an ungenerous man, spoke for the trustees and for himself: "The success [the medical school] has attained, the reputation made, are due in large measure to your efforts and to your wise planning. You brought together a faculty of great distinction, and this body of men is attracting attention throughout all the medical centers of the nation. . . . Please accept this expression of sincere good will on the part of the Trustees, which is accompanied by the best wishes possible for your future career and happiness."[4] What he did not speak but surely thought was a sigh of relief that this particular able but exasperating medical man would soon be safely distant in New York and unable to work any more mischief with Vanderbilt's budgets.

But Robinson's record at Vanderbilt was written not just in budgets, dean's reports, and contentious correspondence with Chancellor Kirkland—for he was dean and professor of medicine too, a part-time administrator and (as Flexner wanted) a full-time physician. As Kirkland had dangled it before him back in the winter of 1919–20, the Vanderbilt prospect had been doubly alluring both as opportunity to conceive a whole new medical school and as chance to practice his trade, which was internal medicine. As things turned out, it was the last such chance he would have to organize his own department and daily to oversee the education of young doctors-in-training.[5] In that job he was perhaps even happier than as dean, for he was at heart not a business manager at all, which was (once the new school had finally opened) what the position seemed increasingly to entail. Serving as a dean was something that fortune had thrown across his path at the right time to tempt his ambition, and he rode three deanships to the pinnacle of his profession.

But by training and by choice he was prepared to do something else. At Hopkins, at the hospital of the Rockefeller Institute, and at Washington University he had learned internal medicine as a student, a resident, and a professor, and he had learned the then unquestioned best ways to educate others in it. At Vanderbilt at last he had the scope and the power to act on those self-evident truths. With typical enthusiasm he instilled there a technique of teaching and learning that fixed internal medicine as the keystone of clinical medical education. The technique long outlasted his own brief tenure, and it confirmed class after class of Vanderbilt medical students, interns, and residents in a sturdy faith in the utilitarian partnership of science and service well suited to the needs of practitioners, which most of them would become.

The inspiration for it all was the somewhat-larger-than-life-size figure of William Osler, under whom Robinson had studied at Hopkins at the turn of the century. Robinson thus belonged to the select company of disciples who had been present when Osler the great physician had walked, talked, and laid on the hands. To Osler many doctors of that era fondly traced their intellectual ancestry, so dubbing themselves "first-" or more commonly "second-generation Oslerians."[6] The title implied more than filiopiety and united its claimants in a fraternity such as few teachers in any calling can claim to have inspired.[7] "Second-generation Oslerians" were well represented among the new members of Vanderbilt's department of medicine in the 1920s and 1930s, and it is no surprise that with "first-generation" Robinson as their chief they developed an organization and a program of instruction wholly faithful to their master's teachings.

To learn by doing is almost a cliché of American culture and history. A practical people bred on the edge of a wilderness, Americans had early learned to value experience as a teacher. They brought with them few formalized authoritarian institutions of education and for years they trained themselves as befit the unsettled nature of their lives. They improvised, and much of what they learned they learned on the job. "On the job" in modern medicine meant in the clinics and on the wards. But because for years there were few clinics and wards, medical education had long made do with lectures, demonstrations, and informed apprenticeships. Didactic though they once were, the old ways were not utterly devoid of clinical application. The clinics then were of course different from what they would become, but for at least a hundred years in Europe and North America physicians had been "walking the wards," faithful in tow, demonstrating at the bedside the manifestations of disease in real patients. Often, though, students got only a glimpse. They missed the exchange between doctor and patient and learned what they learned as passive observers of mysteries to which they were not yet truly admitted. So Robert James Graves had complained of his student experience at Edinburgh in 1819. By contrast, the German method of clinical instruction, which Graves later developed with his student and colleague William Stokes at the Meath Hospital in Dublin, supplied what merely walking in the wards had neglected: an opportunity for students to begin to exercise their own clinical judgment by participating with their mentors in diagnosis and treatment. The procedure involved specific assignment to one student of one patient for whose medical history and physical examination the student was then responsible. Findings, presented at ward rounds the next day, were verified by the teacher, who with the group then retired to a separate classroom to discuss the case. The student was then expected to commit to a course of treatment and, with the teacher's approval, to write the prescriptions that supposedly would accomplish it. By applying similar techniques to dispensary patients (outpatients), Graves concluded that the need for systematic clinical lectures—the great staple of nineteenth- and early twentieth-century medical education—would disappear.

Graves and Stokes were themselves out of place and out of time, but years later in Montreal, Philadelphia, and finally in Baltimore, they found vindication in the person of William Osler, who made their technique his own. From them he was two generations removed, but his teacher at McGill University, Palmer Howard, had been their student, thus making the link a direct one. At Vanderbilt a generation later, Osler's student, Canby Robinson, carried on. A Canadian by birth, Osler graduated from McGill Medical School in 1872, and after a two-year pilgrimage to Europe's clinics and hospitals he returned to Montreal and entered private practice. But mentor Palmer Howard soon invited him back to McGill as lecturer in the fields of physiology and pathology. Although unsure of his qualifications, he accepted and so began his career in medical education. In 1879 as Physician to the Montreal General Hospital, he had his first opportunity to teach at the bedside. He next moved to the chair of clinical medicine at the University of Pennsylvania and, in 1889, settled in Baltimore as chief of medicine at the new Johns Hopkins Hospital. Between then and the opening of the new medical school at Johns Hopkins in 1893 he developed a large consultation practice and wrote the book that would make him famous: *The Principles and Practice of Medicine,* holy writ for English-speaking physicians for half a century. The new Hopkins provided him an ideal setting. The classes were small, the faculty young and enthusiastic (Osler was forty-four in 1893), the students well-trained in the sciences and with a reading knowledge of French and German. Osler himself brought to the job impeccable scientific credentials. He was well-versed in pathology and awake to burgeoning new knowledge in chemistry, physiology, pharmacology, and bacteriology, all of which, with his convictions about the value of the German method of bedside teaching and the importance of the clinical laboratory, set the stage at Hopkins for a new and different approach to the teaching of clinical medicine.

Osler's curriculum became one of the highlights of Flexner's report, which described it as the ideal method of instruction during the third and fourth (or the clinical) years of medical school. Osler himself (a writer as well as a healer and teacher) described the method numerous times, never better than in an address, delivered to the New York Academy of Medicine in 1903, whose title, "The Hospital as a College," aptly summarized its substance. In the third year of medical school he called first for "a systematic course of physical diagnosis . . . in rooms adjacent to the out-patient department." That would be followed in the second half of the year by systematic opportunity actually to examine outpatients. Three days a week the entire class would meet the professor, "each student report[ing] upon a case and keep[ing] track of it." Faculty taught students "how to look up questions in the literature by setting subjects upon which to report in connection with cases they have seen." In clinical microscopy class they received "routine instruction in the methods of examining the blood and secretions, the gastric contents, urine . . ." and became familiar "with the use of a valuable instrument [the microscope] which becomes in this way a clinical tool and not a mere toy." Finally, one day a week third- and fourth-year students attended a general medical clinic in the amphitheater where more interesting cases from the wards would be brought before them. Other than the set recitations in the course on physical diagnosis, there were to be no systematic lectures.

The third-year students learned first-hand the basics of dealing with patients and dealing with disease in the outpatient clinics. The fourth year was reserved for ward work in the hospital. One-third of the class at a time rotated through each of the three major hospital services: internal medicine, surgery, and obstetrics and gynecology. There they served as clinical clerks, those under Osler in medicine taking notes on new cases as they came in, doing blood and urine work, and in various ways assisting the house physicians in the general care of patients. The chief physician was to visit daily with the clerks, listen to them present their cases, and discuss with them proposed treatment. Osler emphasized that such an experience was far different from and superior to a mere ward class—the old ritual of walking the wards—"in which a group of students is taken into the ward and a case or two demonstrated; it is *ward-work,* the students taking their share in the work of the hospital, just as much as the attending physician, the intern or the nurse." If the system had a fault, Osler concluded, it was doubtless that too many students ended not well enough informed theoretically on some subjects. But compared "to that base and most pernicious system of educating them with a view to examinations," it was enough that in his curriculum "even the dullest learn how to examine patients, and get familiar with the changing aspects of important acute diseases. The pupil handles a sufficient number of cases to get a certain measure of technical skill, and there is ever kept before him the idea that he is not in the hospital to learn everything that is known, but to learn how to study disease and how to treat it, or rather how to treat patients." He claimed that this was a true method because, simply, it was a natural one, "the only one by which a physician grows in clinical wisdom after he begins practice for himself—all others are bastard substitutes."[8]

Osler's self-assurance befit the new medical education, whose practical method of learning by doing (which would change little from that day to this) was well-matched to the substance of the new medicine, which was the application of scientific knowledge about disease to the care of sick people. The method demanded certain things, such as enough patients to meet the teaching needs of all the clinical services, and hospitals that granted free access to faculty and their student apprentices. Not many places offered such conditions, as Flexner had documented, but of the few that did Hopkins offered the young Canby Robinson exposure to the master himself and to numerous of his lieutenants. And during the two decades between Robinson's graduation and the time he came to Vanderbilt, he was faithful to all he had learned there. At Hopkins he learned physical diagnosis under William Thayer, Osler's right-hand man, and served in the outpatient clinics under such disciples as Henry M. Thomas, Thomas B. Futcher, Thomas R. Brown, and Louis P. Hamburger. As a fourth-year clinical clerk on the wards, he served under the watchful eyes of Thomas McCrae, Rufus Cole, Charles P. Emerson, and Campbell P. Howard, whose father had been Osler's teacher at McGill where Howard himself would later serve as professor of medicine. Each morning at nine o'clock Robinson attended ward rounds, usually with Osler himself, and on Saturday nights at Osler's house at 1 West Franklin Street he and fellow students gathered around an ample dining-room table to hear Osler talk on the history of medicine, discuss their own work, and suggest future studies they might undertake.

At the Pennsylvania Hospital Robinson served with Warfield T. Longcope, two years his senior at Hopkins and another Osler protégé. In 1910 he was invited to become the first resident physician at the new hospital of the Rockefeller Institute, which was directed by Rufus Cole, the last resident physician to serve under Osler before Osler left for Oxford in 1905. At Washington University Robinson's dean and chief was George Dock, who had been Osler's student at the University of Pennsylvania Hospital before going to Hopkins. Back at Hopkins himself in 1921 and 1922, Robinson filled for a year Osler's own chair and savored, if briefly, a true homecoming.

Robinson's biography suggests how pervasive was Osler's influence among American physicians in the first quarter of this century and how small and collegial was their club. Osler taught at Hopkins just twelve years before resigning to become Regius Professor of Medicine at Oxford, in which time around 1,200 people passed through his wards and clinics as students and house staff. They alone could call themselves "first-generation Oslerians" of Hopkins vintage, but they alone were enough to implant Osler's technique of clinical medical education in virtually all of the medical schools whose reform Flexner and the foundations so artfully coerced. So establishing it at Vanderbilt, Canby Robinson was not unique and did not claim to be. His ties to his mentor, as such ties frequently do, combined genuine intellectual allegiance with increasing sentimental attachment to a figure who grew only more heroic as time passed and things changed. To Osler, as far as the record will tell, Robinson was but another bright and green college boy eager to become a doctor and make sick people well. His name is not prominent in the great man's papers, nor are the names of many students, and there is small reason to suspect that Osler ever heard much of Robinson again. The first event in Robinson's career that might well have stirred much notice in British medical circles—his selection to head the Vanderbilt reorganization—did not come until 1920. But Sir William (he had received a baronetcy at the coronation of George V in 1910), wearied by the war and heartbroken by the death of his son on the western front, had died the year before.

To Robinson, recognition from his old master might have increased the pride he already felt at his Vanderbilt accomplishment. He shared the early success of that accomplishment with two second-generation Oslerians whose younger age removed them further from the great physician but who by education and temperament were fully as faithful to his precepts. Sidney Burwell and Hugh Jackson Morgan were brought to Vanderbilt by Robinson at the very beginning, and with him (and after his departure) they made Vanderbilt's department of medicine into something that Sir William might proudly have called his own. Fully the outsider, Burwell was a Coloradoan by birth, a medical graduate of Harvard (1919), and former house physician at the Massachusetts General Hospital. He then served with the American Red Cross Commission to Poland and Russia in 1920, which would be his only excursion outside the academy. On his return and on the recommendation of his Harvard teachers, Roger Lee and Paul Dudley White, Canby Robinson, then acting professor of medicine at Johns Hopkins, invited the young Burwell to Baltimore.

It was the beginning of a long and happy association for them both, and at Hopkins it was something of a precedent, for Burwell was the first-ever resident physician at the Johns Hopkins Hospital who was not also a graduate of the Johns Hopkins Medical School. But he made his way on his merits and stayed at Hopkins for three years, until Robinson (by 1924 in Nashville

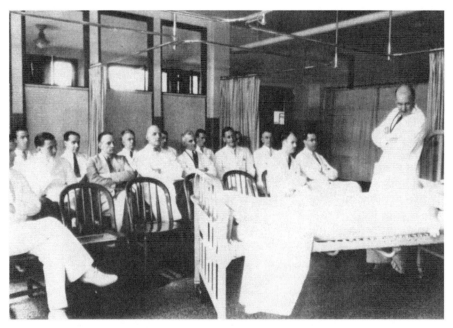

Medicine: rounds with Sidney Burwell (standing) and Hugh Morgan (seated center, bow tie).

at last) offered him the post of associate professor of medicine at a salary of $3,500 with consultation privileges in the Vanderbilt Hospital. (In 1926 Burwell's status was changed to genuine full time and his salary raised to $6,000.)[9] Burwell climbed the ladder quickly, in part because of superior skills both as clinician and as administrator and in part because of the fortuitous timing that took Robinson off to Cornell in 1928 and left Burwell heir-apparent to his departmental domain. Still, his head must have spun at least a little at such a quick passage (just seven years) from humble house officer to full professor and physician-in-chief at a prestigious medical school—in a profession where more than a few talented individuals lingered for years as associate professors. Burwell left Vanderbilt in 1935 to become dean of his alma mater, the final step up. But as he and others recalled, his concern always remained for the school where he had first and without question proven himself as an academic doctor.

Burwell's connection to Osler was through his teacher and professor of medicine at Harvard, Henry A. Christian, Osler's student at Hopkins. Those who knew Burwell attributed to that connection his technique of guiding students to think on their own and of eschewing the authoritarian style common to the professors of his generation. Learning, not teaching, governed Burwell the teacher and Osler's intellectual descendant. He recalled, for example, how the central location of the medical library "allowed his teaching rounds with students to move from the patient to the library and back to the patient with needed information for rational decisions and judgments about patients' problems and at the same time demonstrated the physician's need to seek more information than ever is presently at hand. Such a perspective is clearly one of an asker of questions, not a expounder of fragile facts; an educator, not a pedant."[10] Rudolph H. Kampmeier, who headed the department during World War II and who later became its historian, remembered how, after he was happily ensconced at Harvard, Burwell at the Atlantic City meetings of the American Association of Physicians diligently inquired about Barney Brooks, Paul Lamson, Ernest Goodpasture, and others with whom he had worked so productively at Vanderbilt.[11] There, in the early days when Robinson was still the chief, Burwell, a kindly faced man with thinning hair and small mustache, then only in his early thirties, was a warm and friendly presence to the serious and anxious groups of young students and house staff passing up and down those long hallways. There he was responsible for the physiological division of the medical department's research laboratories and, with Morgan, for the medical ward services of the hospital.

For Hugh Morgan, with whom Burwell worked closely and well, coming to Vanderbilt at Robinson's call in 1925 was like coming home. A Nashville native son and a favorite one at that, he had grown up, gone away twice, and returned with laurels fit for a hometown hero. He had a history to live up to: his grandfather, Henry William Morgan, had been the first dean of the Vanderbilt school of dentistry and in 1875 the first man to receive a diploma (Doctor of Medicine) from the then new Vanderbilt University. The grandson attended the undergraduate college at Vanderbilt and the first two years of its medical school. To friends and the readers of local papers he was "Buddy" and among football fans (of whom Vanderbilt then had many with good reason)[12] he was fondly remembered as a member of "Dan McGugin's terrible gridiron machine" between 1910 and 1914 and the Commodores' acclaimed all-Southern center.[13] But Robinson did not hire Hugh Morgan for his local connections, though they surely added to his attractiveness. He hired him because, by 1925, Morgan was one of the most promising young clinicians in the United States and one who seemed ready for a career in academic medicine. Robinson, who was about as good a judge of other people's promise as were Kirkland and Flexner, judged rightly, with the result that Vanderbilt became the chief beneficiary of Morgan's considerable talents as teacher and healer. He stayed there until the end of his career in 1958, longer than any other of the twelve original new men.

Morgan's local renown was buttressed by solid accomplishments far from home, the first of which brought him into contact with Robinson. He transferred from Vanderbilt's old medical school to Johns Hopkins in 1916, thus assuring himself the best possible credentials for whichever way his career might turn. It turned first to France and the medical corps of the American Expeditionary Force where he served first as a private then as a lieutenant with the Johns Hopkins Hospital Unit. In May 1918 he received his M.D. degree and his officer's commission and, mustering out the next year, returned as a house officer to Hopkins. There he became assistant resident physician under Osler's colleague since the opening of the school, William S. Thayer, who had also taught Robinson years before and who as chairman in 1919 organized the department of medicine on a full-time basis for the first time. By 1921 Morgan had earned a place on the staff as an instructor. That was the year that the Hopkins department was badly shaken by Thayer's resignation and Walter W. Palmer's (Thayer's presumed successor) defection to the College of Physicians and Surgeons of Columbia, a development that led to Hopkins's borrowing Canby Robinson from Vanderbilt as locum tenens while a new head and a new direction were found.

In the shuffle, meanwhile, Hugh Morgan sought his own fortune elsewhere and accepted a position as resident physician at the hospital of the Rockefeller Institute in New York, thus following in the footsteps of Robinson, who had passed that way a decade before. From there Robinson brought him home to Vanderbilt. He came, like Burwell, as an associate professor with private practice privileges in the Vanderbilt Hospital at a salary of $3,500, and when Burwell succeeded Robinson as chief in 1928, Morgan took the title of professor of clinical medicine with the same private practice privileges as before and a seat on the executive faculty.[14] In 1935 he became professor of medicine and physician-in-chief, posts he held until his retirement twenty-three years later, except for a four-year absence during and immediately following World War II. He returned to active duty in the army as a colonel in 1942 and later became chief of the Medical Consultants Division in the Office of the Surgeon General, a post that carried a brigadier's star. The title "general" stuck with him over the years and seemed to suit this imposing, six-foot, four-inch physician in the double-breasted white coat. Command became him and quiet was known to fall over the wards when, with house staff and students in train, Hugh Morgan walked in. Courtesy too became him, and in that hierarchical world where he was demigod, Hugh Morgan's kind word eased the embarrassment of many a reprimanded student and reassured countless bewildered patients. With Burwell he shared responsibility for the medical wards and himself had charge of the infectious disease division of medicine's clinical laboratories.

There were others of lesser rank but with talent that suited them to be junior colleagues of the three chiefs. "A human dynamo" was the phrase Robinson used to describe Tinsley R. Harrison, the first resident physician at the new Vanderbilt Medical School. Like so many of his fellows a Hopkins product, Harrison held an impeccable second-generation Oslerian heritage. During his third year in Baltimore, William Thayer had headed the department of medicine, during the fourth, Canby Robinson. His two years on the house staff of the Peter Bent Brigham Hospital in Boston were served under Henry Christian, and his assistant residency back at Hopkins was under Warfield Longcope. John S. Lawrence and Charles P. Wilson followed him in that role, and all, building on skills as teachers and scientists tried at Vanderbilt, went on to distinguished careers elsewhere.[15] In 1927, in anticipation of the need created by his own departure for New York, Robinson recruited John B. Youmans, whose service at Vanderbilt would be even longer than Hugh Morgan's. Like Morgan he had transferred (from the University of Wisconsin) to Johns Hopkins as a third-year student; he received his M.D. one class behind Morgan in 1919. Thayer was then abroad with the Red Cross, but in his absence the department during Youmans's clinical years was in the good Oslerian hands of Louis Hamman, Hopkins class of 1901. Returning to his native Wisconsin, Youmans interned at the Milwaukee Children's Hospital and spent a year on the house staff at the Massachusetts General Hospital in Boston before returning to Hopkins as an assistant in medicine in 1921 and 1922, the same year Robinson was serving as acting professor. He then joined the faculty of the University of Michigan Medical School, whose department of medicine was then headed by Louis M. Warfield, Osler's student and intern in Baltimore. Warfield's resignation in 1924 afforded Youmans a chance to try his administrative wings as the man in charge of the department's educational activities, talents that later blossomed when he found himself a medical dean, first at the University of Illinois and in the 1950s at Vanderbilt. His skills as a clinician and teacher, as remembered by those who knew him, were quintessentially Oslerian: attention to patients' medical history, meticulous care with physical examinations, recognition of disease and resolution in differential diagnosis, demanding and caring supervision of clinical clerks. In 1929 Seale Harris, Jr. (Hopkins, 1926), joined the department as assistant and was followed seven years later by Rudolph H. Kampmeier, a 1923 graduate of the University of Iowa Medical School and student there of Campbell Palmer Howard, who was assistant resident under Osler between 1902 and 1906 and Osler's godson.[16]

It would almost seem that among Vanderbilt's new faculty in medicine every one of the wonderful Oslerian traits was commonplace. Whether they really were to the degree that they seemed to have been remembered is impossible ever finally to test, but this much at least is certain: Osler's thoughts and techniques about the practice of clinical medicine were then on the leading edge of practical reform in medical education, and they were remembered by those then present as a sacred trust somehow later accidentally forsaken. "In the continued remembrance of a glorious past individuals and nations find their noblest inspiration," department member and historian Kampmeier quoted Osler, recalling a glorious time unexampled for excitement when Osler's men had carried all before them.[17] At Vanderbilt, wrote Kampmeier (who was one of them), they were "first clinicians, astute and competent in the universality of internal medicine, and only secondarily subspecialists," faithful ever to Osler's dictum that "there are in truth no specialties in medicine, since to know fully many of the most important diseases a man must be familiar with their manifestation in many organs." To follow internal medicine as a true vocation, Sir William had said, meant to be a "pluralist—and as [the young physician] values his future life—let him not get early entangled in the meshes of specialism."[18] So Osler and his disciples were honored ever after in form, if not for long in substance. It was a bit like wishing reason upon the sea, so diverse was the specialism then about to crash over the "universality of internal medicine." Indeed, it was a fair question whether the Oslerian technique so well established at the new Vanderbilt was not at once vanguard for a new and better way of thinking about and of doing medicine and medical education (as the young Oslerian physicians truly believed) and, outpaced even then by history and science, rear guard for already aging verities.

Whichever, it was enough for medical faculties of the 1920s and 1930s just to translate what by education and conviction they knew to be true into a practical design for training young doctors. It was hard work that demanded much of the sturdiest constitutions, and it left little time for introspection. Their reward (for few were wealthy) lay in fashioning a pattern of teaching and learning that made of professors and pupils as much a true intellectual community as was then known at Vanderbilt and may have been known since. The curriculum, which remained relatively unchanged for the next twenty-five years, was governed by Osler's principle that to learn internal medicine was "to learn how to study disease and how to treat it, or rather how to treat patients." Some tinkering from time to time was inevitable, but in general the program coached students both in thinking and in acting, supplying tomorrow's clinicians and practitioners with both the means of science and the will to service.

As it was reorganized in 1925 the department of medicine included internal medicine plus the subdivisions of pediatrics, neurology, dermatology, and psychiatry, all of which in time would achieve autonomy.[19] At the beginning only pediatrics was in the charge of a new full-time man: Horton R. Casparis, whom Robinson brought from Hopkins as associate professor. The others then relied on local, part-time practicing specialists. Internal medicine itself, however, was Robinson's domain, and there through him Osler's spirit reigned supreme. It was for that—as much as for the tangible monument of the buildings he designed—that generations of Vanderbilt physicians remembered and lionized him.

Robinson made only one major departure from Osler's blueprint for teaching internal medicine. He set the clinical experience of the fourth-year students primarily in the outpatient clinics, whereas Osler had put fourth-year students to work in the wards as clinical clerks and third-year students to work in the clinics. In the clinics Robinson believed that seniors would have greater independence and that their work, being somewhat more specialized, would resemble more closely the work they would soon encounter in daily practice.[20] Third-year students meanwhile began to learn clinical medicine, closely supervised on the hospital wards. Robinson had seen such an arrangement in successful operation at the University of Michigan Medical School at Ann Arbor. He may have decided too that, newly located as it was in Nashville's prosperous West End, Vanderbilt's clinic would not attract to such an extent as Hopkins's clinic an indigent clientele, but rather low- to middle-income part-pay patients similar to those most young doctors would soon meet in practice.[21] For whatever reasons he made the transposition, it worked well at Vanderbilt and in the end merely rescheduled Osler's plan without changing its nature.

Students' first exposure to internal medicine actually came in the second trimester of their second year when they had completed basic work in anatomy, biochemistry, physiology, and immunology and were in the midst of pathology and pharmacology. Then the department of medicine cooperated with the department of pathology to demonstrate various pathological conditions in actual patients. Also in the second trimester, second-year students began their formal course in clinical pathology within the department of medicine itself. Designed as the key bridge from the preclinical to the clinical halves of medical education, the course set students to work on things that in later years (at Vanderbilt not until after World War II) the hospital would employ technicians to do. Learning practical laboratory technique as they went, they applied their newly acquired knowledge of the basic sciences to the analysis of blood, urine, sputum, gastric contents, and spinal fluids, in

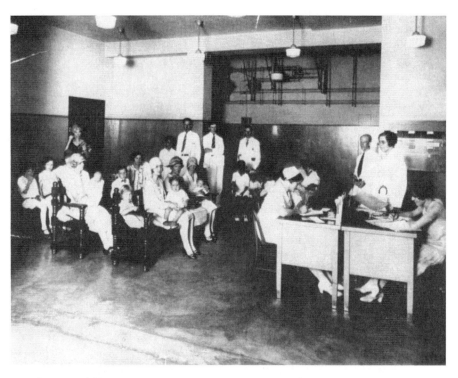

Pediatrics waiting room, ca. 1928

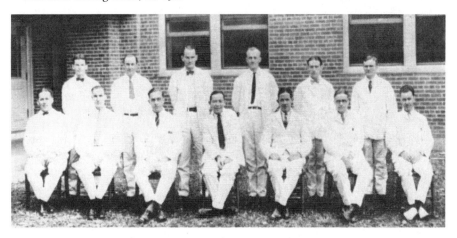

Teaching: the first house staff, 1925–1926. Alfred Blalock and Tinsley Harrison are seated third and fourth from right.

the beginning under the supervision of Hugh Morgan and Tinsley Harrison and over the years under different senior residents in their turn.[22]

The true watershed, however, and the moment that every medical student longingly awaited came not in such laboratory work but with the chance—if not actually to treat—at least to deal with sick people. They began in the second trimester to learn physical diagnosis. They did not, of course, learn on real patients right away but on each other and through a series of lectures, demonstrations, and practical exercises. Of such art as remained in the new medicine much resided in the technique of taking a patient's medical history and in conducting the physical examination as preface to further diagnostic testing. Hardly more than a start could be made in a few weeks in medical school; the course merely introduced students to methods of examining patients and interpreting the information gathered from their observations and their knowledge of their patients' history. They began to sense what questions to ask, what to watch and listen for, and where and how to lay on the hands. Robinson himself first took charge of the course, and as conducted by him and his followers—Burwell, Youmans, Harris, and Kampmeier—physical diagnosis taught Vanderbilt students to observe and to order the things they observed. It taught a technique that invited the constant testing and refining of experience. It invited them always to learn as they went.

So coached to ask the right questions, to see what could be seen and to test in the laboratory for what could not, Vanderbilt students could look forward in their third year to more work with real patients. Through the year's three trimesters, the entire class of fifty rotated by thirds through the medical service, serving as clinical clerks in the Osler tradition. For eleven weeks, sixteen or seventeen students were assigned to the hospital's three medical wards (for white men, white women, and blacks), each student being given three or four of the ward's approximately sixty patients to study intensively. The students took histories, did routine laboratory work, and, after physical examination had been completed by a member of the house staff, also examined the patient. They spent three hours a morning, six days a week, at it, plus whatever other time they could steal. They knew they always had to be prepared, and they knew that their testing likely would be on the spot. For one hour, five mornings a week, at teaching rounds, they and various house officers trailed the professor or an associate professor through the wards. Students were then expected to present the history and other data that had been gathered on the patients assigned to them and to be prepared to discuss with the entire group the diagnosis, management, and treatment of that case. Each student might be responsible specifically for only three or four patients but was nevertheless brought into contact with virtually all patients entering the medical wards. As a follow-up and true to the Osler spirit, the same group of one-third of the class met for an hour once a week with the professor to discuss informally patients who had been discharged, with attention to the social and psychological aspects of a case and its relation to the history and literature of medicine. Although Robinson as professor was the final authority, he left immediate supervision of the ward services and the third-year clerks who learned there to his two associate professors, Burwell and Morgan. When Burwell became chief in 1928, the responsibility devolved increasingly on Tinsley Harrison until Morgan took over in 1935.

As it was all remembered from the viewpoints both of students and of teachers, it was a worthy if a wearing exercise.[23] Even, for example, if a patient was admitted and assigned late in the afternoon, the clinical clerk had to be ready by 8:30 the next morning to discuss the case at teaching rounds, which meant the clerk had to have in hand—and presumably to have drawn the right conclusion from them—the patient's history, the record of physical examination, and laboratory test results (students' histories and test results were for years an official part of patients' hospital records). Interns recorded similar information and within a day or two the assistant resident and the chief resident had made their own notes on a patient's chart. Students' records were constantly scrutinized by house staff, especially the assistant residents, though senior residents and attending staff also enjoyed and sometimes exercised the prerogative of demanding that work be done again. Although not as hectic as it would become in more recent times, life on the ward service was pressured enough and not for the students alone. Members of the house staff were unmarried, or at least if single when appointed had to promise to stay that way for the duration. Hopkins-style, they lived and ate in the hospital, were constantly on call and thus constantly on display to students and faculty alike. Some Saturday nights were free, but, as one veteran recalled, weekends seemed to be made only for more laboratory studies. For an entire summer his sole excursion out of the hospital was to get a haircut.[24] Pay to house staff was meager and the hours long, and day or night it was never hard to find third-year students in laboratory or ward under the tutelage, one to one, of a young house officer.

The entire third-year class came together once a week for a clinical lecture or demonstration by a senior member of the part-time faculty, and throughout the year, also once a week, third- and fourth-year students gathered in the medical school's amphitheater (a room whose largest dimension seemed to be vertical and the one most evocative of the old European operating theaters) for a teaching clinic conducted by the professor or an associate. In both medicine and surgery it was something of a ritual occasion. In medicine it was held each Wednesday from 11:30 to 12:30, the third-year students presenting their cases and fourth-year students being quizzed by the professor on various matters of diagnosis and treatment. Third-year students also attended a twenty-two-week course in medical psychology as an introduction to psychiatry. Lectures and exercises focused on physiological psychology and were tailored to the needs of the medical practitioner. Likewise, twenty-two hours were given over to neurology. And finally, pediatrics (until 1928 a subdivision of internal medicine) also began in the third year with a series of lectures and demonstrations in child nutrition and in the growth and development of infants and children. Small groups of seven or eight students were assigned to the pediatric wards for rotation of five and a half weeks to learn at the bedside, with emphasis always being placed on the physiology of the normal child and various problems of growth and nutrition.

By the end of the third year in medicine students had observed and done much. Although they were not yet perfect at it, they knew the technique of history taking, the methods of physical examination, and basic laboratory procedures. A considerable array of diseases had passed before them, and they had learned something of dealing with the patients who were host to those diseases and something of managing their afflictions. They had learned to be comfortable (as comfortable was) in the wards and corridors of a large teaching hospital and they had learned to learn from the house staff, who though several years older were learners themselves.

During the fourth year, while the purpose and the procedures remained the same, the setting changed from ward to outpatient clinic. Following the third-year pattern, a third of the class rotated every eleven weeks through the general medical clinic and the specialty clinics. Cases were assigned, students took histories, conducted physical examinations, and performed the simpler tests. Their work was then checked off by a staff member who requested needed consultations with other departments. Of the eight students assigned to general medicine, two daily did complete blood count and urinalysis and venipunctures on all entering patients as well as those who for one reason or another had returned to the clinic or had been referred for consultation from other departments. The other half of the group then rotating through medicine could be found scattered in the special clinics for neurology, dermatology, chest diseases, and metabolic and gastrointestinal disorders.

During his Vanderbilt tenure, the outpatient service of the department of medicine and the teaching of fourth-year students there was Robinson's personal charge and a job he said he wanted himself to assure that the clinics did not suffer the subordination to the wards common in many hospitals. It

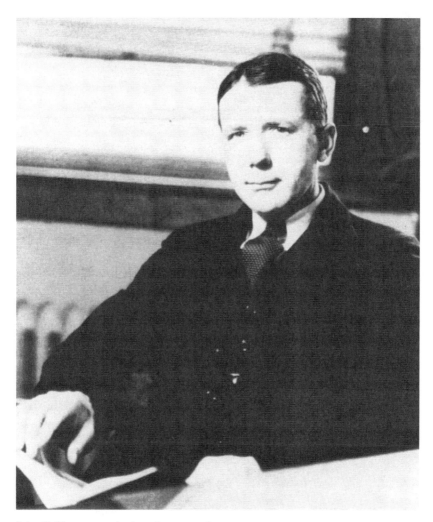

John B. Youmans, who later became a dean

was a problem obviated in part by the design of the plant itself, which physically integrated, one atop the other, medicine's ward and clinic services. Too, in John B. Youmans, Robinson selected an extraordinarily able young physician to become director of the outpatient department in anticipation of his own departure in 1928. Youmans came in 1927 as an assistant professor from the University of Michigan where he had gained experience in outpatient work that prepared him for the job of building up Vanderbilt's clinic clientele and faculty. He succeeded to the point where the Vanderbilt Hospital clinics achieved a reputation out of proportion to their tender age. As with much else that Robinson (and, through him, Osler) conceived, Youmans's expression of their ideas displayed the clarity and the self-assurance that made for good policy. Thoroughness and accuracy in examination, diagnosis, and treatment was mandatory; recognition of relevant social and emotional factors no less so. There was to be a clinic chief, for whom teaching was the main university responsibility, and enough doctors and enough space to assure good work. The size of the clinic had to be in proportion to the size of the hospital wards it complemented to assure continuity of care for patients moving from one to the other and to reap maximum teaching benefit from each patient. Records had to be complete and accurate, for complete records meant complete and accurate examinations. Responsibility for the individual patient had to be fixed with an individual doctor, start to finish; hopscotching was bad for patient, doctor, and student. Students learned most by example, and no example was more important than unfailing kindness toward the patient and respect for individuality and privacy.[25]

So it was at Vanderbilt: senior faculty in charge, representation from pharmacy and social service, meticulous record keeping, and a large and dedicated corps of teachers, many of whom had been senior house officers at Vanderbilt and who had gone into practice in Nashville, or others, newcomers to the city who had had postgraduate training elsewhere in internal medicine. Such were Samuel S. Riven, a 1925 medical graduate of McGill University with graduate training at Michigan; Clarence S. Thomas, Hopkins, 1929, with house officer experience there, at Vanderbilt, and at Stanford; Albert Weinstein and Edgar Jones, both Vanderbilt graduates of 1929; and David Strayhorn, a 1928 graduate who had been first resident physician at Robinson's new Cornell University–New York Hospital and who joined the Vanderbilt clinical faculty in 1936. Stipends for these part-time men were small—$100 to $300 a year—but they gave at least three hours a day, three days a week, to teaching fourth-year students in the medical clinics. Himself not exactly a disinterested observer but a well-traveled one nonetheless who had seen many other places, John Youmans years later judged Vanderbilt between 1927 (the year he arrived) and World War II as having the best volunteer faculty in the nation.[26] Whether the best or just one of the best, in relying on young part-timers (who were trained either at Vanderbilt or at similar modern medical schools) to staff its clinics and thus bear much of the burden for educating fourth-year students, Vanderbilt was in good and familiar company. Hopkins too relied on local help in its outpatient department and likewise lavished on it high praise and little money.[27]

Beyond their clinic work, which was the core of their fourth-year experience, students completed their undergraduate education in medicine with psychiatry and further work in pediatrics. In the last trimester twenty-two lectures covered various mental disturbances that when possible were illustrated by patients from the hospital wards. Because Vanderbilt then had no facilities for psychiatric patients, clinical lectures and demonstrations were held at the Tennessee Central State Hospital for the Insane, where students spent three hours a week for eleven weeks. Not a specialty clinic of course, it focused (as much else did in the undergraduate curriculum) on the types of psychiatric diseases that might most often be confronted by the medical practitioner. Pediatrics, which had been introduced in the ward training of the third year, continued in greater depth in the fourth. The associate professor of medicine, Horton Casparis (full professor of pediatrics after 1928), and the professor of clinical pediatrics shared a series of fifty-five clinical lectures that included demonstration and discussion of the important phases of pediatrics and all the acute infections of childhood. One-sixth of the class at a time rotated through the pediatric outpatient department, where for eight hours a week for half the trimester they worked as clerks much as they had in the general medical clinics, learning by doing. Finally, the department offered various elective opportunities. A limited number of third- and fourth-year students might pursue special projects in the department's laboratories or in the wards and clinics. Until 1932 when all fourth-year students attended Hollis Johnson's chest clinic, groups of six could study tuberculosis at the Davidson County Tuberculosis Hospital. They could participate in the diagnostic and therapeutic work in syphilis in the special clinic established in 1929 to study that disease. Students were also encouraged to work in one of the clinical laboratories, assisting in the research activities of the faculty, perhaps even earning inclusion of their names, as joint authors, of publications.

That much was eminently Oslerian. Talented clinicians grouped around a core of full-time personnel gave themselves over to teaching by example in the conviction that clinical medicine was more learned than taught and that what needed to be learned was less the facts about every disease than the techniques for studying disease. In that process internal medicine was both foundation and keystone. By the 1920s and 1930s, students at Vanderbilt were as motivated and as well-prepared to study medicine as those remembered by Robinson at Hopkins at the turn of the century. And most of them became in those years, also in the best Oslerian tradition, not "ultraspecialists" and researchers, as some critics predicted, but active practitioners of medicine. Of the 495 medical graduates of the school's first decade, just 1 percent later described themselves primarily as researchers, 6 percent were in institutional

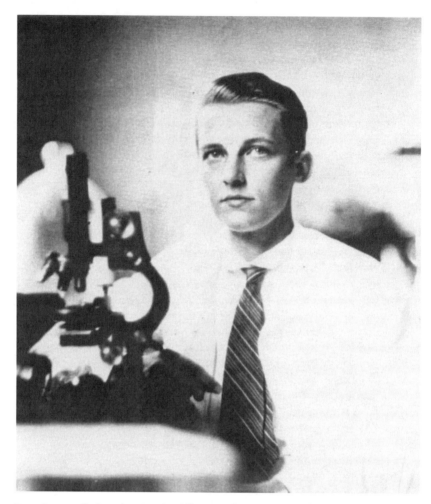

Learning: medical student Louise Allen Beard in 1926, one of the first two women
M.D.'s to graduate from Vanderbilt (class of 1929). Hers was the first class to
complete its work in the new school.

work that included academic medicine, 41 percent were primarily in specialty
practice. That left more than half in some sort of general practice, though
perhaps with some specialty interest. Nor did they all flock to the great cities
(in part, no doubt, because the South had few great cities, and most of these
doctors were southerners who stayed in the South): 104 could be found in
cities of 100,000 to 250,000; 91, roughly a fifth, in small towns of less than
2,500 people.[28]

The students who ran that strenuous clinical course for those two years emerged with habits that supposedly would keep them "student[s] for all of [their] professional life—always questioning, always learning." Or so the educational technique of the department—"inquiring and reasoning rather than didacticism and sophistry"—was designed to assure.[29] Testimony that it did is certainly credible. Historian Kampmeier recalled the astute evaluations of patients' problems given by small-town Vanderbilt doctors requesting consultation with the staff at their alma mater: no floundering recitals of facts learned rote from the textbook, but clear judgments of the clinical situation that marked them as discriminating students still faithful to the techniques of their Vanderbilt masters. To observe, feel, and listen; to gather up the new evidence; to draw upon the large body of scientific knowledge comprehended far back in the first two preclinical years; and finally to make an induction: this was the technique of clinical medicine those masters sought to instill. By most accounts they succeeded rather well.

Thus faithful to the spirit of Osler and under the guiding hands of Robinson and his new faculty, Vanderbilt's department of medicine trained practicing and practical physicians. In that process, however, and in the rhetoric that over the years accompanied it, much could be heard about science and service together. Both were invoked by the doctors and their lay patrons as ultimate justification for all the effort and the sacrifice of those who made it. To students nurtured up under its twin banner, the long march from the first-year anatomy lesson to the serious duties of the resident physician was doubly sanctified, and their subsequent self-esteem and sense of professional worth were doubly buttressed. Most of them became at least credible physicians and some of them became superior ones who applied the techniques of treating disease learned in Vanderbilt's wards and clinics to the job of trying to heal sick people. Of their service there was no doubt. Those who returned to serve for little or nothing on the part-time faculty and to bring to the academy the insights gleaned from practice rendered even more. In the Osler tradition, that should have been enough. Although a well-trained scientist himself, Osler had cared primarily for education and service, for the direct study of patients, which he believed quite rightly promised large dividends for the practice of medicine outside the hospital. And that was what most medical graduates at Vanderbilt and elsewhere did and would do: they studied patients and they practiced medicine outside the hospital.

But many of them also emerged thinking of themselves as scientists, as if by one-time training they qualified for a lifetime as proud replicas of Dr. Arrowsmith. They did not. Between their training, whose foundation was science, and their vocation, which was service, the line had never been perfectly drawn, but the casual identification of the two by many practitioners was as unjustified as it was understandable. What young Vanderbilt students would not naturally choose to see themselves in the flattering image of Robinson, Burwell, Morgan, Youmans, and other true scientist-mentors? Yet it was as likely that in the long run they so deceived themselves and invited their own frustration. They fervently believed that science served, and as its agents they effectively advertised themselves. In the process they strengthened vastly their claims to social legitimacy. What might happen if the supply of service, supposedly fed by ever better science, one day fell below the public's demand for it seemed in the 1930s fairly academic and, at that moment, loose talk about science among Vanderbilt medical students was to be expected and even welcomed. Medical students, then as now, were a driven lot and, while the general pace of life was slower and the scale smaller, few schedules allowed for leisurely contemplation of science in the abstract. The science learned by these practitioners-to-be was the science of the clinical laboratories, which Robinson so carefully had located midway between the north wings, the lair of the basic scientists, and the south wings, the realm of the clinicians. There the members of Robinson's department and their apprentices filled the mandate of modern medicine that owed less to Osler than to the German institutes, where so many young Americans were first exposed to real research, and to such early American counterparts as the laboratories at Johns Hopkins and the Rockefeller Institute. Flexner, the layman, had made research in clinical medicine as well as in the basic sciences a key article in the reformers' creed as set forth in Bulletin Number Four. He was an unabashed admirer both of German scientific prowess and of his brother Simon who, as director of the Rockefeller Institute, had already invested the family name in the cause of true science. Kirkland too, whom Robinson had once accused of being suspicious of research, generally supported its claims and asked only to know how it all would be paid for. Once they were hired, he did not meddle with Robinson's new faculty, who quickly proved themselves faithful to Flexner's and the German model of the teacher of medicine who was deeply involved in research and whose primary interests, in Robinson's words, "would not be interrupted by medical practice outside his departmental activities."[30]

In Robinson's department of medicine, which was the centerpiece for the clinical training of all doctors no matter how they later specialized, the model worked so well that the spirit of research was fondly remembered and extolled by many a practicing Vanderbilt graduate who had long since ceased to do any. Real substance lay behind those memories, however, and the array of research work reported in several hundred publications during the 1920s and 1930s reveals something of the broad interests of academic clinicians before the age of subspecialism. The greater degree to which much of that work is comprehensible to the layman hints that as medicine as inductive science broke itself down into smaller and smaller pieces, it became shrouded in greater and greater mystery, something that was not a little ironic for a profession that claimed and was every year expected to render ever-greater service. But then for a time research was still new, relatively inexpensive, and the researchers, at least in medicine, were Oslerian clinicians who by training and habit actually did shun the "meshes of specialism."

In the original plan Robinson had provided for three research laboratories in the department of medicine: the physiological division under Sidney Burwell, the infectious disease division under Hugh Morgan, and the clinical division under Tinsley Harrison. The research that resulted fit roughly into those categories and reflected commonly enough the established interests of key faculty, the prevalence of certain diseases, and the availability of new tools for combating them.[31] Robinson and Burwell followed their interests in cardiovascular problems. Earlier in his career, as a resident in pathology and medicine at the Pennsylvania Hospital, Robinson had published two papers on heart disease that brought him to the attention of Friedrich Muller, in whose Munich laboratory he then worked in 1908 and 1909. There he met George Draper, with whom at the Rockefeller Institute he continued to study cardiac physiology and to do promising work in electrocardiography. During his year at Hopkins Robinson published a monograph on the therapeutic use of digitalis, and at Vanderbilt (though as dean and chairman his time was more limited) he continued to write an occasional paper on cardiac physiology and therapeutics. His interests, though, were continued in the like-minded individuals he chose to be his new colleagues. At Harvard and Hopkins respectively, Burwell and Harrison had already published on problems of the heart and circulation, and both continued to do so at Vanderbilt. During his tenure there, Burwell turned out papers every year on digitalis therapy, congestive heart failure, and the physiology of circulation during pregnancy. Like many at Vanderbilt in those years, much of his work bore the names of his collaborators, among them Robinson, David Strayhorn, and surgeon Alfred Blalock. The quantity alone of Tinsley Harrison's work proved correct Robinson's description of him as a human dynamo; its quality showed him to be a thoughtful scholar as well. During his first decade at Vanderbilt he continued work in cardiac physiology, exploring the regulation of circulation, congestive failure, and drug action on cardiac output. With a special grant of $1,000 in 1929 he was able to provide an added technician in the biochemistry department to help with his work on the content of total base, chloride, phosphate, magnesium, calcium, and sodium content in muscle tissue. He formulated a "respiration index" that made possible the first quantitative measure of severity of dyspnea, and with Arthur Grollman from Hopkins he tried to discover a successful method of measuring cardiac output during heart failure. Later, Harrison moved on to studies of hypertension and renal physiology, many with the collaboration of Blalock and biochemist Morton Mason. Harrison's book, *Failure of the Circulation,* appeared in 1935.

Research in infectious diseases—the second of Robinson's three clinical laboratory divisions—likewise reflected the interests and experience of its chief, Hugh Morgan.[32] Morgan had returned from the army medical corps after World War I interested in new developments in syphilis therapy, which had continued in the syphilis clinic at Hopkins in the early 1920s. At Vanderbilt under Morgan and colleagues, experimental and clinical work in the disease occupied a large place until in the late 1940s penicillin therapy drastically reduced its importance. Morgan at first worked with colonies of white rabbits, studying (with Edna Tompkins in anatomy) cellular reaction to experimental disease and the effect on it of trypan blue, and probing for the dosage of infecting organism required to produce the disease. Over the years he published numerous papers on syphilis and contributed sections on aortic disease and the treatment of spirochetal infections to several medical textbooks. With the appointment in 1936 of Rudolph H. Kampmeier, who took charge of the syphilis clinic, epidemiological and clinical research continued. A year later Vanderbilt was selected by Thomas Parran, surgeon general of the United States Public Health Service, as one of the centers to be established with federal funds at academic institutions to help educate health officers and public health nurses in syphilis control. Following from that experiment, the wartime Office of Scientific Research and Development in 1943 chose Vanderbilt as one of the centers for the testing of penicillin therapy in syphilis. Kampmeier's book, *Essentials of Syphilology,* appeared that same year. Tuberculosis, an infectious affliction that caused more deaths by far than syphilis, was studied by Hollis Johnson, who at Robinson's invitation had established a chest clinic at Vanderbilt. After extensive clinical study he wrote on artificial pneumothorax (therapeutic collapsing of a lung) in the treatment of tuberculous in pregnant women. With pathologist Roy Avery and others, he reported on the use of streptomycin for advanced chronic pulmonary tuberculosis and on a variety of other thoracic problems.

Hematology and nutrition were two other areas that received early attention from Vanderbilt's investigators in clinical medicine. R. Sidney Cunningham and Edna Tompkins in anatomy studied leukocytes from the very opening of the new school; involved in that work were students Frank Luton and Edgar Jones, both of whom later would join the department of medicine.

Studies in nutrition, something for which Vanderbilt would earn considerable renown, rightly began with John Youmans, the young Hopkins doctor whom Robinson imported in 1927 to take over the medical outpatient department. He came from an area of Wisconsin afflicted with endemic goiter, had studied the problem while at Michigan, and in Nashville continued to pursue his interest in thyroid dysfunction. In the 1930s he securely established himself in the field of nutrition (with papers on serum proteins and nitrogen balance in endemic edema) and in the field of vitamin deficiencies. With collaborators he began in 1936 a series of studies of vitamins A and C and thiamine, work that led to his development of a program assessing the nutritional problems of the rural population of Wilson County, Tennessee, near Nashville. That work, which was funded ($50,000 over five years) by the International Health Division of the Rockefeller Foundation, was described in half a dozen papers published throughout the 1940s, and on it were patterned numerous nutritional surveys conducted in many countries after World War II. On leave from Vanderbilt in 1940 and 1941, Youmans made similar nutritional surveys in unoccupied France and in 1941 published his textbook on the subject, *Nutritional Deficiences: Diagnosis and Treatment.*

There were, of course, others who in those years made their mark through research in one field or another of clinical medicine. Their work reflected the still broad interests of these early academic internists whose careers were shaped to the canons of Osler, Flexner, and Robinson. Compared with that of their predecessors at Vanderbilt before 1925, their work seemed to anticipate the antimicrobial revolution of the 1940s and the resulting shift in clinical research toward degenerative disease and in the development of tools better to study physiological process.[33] Not only were they thus moving in the right direction but in so doing they seemed to vindicate Robinson's hopes for a truly coordinated medical school and hospital. Shared labors and joint authorship with members of other departments, especially surgery, anatomy, and biochemistry, made much research at Vanderbilt interdisciplinary years before such became an educationist's cliché. The faculty and student body were small; doctors dined together daily; the doors to laboratories were always open. How much those things helped, along with Robinson's design that put the clinical laboratories at the center of the grid and across the paths of scholar and student alike, can never be known for sure. But none of it hurt and surely all of it invited the kinds of collaboration that in fact became common. The amount of research generated in this keystone clinical department, measured by crude arithmetic alone (344 publications between 1925 and 1945), suggested that here was the community of producing scholars that reformers had said was the foundation of medicine as science. Although, as one of those scholars, John B. Youmans, warned, publications do not necessarily measure excellence or even competence, they do at least measure curiosity and perhaps ambition. The costs by later standards were ridiculously low and were largely covered in the early years in the department's budget, supplemented during the 1930s by a fluid research fund provided by the Rockefeller Foundation.[34]

Deliberate, sustained, and prolific research—once the exception but later the expectation—was becoming the routine. As it did, it promised and produced new and useful knowledge. It also helped change the solid core of Osler's old art into something new. In such departments of internal medicine as Vanderbilt's (which was a good example of how medicine was supposed to be taught and worked at in modern medical schools of that era) Osler's practical precepts long commanded the allegiance of teacher and student alike. But the great physician's sagacity was being blended with clinical research that was both exploratory and instrumental. The clinicians' research was enlarging and changing the body of acknowledged truth whereby others would judge the doctors' science and art. Instrumental as it was, their science touched the popular imagination by its tangible results and thus conformed to the American canon (still then ascendant) of historic progress in material things. Inviting medicine to be viewed as a commodity, their kind of science seemed to suit Americans well.

Osler would have been pleased with these new people and their research. His own hopes for science had been high in two respects especially, even though he knew science could fulfill them only imperfectly. A Victorian at heart, he was proud of the practical progress, the simple increase in physical well-being that even in the nineteenth century science had accomplished in medicine. "Think of the Nemesis which has overcome pain during the past fifty years," he wrote in 1894. "Anesthetics and antiseptic surgery have almost manacled the demon, and since their introduction the aggregate of pain which has been prevented outweighs in civilized communities that which has been suffered. Even the curse of travail has been lifted from the soul of women."[35] Science through medicine had done much and would no doubt do more to improve the condition of humankind. Thanks to science, medicine rendered service that was better than ever before. But, scientific physician though he was, Osler knew that most human despairs were not amendable to the mere physical remedies that scientific medicine had to offer. He knew that medicine, however scientific or however artful, had limits. "We are apt to forget that apart from and beyond her domain lie those irresistible forces which alone sway the hearts of men. . . . With feeling, emotion, passion, what has she to do? They are not of her; they owe her no allegiance." Benjamin

Franklin, he wrote, had "chained the lightnings, but who has chained the wayward spirit of man?"[36]

Proud though he was of the science that had made for great progress, he defended another science that always had not. He acclaimed a researchers' world where "no secondary motives sway their minds, no cry reaches them in the recesses of their laboratories, 'of what practical utility is your work?' " To those few individuals blessed with the powers actually to do science—"the last gift of the gods"—it imparted, like religion, "imperturbability amid the storms of life, judgment in times of perplexity." Would that it did, for the future held perplexity aplenty. How vexing, for example, that in the process of working out new truths through science, Osler's and Vanderbilt's researchers should hasten the obsolescence of their practicing colleagues. As Osler borrowed from Keats's "Hyperion": "So on our heals a fresh perfection treads / . . . born of us / And fated to excel us."[37] "Fresh perfection" did not come all at once but, with the probability that it would come, medicine's new people were learning to live. It was not an easy lesson.

Surgery

8

Osler never saw Vanderbilt. Robinson stayed there only eight years. But through their many followers they marked the new school as few others would. They shaped not just internal medicine, which was their own particular calling, but the whole school, from a building designed to coordinate the basic sciences with medicine's clinical branches, to the function of a daily round of teaching and learning where masters taught apprentices to learn by doing. That technique aimed to produce practicing generalists who, though taught to think as scientists and therefore inductively, held with Osler that to study medicine was to study the whole person. As practical clinicians, science was for them ever wedded to service.

But in the world of internal medicine, science in the early twentieth century did not render so quickly the service a later generation would come to expect. Careful fact gathering and cautious induction took time, and foundation subsidy and the full-time system guaranteed among the scientists no imaginative leaps or instant discoveries. As agents of change sometimes do, science for the physicians demonstrated first and most clearly what was wrong with the past. Only more slowly did it work out what the future would be like. Thus all the new doctors produced by Hopkins and the other reformed medical schools of the early twentieth century knew this much for sure: that the pills, potions, and plasters of their nineteenth-century predecessors were wrong. They did not yet have much to substitute, too small still was their new knowledge of the biochemical mechanisms of disease. But they took their oath seriously. To do no harm, they forsook the therapies of their predecessors and did what little their new science then said they could do to mitigate the effects of disease. In the meantime, through research, they sought understanding of its causes, from which true therapies someday might come. Their service for many years lagged behind their science, something that required of the early scientific physicians considerable patience and faith that in the end science would not betray them.

For the surgeons, the transition from the past to the present was easier. With them science in the nineteenth century had indeed wrought some immediate and practical changes in an old craft. Anesthesia had removed much of surgery's terror. Asepsis and antisepsis had made much greater the prospect of happy endings. Before ether, the best surgeons had worked with dazzling speed. They made their incisions and removed or repaired the offending parts. Students looking on were suitably awed. They were master anatomists whose errors could be charged up to the accident of living too soon to know that pain could be conquered or infection stymied. If in haste they handled precious tissues roughly, they did so with the good intention of shortening the suffering of their poor patients. If they operated with bare hands and bloody aprons, they did so without knowing that they thereby introduced more evil than ever they excised.

Pasteur, Lister, Koch, and germ theory in time changed the way they dressed. With anesthesia came the time needed to be gentle. With surgical pathology came knowledge of what surgeons were actually looking at. But unlike the old physicians, whose theories and much of whose practice of medicine the new science repudiated, the old surgeons whose manual skills had often been unexcelled still inspired intelligent awe among their younger and more scientific heirs. It is common for doctors to speak reverently about medicine's past, but surgeons more than others can evoke a genuine communion. Moreover, in the first decades of this century intervention of the knife seemed able relatively to do more than medical therapies. It was not that medicine and surgery competed but merely that surgery rested more comfortably on its past and enjoyed for a time a more even and visible progress.

Surgeons and physicians shared the old aim of healing, and in training the young they shared fundamental techniques of teaching and learning. At Vanderbilt in medicine, the spirit and technique of Osler in the 1920s and 1930s was transmitted through the administrations of three men: Robinson, Burwell, and Morgan. In surgery, dominion for those years belonged to one man alone, Barney Brooks, who like Morgan and so many of his other medical colleagues was a second-generation Oslerian. Brooks's biography reads like a self-help novel of the late nineteenth century, something that may have had not a little to do with his ability to propel his young department to a point of eminence fully equal to medicine's.[1] In the hierarchical world that medical schools then were, he fit the role of the authoritarian professor in a way that may be attributed to his having earned success over long years. Unlike his counterparts in medicine, he lacked the regal imperiousness of "General" Morgan and kept hidden in his official self the warmth and geniality so natural to Burwell and Robinson. Some said the feisty little Brooks ruled by fear alone (he surely ruled by fear at least in part); others said that he ruled simply through integrity and talent as a surgeon and medical educator. He did rule absolutely, inspiring the fear of his students at the time and, typically, their reverence later on.

Brooks was born in 1884, while Kirkland was studying in Leipzig and while Robinson, nine years his senior, was a boy in Baltimore. He was a son of the rural West (Jacksboro, Texas) and like many such sons he seemed, when the chance came, eager to leave it. In a humble upbringing (a two-room shack for a home, days spent punching cows, frequently interrupted schooling, time served as a high school science teacher—and, from boyhood, the ambition to be a doctor), those who have memorialized him spied the early seeds of greatness—of strong character made stronger by hard work and hard knocks. At the very least, life had not always been easy for him and, as with thousands of other young Americans, early hardships had taught him the virtues of self-help through education. Through schooling he set out to enter a profession. Neither then nor later was he ambitious for material things, and though in surgery he chose a profession that could promise munificent returns, he seemed satisfied that the sacrifice of relatively low academic pay bought him the privilege of teaching, of doing research, and of being left alone.

His four years at the University of Texas emptied the family exchequer, and it was not until 1907, two years later, that he was able to finance his entrance into the medical world at Johns Hopkins. Osler had left for Oxford two years before, but there remained the distinguished array of Osler's students to impart to Brooks and his classmates the true religion of their master. He worked hard and did well, graduating in 1911 fifth in his class. That was better than Robinson, who had ranked only in the middle of his class of fifty in 1903, but it was not quite good enough to qualify him for one of the coveted Hopkins medical internships reserved for the four top students. As number five, Brooks became a surgical intern under William S. Halsted, himself one (with Welch, Osler, and Howard A. Kelly) of the Hopkins "Big Four" immortalized in John Singer Sargent's famous painting. Although Brooks presumably continued to work hard and do well, he was not rewarded at the end of his internship with a place on Halsted's resident staff, then probably the best and surely the most prestigious training ground for young doctors wanting to become surgeons. Instead, he continued his training on the staff of Barnes Hospital, the teaching hospital of the newly reorganized medical school of Washington University in St. Louis. There, in caring for patients and in the beginnings of serious investigative work, he put aside his disappointment at not being able to finish what he had begun at Hopkins. During his thirteen years in St. Louis he established a considerable reputation for his work on bone regeneration, intestinal obstruction, Volkmann's contracture, arteriography, and vascular disorders in general.[2] Between 1912 and 1925, when he came to Vanderbilt, he passed steadily up the ranks of Evarts Graham's department from assistant resident to associate professor, refining as he went his research skills and his considerable talents as a teacher. He organized a laboratory and a course in surgical pathology that became a model across the country, and he won the recognition of Halsted, his old teacher, who seemed to have regretted not keeping the talented young Brooks for his own department at Johns Hopkins.[3]

It was also at Washington University that Brooks first crossed paths with Canby Robinson, then associate professor of medicine there and after 1917 dean of the medical school. But when he set about recruiting for his new Vanderbilt faculty a few years later, Robinson did not rely on his own memory and judgment alone. For advice on the key post of surgery, he went to the very top, which was of course to alma mater Hopkins and to former teacher and dean of American surgeons, William Halsted. Robinson recalled that Halsted directed him especially to "little Brooks."[4] Halsted died in 1922, before Brooks at Robinson's invitation had the opportunity to prove himself as head of his own department and chief surgeon in a modern teaching hospital. But had he lived, he would have seen "little Brooks" build at Vanderbilt a department of surgery and a surgical service suited to Halstedian specifications that together with the general influence of Osler throughout the school brought to the training of Vanderbilt surgeons a certain balance and gave to the surgeons themselves double the heroes to worship.

Like Osler, his medical colleague in early years at Hopkins, Halsted had the good fortune to live at a time and in a place congenial to his ambitions. Also like Osler, his was the eminence of a man who had excelled not by intrigue, cleverness, or luck but by true talent and the power of his ideas. In that, Canby Robinson, Barney Brooks, and others shared fully. To know those ideas is to know much of the substance and of the limits of the schools and departments that the young missionaries like Robinson and Brooks created in the image of the great masters. Osler, less the laboratory man than the clinician and teacher, left to his followers a general technique of learning by doing that was embodied in the new institution of the clinical clerkship. Halsted, much the laboratory man and more remote as teacher and healer, left a new technique of making young doctors into surgeons, a technique that was embodied in the institution of the postgraduate residency.

Halsted was a native New Yorker, born to a prosperous family in 1852, which left him well-positioned in the 1870s and 1880s to enter the exciting new age of bacteriology, embryology, histology, and pathological anatomy.[5] Though at Yale he had distinguished himself more as an athlete than as a scholar, he went on to medical school at the College of Physicians and Surgeons at Columbia, and there he became a doctor in 1877. During the internship that followed he met William Henry Welch, who later would recruit him for the new Johns Hopkins, and in 1878 (the year Robinson was born) he set off for two years of study on the Continent. In Vienna, Wurzburg, Halle, and Leipzig (where Kirkland too would go a few years later) he took in the teachings of Volkmann, Billroth, Thiersch, Bergmann, and other German scientists. Those were also the years when Lister's teachings about antiseptic and aseptic surgery were gaining wide acceptance in Europe and more slowly in Halsted's native America as well. When he returned home to New York in 1880, intelligent, well-trained, and socially well-connected, he seemed ready for an exceptional career as a practicing surgeon. It could have been his for the asking.

Indeed he did prosper, enjoying appointment as visiting surgeon to many New York City hospitals. But it was also in the 1880s that he turned to investigative work, at first on the anesthetic properties of cocaine. It was fitting work for a surgeon whose later contributions relied on the luxury of time that came only with effective anesthesia. In experiments with cocaine he achieved a major advance in the infant science of anesthesiology by demonstrating the neuroregional method of anesthesia. But he had used himself as a guinea pig, and the discovery cost him temporary addiction to cocaine. In 1886 he joined Welch in Baltimore but without yet appointment as head of surgery at the new Johns Hopkins Hospital. That offer went first to a foreigner, William Macewen of Glasgow. When Macewen declined, Halsted was appointed, though at first only on an acting basis for one year. In Baltimore he found, as did so many others, the medium his talents and temperament needed. In the years before the medical school opened in 1893, Welch's pathology laboratory gave him the leisure and opportunity to win back his own health and self-confidence, and with such men as Franklin Mall, Walter Reed, and Simon Flexner he found intellectual company that confirmed his scholarly ambitions.

Then beginning the work that would later make him famous and that would help immensely to advance surgery as a science in the early twentieth century, Halsted studied the basic questions of operative procedure and wound treatment. He read all of Lister's papers and copied his methods. And with the advantage that advances in bacteriology gave him, he refined the Englishman's general principle to a point that vastly increased its practical usefulness to surgery. William T. Councilman, later professor of pathology at Harvard and present then in Welch's laboratory, remembered: "Halsted showed that cultures made of wounds treated after the meticulous use of Lister's methods slowed the presence of bacteria on the surface. This led him to a careful microscopic study of wounds and the realization that care in operating, the exact approximation of surfaces and the avoidance of dead spaces was as important for results as the supposed avoidance of bacteria. . . . The study of hand disinfection was no less thorough and this led to the realization that the hands could not be sterilized, and finally to the use of rubber gloves in operating. . . . It is difficult to think of surgery more carefully conducted than was the experimental surgery of Halsted. . . . Probably not since the time of John Hunter had the experiment been so fully utilized in the development of surgery."[6]

Osler had conceived of the hospital as a college for physicians and physicians-to-be. Halsted conceived of the operating room as a laboratory for surgeons. There, in the path of Hunter and Lister, he worked out basic general principles that later had wide application in many branches of surgery: gentle handling of the tissues, meticulous control of bleeding, rigid asepsis. These were things that with Lister's principles, with better anesthesia, and in time with antibiotics made a science of the old anatomist's craft. To teach such things to young doctors who would become surgeons required, to Halsted (as it did to Osler and Kelly in their fields), a postgraduate residency. In the German fashion, such a residency blended the work of the clinic with the basic sciences and provided an extended training period of several years for only the most promising candidates fresh from their internships. The number of residents directly so trained under Halsted was not large (indeed the system was so competitive as to exclude Barney Brooks, who ranked fifth in his class and who had done well as an intern). Senior resident physicians at Hopkins retained their positions for as long as four and a half years in one case, and a total of only seventy-two people passed through Halsted's service at all levels. It was a fiercely pyramided system, but those who were not chosen for the select senior posts, or those who like Brooks were not selected at all, often went on to finish their training elsewhere under others who had served as Halsted's residents. Still the numbers were small, which makes all the more amazing the way Halsted's students seemed to carry all higher academic and professional surgery before them. Through them Halsted created, in the judgment of William Welch, his mentor and colleague, the first genuine school of surgery in the United States.[7]

As its builder, Halsted begat for his pupils a philosophy of surgery whose considerable power stemmed from a happy alliance between history and enlightened institutional arrangements.[8] Modern surgery was of a piece with its past, resting as it did on a few general principles worked out over long stretches of time and whose value seemed permanent. It rested first on knowledge of the structures of the human body that over the centuries the anatomists had made possible. To know what things looked like, and quickly to be able to recognize what form it was that the knife had uncovered, mattered as much to new surgeons at Hopkins and Vanderbilt as it had to their surgical ancestors who knew just that and nothing more.

But not until William Harvey in 1628 demonstrated the true course of the blood could surgeons begin to understand the physiological principles underlying the control of bleeding by the ligature, a technique employed empirically from Alexandria to Rome to Renaissance Europe. Operations once studiously avoided for fear of hemorrhage and the absence of means to control it could at last then be contemplated, which itself invited refinements on the principle. "In all times, even to the present day," Halsted wrote in 1904, "the surgeon's chief concern during an operation has been the management of the blood vessels. The fear of death on the table has deterred many a charlatan and incompetent surgeon from performing otherwise perilous operations"—to say nothing of the competent surgeons also deterred. Harvey's knowledge, however, solved such problems incompletely; he did not understand, for instance, the path by which the veins and arteries were connected. But the general principle of circulation through the whole body, powered by the heart, shortly led the Italian Marcello Malpighi in 1661 to demonstrate microscopically the existence and function of the capillaries.[9]

To Halsted, the next great principle of surgery came with the studies of John Hunter and dealt with the healing of wounds, inflammation, and the ligation of arteries. Halsted revered no surgeon more than Hunter (1728–93), giving his name to the surgical experimental laboratory at Johns Hopkins and ever holding up to the admiration of young surgeons not just the fruits of his investigations but also Hunter's confessions of "honest doubt." "I am not able under such circumstances," Halsted quoted one example, "decidedly to say which is the best practice, whether to leave the slough to separate, or to make a small opening and allow the blood to escape slowly from the cavity." Or, groping with observations that later could be seen to point to the principle that the blood was a power for good, that clots had value, and that dry scabs, usually desirable, were sometimes harmful: "But this operation of nature [scabbing] reduces the injury to the state of a mere superficial wound, and the blood which is continued from the scab to the more deeply seated parts, retaining its living principle, just as the natural parts do at the bottom of a superficial wound, the skin is formed under the scab in one case as in another; yet if the scab should either irritate or a part underneath lose its uniting powers, the inflammation and even sometimes suppuration may be produced."[10]

To anesthesia in the mid-nineteenth century Halsted next ascribed the status of a great principle as he did shortly thereafter to the discoveries of Pasteur and Lister. In 1876, the year he had first walked the wards at Bellevue Hospital in New York City, Halsted recalled that so recent was the dawn of modern surgery in the United States and so recent was the usage of ether that vestiges of the old surgeon's rule of *cito, tuto, jucunde* still lingered among the lightning-quick operators of the preanesthetic age. Yet times did change and, as general anesthesia was more widely accepted, the cautious and conservative surgery of which Halsted became the greatest advocate wholly supplanted the spectacular displays of speed that once measured surgical prowess. Slowly, bones and joints yielded to the knife for purposes other than amputation, and the abdomen was explored in the leisure that came only with a sleeping patient. Even so, anesthesia alone went half-way at best. By tempting surgeons to probe deeper and stay longer in the body's hidden places, it also tempted the infections that so commonly killed patients who had survived mechanically perfect operations. Only after Lister had made the vital connection with the work of Pasteur and had demonstrated the prophylactic effects of carbolic acid in wound treatment was the scene set for the nineteenth century's two great surgical principles—anesthesia, and antisepsis and asepsis—jointly to ring open a new era in surgery.

For Halsted the most recent of the great surgical principles—antisepsis and asepsis—related intellectually to those few others that had preceded it. The history of those principles demonstrated surgery's cumulative evolution: to the structural knowledge of the anatomists were added the insights of individuals who had begun to think as physiologists and, after Pasteur, those who thought as pathologists. So select and so few were such basic principles at any point along surgery's time line that to Halsted none had been repudiated in surgery's advance as a science in his lifetime. To the contrary, the more the general principles were refined by modern surgeons with better tools and techniques that yielded ever-happier results, the more compelling the thinking of surgery's old masters became.

The circumstances surrounding the acceptance and proliferation of Listerism, the latest principle, led Halsted and those who afterward labored in his shadow to a certain conviction about how modern surgeons—the lucky heirs of the Harveys and Hunters—could best be nurtured to carry on. Lister's ideas about clean wounds and antiseptic techniques first took hold not in his native England and surely not in the United States, but in Germany. "Why did almost every surgeon in every German university," Halsted wondered, "embrace Lister's system almost at the same moment and as soon as it was clearly presented?" The answer, he believed, lay in the special character of the scientific and clinical training of German surgeons—not the introduction to surgical principles that medical students received in the undergraduate curriculum, but rather the requirements set for those young doctors who had chosen specifically to make their career in surgery. As an example of the contrast between his own experience with both German and non-German medical education, he recalled that at a meeting of the Congress of German Surgeons in Berlin in the 1870s he had heard discussed the subject of hip joint tuberculosis, with one surgeon alone reporting on some 600 cases, some of which he had been able to follow for twenty years. Two weeks later in the United States, Halsted attended a meeting on the same subject "of a very superior 'surgical society' in one of our large cities, only to find that one of the surgeons had had experience with all of twenty-eight cases and knew little of their subsequent history." The German group, the renowned *Deutsche Gesellschaft für Chirugie,* admitted to its membership qualified surgeons from around the world. The American society, rather more a professional club than a scientific organization, limited its members to twenty and at meetings typically counted fewer than that.[11]

The contrast illustrated for Halsted two fundamentally different habits of mind and approaches to medicine. The Americans were easily enough dismissed as the sad product of commercial and democratic medicine in an expanding, unsettled nation whose political culture nurtured suspicion of many authoritarian forms and institutions. The Germans suffered under no such cultural handicap. Indeed, Bismarck's Second Reich warmly embraced medical research and education, making them in time the wards and clients of the state. Specifically, the German surgeons were products of an educational system that had as its single business the training of a few to be the best. Worthy of the great principles they had inherited, such scientist-surgeons were equipped to make refinements on them and perhaps even, with hard work and much imagination, to work out new principles entirely. The residency system that Halsted brought to Hopkins owed much to that German example. Members of the surgical staffs-in-training in the great university clinics in Germany enjoyed excellent facilities for learning technique and doing research. They spent long hours in wards and outpatient departments carefully supervised by senior faculty. Patients when dismissed were diligently followed up. Pathological material obtained at operations was carefully studied and if significant was preserved in the museum of the surgical department. Above all, there was always abundant clinical material.

It took time—eight to twelve years of hospital service as assistant in a university clinic—before the German surgeon was ready to venture out. But so prepared, the German surgeon could expect much, not in money but in reputation. "He now longs to prove himself worthy of the new position," Halsted wrote, "he has the incentive to inspire others to achieve, he measures himself by a new standard, and there is born in him the desire to rise higher, to sow the seed which will produce a bloom worthy of the greatest universities, possibly even of Berlin."[12] In that spirit and in contrast to the typical American surgeon, who underwent only a year or two of hospital training beyond medical school, Halsted proudly reported that at Hopkins "the average term of service for the intern on the surgical side who succeeds to the house surgeonship in this hospital is at present eight years—six years as assistant in preparation for the position and two years of service as actual house surgeon." Added to four years of medical school and the junior and senior years of college given over to premedical preparation, anyone who aimed to be a Hopkins house surgeon could look forward to "twelve or fourteen years of hard work, very hard work, in order to secure this prize to which in this country of necessity only a few at present attain."[13] To those who objected to so long an apprenticeship, Halsted said simply that the young surgeon whose enthusiasm for the profession was likely soon to go stale should not apply. There were plenty of others who, he was sure, would gladly serve ten years in training to become the Hopkins house surgeon. He was probably right. Those few who were chosen could look forward at the end to much prestige, and some could look forward to much money besides. For it they paid with their youth.

That was something they shared with other modern doctors trained according to the new scientific standards. Both Osler's students and Halsted's students gave up their twenties to their future. Their personal sacrifice, however, more concerns their individual biographies than the history of their profession. Yet, long residency training as Halsted developed it shaped the profession too. It meant that only a few (only the few with real promise of mastering the great general principles and of partaking of the spirit that went into their discovery) would be so trained. From their knowledge and skill would come the only kind of service that to Halsted mattered. It mattered because it was the best. The educational standard, borrowed from Germany and elaborated at Hopkins, rose as surgery itself progressed—a progress that science seemed now to assure. But history too—the surgeons' history at least—reinforced the mandate of science. Their history seemed happily cumulative; on what had come before, younger doctors or medical scientists had directly built their own great things. Thus all surgeons had built on the knowledge of the anatomists. Thus modern surgeons in future would take great principles—developed by the conquerors of pain, hemorrhage, and infection—and build on them. With the gift of time, conservative surgery became possible and overnight became the rule. On conservative techniques were pinned new hopes for discovery of other great principles. With time and new knowledge born of experimental work, especially in physiology and pathology, the operating room truly became the clinical laboratory and a seat of learning, healing, and progress. No longer mere operators skilled with the knife, the Halstedian surgeons had become inductively thinking scientists and medical generalists. Their careers would write a new and happy chapter in surgery's long history.

Although Halsted was probably the world's preeminent surgeon by the time he died in 1922 at the age of seventy, he only sketched the outlines of that chapter, and to the next generation fell the work of filling in its substance. Whether veterans of his residency, those who had served as interns, or those who as mere undergraduates had briefly brushed against him, his students now in their own departments of surgery in reformed medical schools across the country made surgery in the 1920s and 1930s an enviable art, redeeming once and for all their craft's lowly origins among the barbers of past centuries. The great manual skill of the past remained and with better tools and instruments was even improved upon. Surgery had also become an experimental science, or was fast becoming so in the university hospitals, and that was something new. Barney Brooks was one of those new surgeons whose job it was to work out in a new place Halsted's principles. As is not surprising, the working out of new principles in new places by new people entailed a certain amount of adjustment, compromise, and some complaint, no matter how confident they were of the ultimate correctness of their course.

Brooks came to Vanderbilt in 1925 for much the same reasons as had the rest of Robinson's new staff. The prospect of being part of a new school, blessed by Flexner and the foundations, stirred idealism and tempted ambition. Robinson, more even than Kirkland above him, believed in giving good individuals free rein to do the good work for which they were best qualified. And though the fundamental heritage of Osler bound Robinson and his new staff more closely than later generations of doctors in different fields, the heads of departments enjoyed wide freedom to establish and govern their domains with little outside interference. Nowhere at Vanderbilt was this more true than in surgery. Like Halsted's at Hopkins, the reign of Brooks was long and uninterrupted.[14] For more than twenty-five years, Brooks trained a whole new generation of surgeons to his own self-assured specifications, through a process that was a model of enlightened despotism in medical education. Brooks was a man of absolutist convictions and as such was hard to satisfy. So was Robinson, whose own ideas had once led Kirkland to accuse him of extravagance and to have second thoughts about their partnership. When Brooks arrived at Vanderbilt he had as large hopes for surgery as Robinson as dean had for the whole school, and over the long years that he stayed he made many of them come true. Brooks's ideas about a university department of surgery reflected both his training and experience as a young academic surgeon and his ambition to make surgery at Vanderbilt a leading department and a leader in the country. The heirs of those ideas, many of them at least, still staff the operating rooms at a newer Vanderbilt Hospital that in 1980 replaced Robinson's 1925 creation, and in them Barney Brooks has achieved his best memorial.

It was not easy work. Shortly after Vanderbilt opened, Brooks wrote that "the greatest deficiencies in university medical schools in this country at the present time are to be found in the departments of surgery." Although surgery's budgets always ranked at least with medicine's and were usually greater, to him it seemed obvious that surgery by nature required more—in equipment, teachers, laboratory facilities, and, above all, patients—than other departments and that therefore the building of "institutions of medical education should not be undertaken without advice from those familiar with the operation of a surgical department." In the face of what he perceived as the lingering traditional distrust of surgeons by basic scientists and by internists, he sought to establish surgery's intellectual independence as a science, something that he knew demanded as much reform among the surgeons themselves as it demanded trust and good will among other kinds of scientists and doctors. Were surgery not so established, it had no rightful place in the university, which should not accommodate mere craftsmen. The old assumption, for example, that all patients must first pass through the hands of the internist before referral to the surgeon, Brooks attributed to a generation of surgeons content to be only skilled operators who were uninterested in and unwilling to do the thinking necessary intelligently to determine the need for surgical therapies to begin with. They are "too much content to deal with organ rather than the organism."[15] Anyone who ever saw Barney Brooks soothe an anxious patient in clinic or ward with talk of the crops back home knew how strong that indictment was. By independence he did not mean a fiefdom insulated from the rest of the medical school; far from it, he invited reciprocity and cooperation. But he did demand that surgeons and surgeons-to-be think and act like true medical scientists and that once they did they should be respected for it.

It is an old saw that among doctors the physicians (internists) are the thinkers and the surgeons the doers, and like most clichés it contains some footing in truth. It did for Brooks, whose life work was to make the surgeons thinkers as well as doers and thus true modern scientific doctors. Again, as in so much of surgery, history seemed relevant. Surgery to Brooks had abounded in great leaders skilled "as artists as well as philosophers." Students of surgery in the past almost always had flocked to the surgical teachers most skilled in the practical application of what they taught, with the result that even "the skillful operating surgeon with unsound principles will often have a greater following than the clumsy philosopher." Surgeons less skilled with the knife might indeed make important contributions, but initially their audience would be smaller. Lister, Brooks believed, had he been regarded as a skilled operator (which he was not), would have faced less of a battle to win acceptance for his principles of aseptic surgery. It helped, simply, to have a following first and a great idea second. That, however, was not the major problem: excellence in operating skills was not difficult to find (for instance, among the practicing surgeons in Nashville who served in Brooks's department on a part-time, clinical basis); great principles or at least the will to seek them were. If the function of the university teachers of surgery was not only to impart all of what they knew of surgery today but also to prepare students to be surgeons tomorrow, then the teachers had also to be scientists equipped to keep pace with the changing profession. They had to be trained in the atmosphere of the laboratory and imbued with the spirit of research. Surgeons like other academic doctors had to wear two coats at once or fail as effective instruments of both science and education. "If surgery is ever to be more than art and if teaching is leadership," spoke Brooks the scientist-teacher, "then the teacher of surgery must be a leader in investigation and research. Leadership in practical surgery is necessary to obtain an audience. Leadership in investigation and research is the main object striven for when the audience is assembled. True progress in surgery comes from the laboratories, and it is the man who is trained in its laboratory methods who will ultimately contribute to the advancement of surgery as a science."[16] Although he himself was comfortably competent at both, Barney Brooks was neither the most brilliant operator nor the most brilliant investigator ever to grace his profession. But he did combine both and so personified the new total technique of doing surgery as a science. He knew what he was about in the operating room and so was equipped to render the service that made of him a physician and a healer. But home was the laboratory—which could be either the operating room (which, as Halsted had said it must be, was the surgeon's laboratory) or the experimental laboratory—where he sought the truths, the general principles, that made of him a scientist.

Barney Brooks, despite a much too small teaching hospital, made surgery at Vanderbilt work and work well, even at the beginning. That success grew from an understanding, comprehensive at the outset, of how a university department of surgery should function. He demanded first that a patient entering the surgical clinic be assigned in such a way as to match the disease with the interests of the faculty and so best serve the teaching and research interests of the school. He also believed that the best care would thereby be achieved, but he never forgot that, foremost, he was running a school or a part of one. Objecting to old procedures by which staff members had charge for certain periods of time of whole wards and thus were responsible for care of all sorts of conditions, he insisted that clinical material be sorted continuously and assigned to those surgeons whose previous work had demonstrated that they were the best qualified to make use of this material for teaching and for advancing surgery. There should be a feeling of confidence in all members of the staff that they would be given the patients to whom they had gained the right by reason of their having advanced the knowledge of surgery as it related to a certain disease. Brooks said such a policy made for better teaching, promoted better use of patients, and aided in establishing the reputation of the teacher as a surgeon. It also meant that the surgical staff member had first to have a proven reputation as an investigator: research earned patients. Brooks dismissed the objection that such a policy abetted the growth of narrow specialism—anathema to the true Oslerian and Halstedian—by seeing that all patients were first held on the general surgery service and thoroughly studied there before specialty sorting. In that way several surgeons of varied interests would examine every patient, with frequent consultation familiarizing the one surgeon who ultimately would get the case with all its aspects.

Science, said Brooks, also demanded that a properly conducted department of surgery have two different kinds of laboratories. Surgical pathology was one of the things that distinguished surgery as a science from the older anatomical craft and that gave modern surgeons a clearer understanding of the manifestations of disease in body tissues. In its laboratories they learned what they were looking at. At Vanderbilt all the material removed at operations was studied and kept in the surgical department, routine description of gross and microscopic examination falling to the assistant resident surgeon who, before filing the final diagnosis of the disease, consulted a member of the department of pathology. It was a satisfactory arrangement that relieved

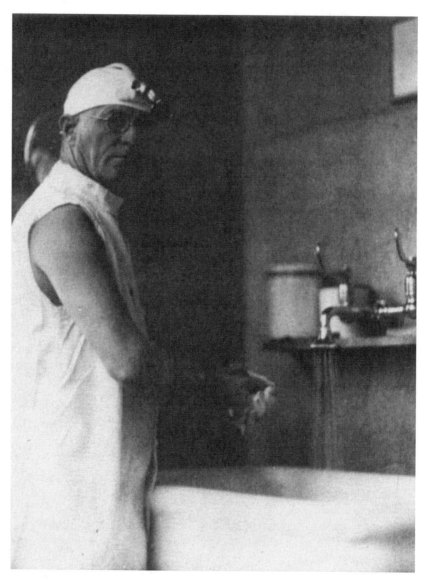

Surgery: Barney Brooks scrubs.

the pathologists of the tiresome routine of doing it all themselves, and it began to teach the young surgeons about disease processes. "There is nothing so damning to surgery," wrote Brooks, "as a surgeon who has to have a pathologist stand by and tell him the nature of the processes of disease which he is uncovering with the knife."[17] Long ago surgeons had excuse for their ignorance, but no longer. Every surgeon who performed an operation had to follow the specimens that came from it through final judgments in the surgical pathological laboratory. From those specimens, preserved all together in the laboratory, students in a single afternoon could see before them years of experience with many surgical diseases.

In addition to a laboratory in surgical pathology that was both a clinical tool for the surgeon and a means to help the resident surgeon learn by doing, experimental study required its own space. In a separate laboratory there should be facilities for conducting animal experiments in aseptic technique with such physiological and chemical apparatus as the experiments required. At Vanderbilt experimental surgery was conducted in a large common operating room and several smaller rooms located on a corridor adjoining general physiology on one side and the surgical wards on the other. Brooks believed that "research can never be requisitioned, as some seem to think." Therefore, if the research of any member of surgery required any more than routine assistance from other departments (bacteriology for example), then the facilities for that bacteriological component of the surgeon's research should be provided in the surgery department. Brooks did not intend such a policy to work in a contrary spirit to the cooperation among departments that Robinson had tried so hard to foster. With many others, Brooks lauded the great advantages realized through an arrangement of physical space that brought all departments into close association. For surgery in particular, advantage came from the proximity of surgical pathology and general pathology, of experimental surgery with general physiology, and of operative surgery with anatomy. He believed only that no department had the right to ask another department to do its research. If the large amount and impressive quality of research that came out of Vanderbilt's experimental surgical laboratories in those years is any measure, it was probably a wise policy.

With those laboratories, the outpatient department, and in future more hospital beds, Brooks felt that his university department could fulfill what he believed were the three functions of academic surgery: teaching the fundamental principles of surgery to medical undergraduates, training doctors to be surgeons through the postgraduate residency program, and the advancement of surgery as a science through clinical and experimental research. The teaching of undergraduates should differ from that in internal medicine only in that the student was acquainted with methods of examination peculiar to surgery and introduced to a surgical point of view. The object of instruction at that point, however, remained, as in medicine, to train students as medical generalists. The real training of surgeons took place only later, with those young doctors ready to commit another four, five, or six years to rigorous apprenticeship. At Vanderbilt and certainly elsewhere, it was these house officers whom the chief came to know best, and they him. To many of them the irascible little Brooks got very close, and he was known to take care of his own. But like even the best father, he sometimes found them hard to control. The temptations were strong and normal and have changed little over the years: "They are impatient young fellows who are prone to feel that they must begin to do operative surgery with their own hands." A talented and ambitious lot, they were hard to convince that by being good assistants they would advance more quickly, and it was only a man such as Brooks, who had himself been trained in the shadow of great masters, who would say: "The truth is that if conditions are such that the young house surgeon can learn more from doing an operation himself than from assisting his chief, the chief is not a good surgeon or else the student is already trained."[18]

Young people have always wanted to be now what they have long studied to become, and the eagerness of young residents actually to wield the knife measured their youthfulness as well as the youthfulness of surgery as a science, whose doctrines did not yet have the authority that age and tradition would in time bestow upon them. The point was that surgery, as Brooks would teach it and as all Vanderbilt students since would learn it, was more than operating alone, more than the practical application of knowledge and skill that young doctors typically yearned to indulge. Certainly it required great manual dexterity; its proximate tools were the hands and the knife, whose use could in the end be perfected only by practice. And young surgeons in training, like other kinds of doctors in training, looked to see useful results in the healing of the sick. Young surgeons, perhaps more than the others, looked to see those results quickly. In that, Brooks the scientist and the surgeon saw a twin danger, both in impatience and in too easy a satisfaction—for the surgeon who was content only with healing today was lost to science. So at Vanderbilt Brooks strove to do what Halsted had done at Hopkins: to employ the university clinic simultaneously to educate practicing surgeons and to advance the science of surgery. He took seriously the connection between medical school and university and thus saw it as his job to teach more than surgery as a vocation or as a trade. "The department of surgery must be engaged as a whole in endeavoring to solve the problems of medicine, because it is only in such an atmosphere that good teaching can endure."[19] Good teaching and good science meant intellectual seriousness and forbearance both with the impatience of youth and with the stubbornness of nature to yield up the secrets of health and disease. To teach doctors to be surgeons who were more than technicians was to prepare their minds to accept the invitation, implicit in all clinical problems, to investigation of fundamental questions. Of himself and those under him, Brooks demanded research into the principles of pathology and physiology as they rose out of surgical problems. Thus with their science they continuously earned the right to be surgeons.

With all of the new Vanderbilt doctors—surgeons, internists, and others— there was a new confidence that they were about to redeem the wonderful promise of science as it had been given to medicine by early pioneers who had lived ahead of their time. In the 1920s and 1930s the surgeons probably did more practically to redeem that promise than other kinds of doctors, something that was more a matter of historical accident than anything else. But it meant that the surgeons were in the vanguard of a process to which all doctors and the laymen they served would soon be partners. The excitement over new ideas and over research generated by largely internal scientific imperatives that so marked those years was fragile and flourished only briefly—for there came shortly to be no dark and benighted immediate past to contrast with present enlightenment. Thus was lost a prime means of measuring success and of bestirring youth to take up science in quite the old way. Progress, which so handily had dispatched the past and of which now all doctors were agents (and were perceived as agents), was being reduced from an aspiration to a schedule.

In surgery the young people who trained under the regime of Barney Brooks were among the last to know that excitement. They trained or were just entering practice during the Great Depression, before surgery could universally be expected to promise large material reward. For other reasons— the childhood dream of being a doctor, the desire to follow in a parent's footsteps, the need quickly to see the results of the work one did—they struggled hard for coveted places in a department that taught, along with the techniques and principles of surgery, the meaning of asceticism. On that the memories of those who passed through, whether just as students or as house officers too, generally agree: Brooks ran a one-man service, he ran it like an autocrat, and he took care of his students, who endured a years-long daily routine of very hard work, watching as they went responsibilities gradually grow as their skills increased and their judgment matured. Later most of them returned to Brooks the sincere thanks and admiration typically accorded great chiefs of surgery. Certainly few if any of them later in life, when surgery had changed greatly, ever regretted that they had not had some other training under some other master.

Those who stayed the longest—those who worked their way up the ladder to become resident surgeons—got closest to Brooks and usually recalled him the most warmly. But even as undergraduates they had more contact with him than their counterparts ever did with Halsted at Hopkins. The process began when as third-year clinical clerks they rotated through Brooks's service, did most of the worst work, and began to see what surgical science was like. For the three months they served, they were assigned newly admitted patients in the surgical service and were responsible for the patients' routine physical examinations, for taking medical histories, and for simple laboratory work on blood and urine. The results of those "work-ups" all went onto the patients' charts, and on the work-ups the students were checked and rechecked and checked again. Even if a patient had been admitted only late the previous afternoon, students knew that by the time of daily ward rounds the next morning they would have to be prepared to present the case. The ritual was by then a familiar one in the medical school world and in it surgery differed little from medicine: the professor (Brooks performed once or twice a week) in the long white coat over his street clothes, house staff in solid-whites, third-year students in short white coats over their street clothes, all moving quietly along the wards. For demonstration Brooks picked cases that had clear teaching value; arterial and bone diseases especially interested him. The juniors first presented the case based on their work-up of the patient probably the night before; Brooks then asked questions and led the discussion about it. If a student's patient was due for surgery, the student too was expected to scrub and be present in the operating room to watch, perhaps hold the retractor, and, with luck, cut a suture or two.

Surgical grand rounds, the other great fixed ritual of the undergraduate experience, brought third- and fourth-year students together twice a week. On Tuesdays and Fridays—Tuesday was Brooks's day; on Friday W. D. Haggard, the senior clinical man, presided—everyone then on the surgical rotation assembled in the amphitheater, which was located on the corridor between the surgical wards and the experimental surgery laboratories. There a third-year student again presented a case and then sat down to watch a bit of theater-as-teaching that the third-year students knew next year they too would have to endure: for Brooks then called on a senior who, in the pit and in front of everyone, stood the storm of the master's questioning. Some accused Brooks in that setting of teaching by embarrassment only; students were known to faint and to cry under the pressure. It was also the place where, as many later recalled, Brooks most stood out as the master teacher.

He seemed able to distinguish between students who had simply not done their homework, and who could expect no mercy, from those who truly did not understand and who had made an honest error in judgment. On the cases themselves, Brooks typically broke big problems into their anatomical, physiological, and pathological parts. Whether it was a stab wound, gall bladder disease, or osteomyelitis (one of his specialties), he brought the ordered and analytical habits of the laboratory to this teaching clinic. There too he struck his most characteristic pose: the bald bespectacled little man seated with one elbow propped on the raised bed of the patient, one finger pointing. How those patients reacted to all the medical mumbo-jumbo flying around them is seldom recorded, though we do know that the same Brooks who seemed almost to thrive on the fear of his students was a model of gentleness with the sick people whose affection he needed quite as much.

As in medicine, the fourth-year students rotating through surgery worked mainly in the outpatient department and not on the wards. The procedure and the principles, though, were much the same. In between morning and afternoon lectures, they worked up new patients assigned to them, checked on returning patients, learned to do dressings, and had all their work meticulously checked off by their numerous superiors. Afternoons might be spent in one of the subspecialty clinics: orthopedics, urology, ophthalmology, or ear, nose, and throat. Because they did not work the wards as the juniors did, seniors might count on more after-hours to themselves, but all undergraduates knew that the more they saw and heard, the better off they would be. Because of the acute and fleeting nature of many surgical problems, it was the students who were on site who learned and saw things that no service as small as Vanderbilt's could guarantee to demonstrate regularly. Brooks believed in utilizing every possible opportunity, which for third-year students meant his admonition to be on the wards every minute when not eating or sleeping and to learn as much as possible from all patients, not just the ones assigned.

For those who went onto the house staff after graduation, the brief and modest respite of fourth-year outpatient duties was quickly forgotten. As at Hopkins, internships and residencies at Vanderbilt constituted the final arduous rite of passage to the prized profession. It was a system of checks and rechecks designed to keep everybody mad at everybody else part of the time and thus everyone on their toes all of the time. It was also a system where the young interns and residents learned as much basic material from their fellows, usually those immediately above them in the hierarchy, as from the chief. All of a sudden, in the summer after their graduation, fresh young doctors whose age hovered around twenty-six found themselves with a new uniform—full whites now—and with additional responsibility. As clinical clerks during medical school, they had begun under close supervision to exercise responsibility for sick people. As house surgeons ministering to the needs of sick people, they were responsible also for representing their chief. Barney Brooks wanted to be represented right. As interns the physical stress was probably the greatest. That first summer they did all the work usually done by the medical students who had the summers off, and for the rest of the year many did not go outside the hospital for days and nights on end. Like the other house staff, they lived and ate in the hospital and were permanently on call. And as the ward nurses' doctor of first resort, they were called often. Beyond, there were three more years of fierce competition leading finally for those who survived to the chief surgical residency.

The nature of the work beyond the internship changed slightly, even if the pressure did not lessen. These young doctors no longer had to do the full patient work-up but only a note on facts pertaining specifically to diagnosis of the surgical problem. Routine laboratory work was left to the students and interns, which meant that for the first time in at least a year the new resident had at least a little time for reading. Still, like the interns, the assistant residents and residents spent most of their time in the hospital. Under Barney Brooks, who believed that training to be a surgeon and being a young spouse were both full-time jobs (and who was a happy family man himself), none was allowed to marry. The few who were offered posts and who had already married lived in the hospital anyway, with spouses keeping lonely house elsewhere. Residents also spent more time in the operating room and thus more time directly in the shadow of the chief. As interns, they might have excised an occasional lipoma or benign tumor, by the end of the year perhaps have done even a hernia or an appendectomy. But the assistant resident was the second assistant to the chief when he operated, and first assistant when the chief resident was in charge, and thus saw more and gradually did more too. Yet Barney Brooks was not one to turn his house officers loose in the operating room, and he was vain enough about his own skills to set much by their example. He kept his office directly across the hall from the operating suite and frequently appeared unannounced, both to supervise and encourage and to be close by if one of his staff got into trouble.[20]

Some of his staff no doubt yearned for the day when they would be out from under his ever-watchful eye and ominously pointing finger. Some no doubt interpreted his technique of teaching, which was domineering if it was anything, as the technique of a little man fixed in his ways and unwilling to change. But if it seemed small to some, the more discerning residents saw in Brooks's apparent dogmatism assurance that under him they would master

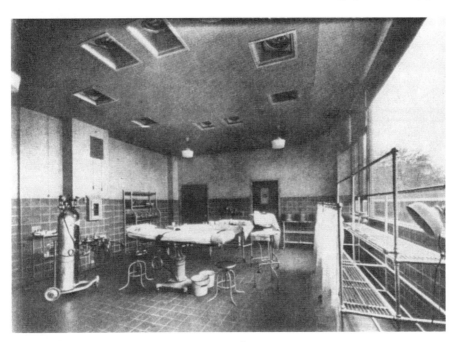

Fourth-floor operating room facing the north court, ca. 1928

at least one good way of doing things—for surgery had not yet then grown so specialized or the kinds of operations so numerous that one good person like Brooks could not still be master of teaching at least one good way in several areas. He certainly had help from able lieutenants: Edward Barksdale in urology; Guy Maness in ear, nose, and throat; Eugene Regen in orthopedics; Cobb Pilcher in neurosurgery; and Alfred Blalock in thoracic surgery. But Brooks's hand was evident in them all.

The first operation logged in the new hospital was performed by Brooks on September 16, 1925, and was, prosaically enough, an appendectomy.[21] The second occurred a day later when Blalock made an incision for an infection of the hand. Selected at random from the late 1920s and 1930s, operations performed at Vanderbilt fairly well reflected the current state of the art. On December 3, 1928: resection of the stomach, drainage of the abdominal cavity, skin grafts. On August 10, 1933: tonsillectomy and adenoidectomy, cholecystectomy (gall bladder), herniotomy, osteotomy of the humerus, clavicle, and ankle. On April 1, 1935: thoracoplasty, 500 cc blood transfusion, mastectomy, appendectomy, salpingotomy. On November 15,

1935: mastoidectomy, exploration for brain abscess. On August 12, 1939: ureterotomy, osteotomy of the toes, radium implantation. In 1926 an average of 77 operations were performed a month; in 1928, 100; in 1933, 158; in 1938, 176. Primarily in the belly, the throat, and the extremities, Brooks's house staff learned their surgery. Some of it was new (some of Blalock's chest work and Pilcher's neurosurgery, for example); much of it was not. But the old things were being done much better than they had been done before, and the surgeons and their apprentices could boast of clearly better results. It was progress due less to the application of new discoveries than to the meticulous refinement of the kinds of general principles that Brooks and Halsted before him had preached: general thoroughness, careful control of bleeding, gentlest possible handling of living tissues, avoidance of surgical trauma, use of small clamps and fine ligatures, rigid asepsis. Such techniques, rigorously applied, made of Brooks's young protégés fine operative surgeons in the Halsted tradition of conservative surgery. But Brooks, whose "one good way" of operating may to some have verged on pedantry, aimed to produce modern surgeons and not just skilled technicians. Rare was the young person who did not emerge from Brooks's service skilled both as an operator and as a surgical diagnostician, who needed no longer solely to rely on the judgment of the internists. Brooks's students were among the first to enjoy membership in a new profession of scientific surgery that was both technically much improved and intellectually newly independent.

To Brooks everything rose out of general surgery, a phrase of somewhat broader meaning then than now, and until late in his long tenure he kept all the surgical subspecialties under his own umbrella. Partly it was vanity, but partly it was his conviction that if he left his students and staff with proven principles and sound judgment he would then have done the best he could. All of them, whether they went on to specialize in bones and joints, in hearts, brains, or stomachs, would need principles and judgment. Neither Brooks nor many of his fellows could then foresee, however, the vast changes that would overtake surgery in the not-too-distant future when the chest and the skull—then as forbidding as the abdomen once had been—routinely would be penetrated with safety and with wonderful results. Few could know of the improvements that would be wrought in anesthesiology and the new boons it would hold for surgery (anesthesiology at Vanderbilt became a separate department in 1946). Few guessed at the possibilities for organ replacement and transplantation. They could only hope, expectant generally that the future would hold large things and that their general principles and habits of judgment would stand the test. In the judgment of some of those who were so trained and who lived longer than their teacher, Barney Brooks, those things wore well enough.

They wore well because Brooks's style of thought was fundamentally experimental. Sure as he was about some things, he did not need to protest newness in order to maintain his self-esteem as a surgeon. That he hammered relentlessly about basic principles suggests merely that he knew their worth and how hard they were to come by. He knew that as time passed and surgery became more complex, its advance depended on ever-greater investment of time and talent in research. But only as research elucidated new general principles was the result progress for surgery. Ever more skillful knot tying and incision making were matters of improved manual dexterity that came with practice. Elaboration of general principles was a matter of the mind that came with hard intellectual work. To earn its place among the sciences, surgery had to transcend mechanics. Its subject had to be the truth about health and disease, and practice alone seldom made truth more apparent. Surgeons trained by Brooks had the power to give the lie to the cliché about doctors who thought and surgeons who only acted. At that particular moment in the 1920s and 1930s they had perhaps more power to act than most doctors and results proved the beneficence of that power. Just as important, some among them seriously took up Brooks's charge to become, as he liked to think of them, surgical physicians whose research, not whose results, made them scientists.

Brooks was proud of them and saw in their work Vanderbilt's best hope to become a truly important university clinic in the Johns Hopkins and German tradition. Before World War II, clinical investigation (whose method was the observation of disease together with its treatment in real patients) ranged widely and resulted in sixty-four articles published in a variety of surgical journals.[22] In such clinical research the names of the part-time or clinical faculty predominated, something that Brooks welcomed as a sign that Vanderbilt was attracting to its part-time staff the right kind of practicing surgeons. It also seemed natural that clinicians tended to do clinical research. Operative surgery was their daily world—and a busy one that allowed little time for extended laboratory study. Its technique was essentially the same as that of the experimental researchers: intensive study of one particular problem, the gathering of information about it from which in time a valid induction might begin to point toward a general principle. With the clinical researchers, the information was gathered, more strictly speaking, through observation and less through experiment.

Among the laboratory researchers, the names of the full-time faculty were most prominent, and while virtually all of Brooks's faculty and house staff heeded their chief's admonition to do some piece of research in the laboratory, the names of just three accounted for the lion's share (over a hundred) of the publications turned out by the department between 1926 and 1940. Brooks

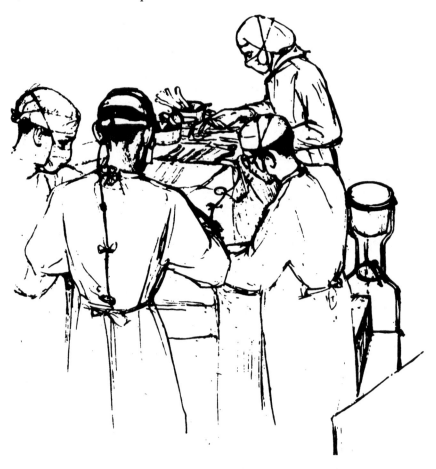

Surgery: Susan Wilkes's illustration of neurosurgeon Cobb Pilcher operating, 1946

himself, though a busy teacher and the administrator of a large service, averaged one publication a year, most on vascular problems, his specialty. Cobb Pilcher, a young Vanderbilt M.D. (1927) who came up through the ranks of the house staff, was beginning impressive work on various aspects of neurological surgery and by the end of the 1930s was author of ten publications and coauthor of nine more. Pilcher was something of the local archetype of the brilliant and driven young surgeon whose promise was easy for all to see. For him Brooks arranged special fellowships to study in Chicago and St. Louis, grooming him to run the neurological subspecialty at Vanderbilt. Had he not died young, his reputation both as an operative surgeon and as a surgical thinker might have equaled even that of the one other Vanderbilt surgeon whose talents truly did put him in the company of the great surgeons of that era. But if numbers mean anything (and with him they were indeed impressive), Alfred Blalock alone and in collaboration produced in his years at Vanderbilt some ninety-five articles dealing with experimental research and some twenty-six dealing with clinical matters—an incredible eight per year.

Though fifteen years younger than Brooks, Blalock qualified as one of the original new Vanderbilt men. He came as the first resident surgeon at the new Vanderbilt Medical School in the fall of 1925 and, except for time off in the late 1920s to recover from a bout with tuberculosis and to travel in Europe, he worked there without interruption until 1941. Unlike his chief, in whose shadow he did not long remain, he was a warm and genial man to students and colleagues alike, a demanding and understanding teacher, but one whose true home was the laboratory and not the wards. By 1938 he had become a full professor, though still subordinate to Brooks, who was then only in his fifties and showing no signs of retirement. Blalock's career would peak elsewhere. But during its first fifteen years at Vanderbilt, he built well. If in Blalock, who was probably his intellectual superior, Brooks saw a threat, he hid well his fear. For the years they were together they worked well enough as a team, though by 1941 the time had clearly come for them to part company and for Blalock to achieve the eminence his work had earned.

Blalock's experimental research on the nature of shock and his resulting doctrine of full fluid replacement came in the decade before World War II. Later in the 1940s and in the 1950s he would win popular acclaim accorded few surgeons for his so-called blue-baby operation and other work in thoracic and cardiac surgery. With both, his place in the history of medicine was secure, and for both the foundations had been laid at Vanderbilt. Blalock's domain was the department's experimental laboratory in the middle of the school's west corridor next to the amphitheater, where his and Brooks's portraits would one day hang. There, on countless dogs and other sacrificial beasts, Blalock the scientist and his faithful assistant, Vivian Thomas, painstakingly divined the secrets to one of the surgeon's greatest nemeses—shock—and slowly worked out in the path of Harvey, Hunter, Lister, and Halsted a new general principle.

Blalock's bibliography was enormous—approximately 228 papers and articles, many of them dealing with the problem of shock, and one book, *Principles of Surgical Care: Shock and Other Considerations* (1940).[23] Although, like most scientists, he had other things to do than expend limited time and energy on the construction of perfect paragraphs, by the standards of the genre his writing is remarkably clear. For him, writing's function was to convey information sprung from observation and experiment. Its purpose was not to argue but to report it; it replicated for others the information-gathering procedure of the individual scientist pursuing induction. If it was to be any good, that procedure usually also was long and tedious, repetitive, and perhaps even at times a bit boring—as was much of Blalock's work. His classic paper, "Experimental Shock: The Cause of Low Blood Pressure Produced by Muscle Injury," which appeared in the *Archives of Surgery* in 1930, has, along with the many others that explored the subject further, the simplicity and neatness of a high school term paper written to an exacting and obligatory outline. That outline, evident enough in bold subheads, might have been an outline for the scientific method itself: problem, method, observations, comment, summary.

For Blalock the clinical problem of shock had been aptly described by Samuel D. Gross in 1872:

The person, although severely injured, congratulates himself upon having made an excellent escape, and imagines that he is not only in no danger, but that he will soon be about again; in fact, to look at him, one would hardly suppose, at first sight, that there was anything serious the matter; the countenance appears well, the breathing is good, the pulse is but little affected, except that is too soft and frequent, and the mind, calm and collected, possesses its wonted vigor, the patient asking and answering questions very much as in health. But a more careful examination soon serves to show that deep mischief is lurking in the system; that the machinery of life has been rudely unhinged, and that the whole system is profoundly shocked; in a word that the nervous fluid has been exhausted and that there is not enough power in the constitution to reproduce and maintain it. The skin of such a person assumes an icterode, or sallow, cadaverous appearance, feeling at the same time doughy and inelastic; the extremities are deadly cold; the pulse makes a desperate effort at reaction, but is, at best, weak and tranquil for one who has sustained such an amount of violence. The system does not seem to be conscious of what has occurred; its sensibilities are blunted, and it is incapable of suffering. Nature, to use the language of Hunter, does not feel the injury.[24]

Since Gross's time there had been several attempts at explanation of what was known clinically as secondary shock, in which an hour or more separates an injury from a marked decline in blood pressure. Particularly after the experience of World War I, when treatment of shock had achieved only poor results, scientists in the United States and Europe had advanced several theories and had done considerable experimental work to test them. Prominent among them was the so-called toxemia theory, which held that the lowered blood pressure associated with severe injury "was due to the absorption of some depressant substances from the injured area into the general circulation,"[25] probably a histamine. Blalock suspected otherwise, and at Vanderbilt he began a years-long series of experiments designed to supply the information that would establish another explanation.

Nearly all of his experiments were conducted on deeply anesthetized dogs, on which he produced symptoms of secondary shock by severe injury to the extremities, by manual manipulation of internal organs, particularly the intestines, and by burns. Having obtained the proper symptoms, he then looked for causes. The first came in comparing in autopsy the weights of a dog's rear extremities, one of which had been severely traumatized (hit with a hammer), one of which had not. He observed that "approximately one half the total blood volume had been lost into the injured part, which was sufficient by itself to account for the decline of pressure." In cases where a dog's intestines were roughly manipulated with the finger, he observed that the fluid that consequently escaped into the peritoneal cavity contained approximately the same composition in protein as blood plasma. And he knew that protein acted to attract fluid to the blood stream and hold it there and thus was an important mechanism in maintaining blood volume. In cases where severe burns were produced, fluid that was blood plasma also accumulated in the subcutaneous tissues. Burned areas when compared with normal ones were always found to be heavier. He studied the effects of hemorrhage and muscle trauma on cardiac output and blood pressure. Upon drawing off blood equal to 27 cc per kilogram of body weight, simulating a massive hemorrhage, the output of the heart was found to decline markedly, but not the blood pressure. Likewise, forty minutes after injury to an extremity, cardiac output declined but not the blood pressure. Contrariwise, the artificial administration of a histamine (thought by the toxemia theorists to be the toxic agent causing shock) led first to reduced blood pressure and only later to reduced heart output.[26] •

Such observations were leading Blalock to see the connection between shock and hemorrhage and to suspect that it was the hemorrhage of tissues caused by injury and the subsequent fluid loss into those tissues through the broken capillaries that accounted for the symptoms of secondary shock. The key seemed to be physiological, not chemical. At least, to changes in circulation he could ascribe experimentally all of the symptoms and in the proper sequence. First, as a result of injury or perhaps surgical trauma, total body blood volume was immediately reduced as fluids rushed into the injured area and were lost to the system through broken small vessels. If the injury and blood loss were not too massive, the vascular system attempted to compensate and maintain pressure by constricting the arterial blood vessels: a smaller amount of fluid flowing through a smaller vessel will yield the same pressure as a larger amount in a larger vessel. That was natural, but as Gross had put it, "the machinery of life had been rudely unhinged" to the extent that nature's own compensatory measures could be maintained only so long. The blood lost into broken tissues at the site of the injury obviously could not be returned to the heart, which explained the observed reduction in cardiac output. As the total volume of circulating blood thus fell, blood pressure eventually declined too, despite constriction of the vascular system. If blood pressure remained low for any considerable time, that mechanism too must fail. At that point problems multiplied: tissues received insufficient supplies of oxygen, the blood became more viscous, capillaries became more permeable, and toxic products accumulated.

It took countless hours and countless dogs, but finally it all fit and in the end seemed so simple. Secondary shock meant internal hemorrhage. Hemorrhage meant loss of blood into the wounded area and out of the circulatory system. Blood loss meant in time reduced pressure and circulatory failure. The therapeutic solution too seemed simple: fluids must be introduced to increase blood volume. It took even more time fully to elaborate the techniques for doing that—for deciding what kind of fluids were best. Blalock himself experimented with saline solutions administered intravenously but found that when they escaped through the broken places they carried with them from the plasma a great deal of protein that was a needed stabilizing agent. Whole blood was clearly ideal. It could be used to combat fluid loss that occurred in operations for any number of reasons: sweating, hemorrhage, plasma loss through exposed surfaces, blood loss through vessels dilated as a result of manual irritation. But in the 1930s blood banks were still rare and techniques of direct donor-to-patient transfusion were awkward and required hospital-like conditions for reasonable safety. Efficient means of whole blood storage in time solved the problem of shock in the operating room but not elsewhere. The answer ultimately was blood plasma, which could be dried, stored for long periods, and quickly reconstituted and administered anywhere it was needed. Happily, that technical refinement arrived in time for World War II, when on battlefields from France to Okinawa, Blalock's new principle of full fluid replacement proved its utility on the shocked and shattered bodies of countless young soldiers.

A modest man, Blalock never claimed to have done it alone. His papers are studded with the names of predecessors and contemporaries, included probably less out of the scholarly habit of establishing one's familiarity with the literature than as genuine salute to other scientists on whose work he built. Likewise, years in the laboratory had taught him caution and the care to claim too little rather than too much for what he learned there. Others, perhaps he knew, would see to his promotion. At Vanderbilt, they graced a wall with his portrait, named a paneled conference room after him (on the site of the old doctor's dining room without, alas, the windows), and from the day he left they remembered him reverently as fine teacher, warm friend, and model scientist. But leave he did, in 1941, just as his new principle was about to be put to the test. He answered the coveted "call" (as doctors then commonly described job offers) to mother Hopkins, where as chairman and chief of surgery he served out the twenty-three years that remained in his career and in his life. He had been gone sixteen years, a time he used to grow from a fairly anonymous resident surgeon to a great man, and his return there restores to the history of Hopkins-Vanderbilt relations a certain symmetry. Although he was a Hopkins man to begin with (M.D., class of 1922), the Blalock who returned in glory in 1941 came on the weight of merit earned at Vanderbilt, which for a change gave to Hopkins more than it got.[27] Blalock probably would have achieved greatness anyway, but the fact remains that the crucial middle years of his career were passed in the long corridors and in the austere laboratories and wards designed by Canby Robinson as the first dramatic proof in brick and mortar that science and service were one.

If ever science served, it did with Blalock. It did not, ironically, serve surgery alone. That was just the way Barney Brooks said it should be. Brooks had wanted to make surgery intellectually independent and intellectually respectable. As long as surgery had been pursued only as a craft, it had had small intellectual dimension at all. When, beginning in the late nineteenth century, it began to be pursued as a science, it gained in respectability to the extent that it concerned itself with the problems of scientific medicine generally: with diagnosis, physiology, biochemistry, and pathology. It would not thereby risk absorption by medicine; the dramatic nature of the surgeon's intervention forever prevented that. But surgery would affirm its fraternity with the other sciences whose method was to observe, to experiment, and to induce and whose purpose was to seek general principles. Blalock's research on shock was one example of that kind of scientific surgery leading finally to a general principle—full fluid replacement—with broadly medical implications. Brooks trained all his students not as skilled technicians but as surgical physicians, who made of the operating room their clinical laboratory and whose experimental research qualified them as scientists. Blalock embodied as well as any and better than most the model of the surgeon as scientific generalist whom Brooks believed modern medicine had called forth.

Much then seemed possible that time proved illusory. In the impatience of his own subordinates for separate specialty departments (which finally did appear after World War II), Brooks glimpsed a future rather unlike the days of his own training and rise to influence. Blalock, who lived a dozen years longer, must have seen it even more clearly. No sooner, it seemed, had the new science of surgery established itself than general surgery, its once stable and fortified center, began to crack. Brooks had always said that only broad training made surgical physicians out of young persons craving to be operators. As the products of induction accumulated and demanded ever-greater depth of training, his worries surely multiplied over its diminishing breadth. Likewise with Blalock's return to Hopkins and the chair of Halsted comes the poignance of a man, the two ends of whose biography seem separated by more than the usual evolution. The science of surgery like the science of medicine generally had speeded things up, which was just what everyone claimed to want, but its agents, who had started out in its early expectant years, sometimes were left far indeed from where they had begun.

Surgeons who were also physiologists, biochemists, pathologists, and radiologists, in their increased knowledge of conditions in the human body, enjoyed untold advantages over their anatomist predecessors. But in a profession dedicated to service, ever-changing knowledge bred a temper at once arrogant and self-critical. An orthopedic surgeon once asked Brooks to look at X rays showing the good results he had achieved in treating a series of leg fractures. "I am quite sure he did not understand me," Brooks remembered, "when I told him that I would much rather see his patient walk, and it has often occurred to me since to wonder if treatment of fractures of the leg were not more successful when it was the purpose of surgeons to make the external appearance of the fractured leg correspond as nearly as possible to that of the unfractured leg than at the present time when surgeons attempt to secure perfect anatomic restoration of the bone fragments by the use of one or more of the several mechanical appliances which sometime remind me of an exhibit which I once saw of the instruments used for torture at the time of the Spanish Inquisition."[28] Young surgeons trained as Halsted and Brooks and Blalock trained them, in the new methods of obtaining ever-better knowledge of the abnormalities of anatomy and physiology, became of necessity materialists. They dealt with facts accumulated through methods that were increasingly impersonal, and they learned, Brooks continued, to "conceive of each human being as compared to a standard human being, a sort of John Doe." The price paid for better knowledge about John Doe and how to make him better—that is, that fewer surgeons any longer bothered "to get acquainted with John Thompson, III, Michael O'Flaherty, Johann von Ribbentrop, Victoria Angelucci or Abie Cohen"—was charged up to progress. As knowledge mushroomed, the natural human tendency to be more comfortable when it was neatly sorted and labeled asserted itself. As tests available for diagnosis multiplied, it became easy, perhaps too easy, to rely wholly on them. As young surgeons were compelled "to acquire such an ever increasing amount and complexity of objective information. . . there was little time or incentive for understanding or appreciating an individual as something more than a machine gone wrong." Would surgeons not be better surgeons, Brooks asked, if they could in addition to acquiring scientific knowledge also be "stimulated to discover before roentgenologic examination that a man complaining of abdominal discomfort, loss of appetite, weight and strength may have these symptoms because his only son is in the Solomon Islands?"[29]

It was not meant as a rhetorical question. Brooks in fact thought the answer might lie with acquainting apprentice surgeons with psychiatrists and psychologists, several of whom he actually brought into Vanderbilt's surgery program in the 1940s. It was neither an especially popular nor an especially successful innovation, and for Brooks the scientist-teacher of surgery the problem went unsolved for the ten years that remained to him. To become intellectually respectable surgery had been made scientific, which meant practically that it concerned itself with things that were also the concern of general medicine. As a science, surgery like medicine rested on sound general principles established inductively through much observation and careful experiment. Through comprehension of more general principles came progress. It became more useful. Its results got better, to much general applause. So science served. Earlier than most other kinds of doctors, surgeons knew the happy feeling that came from being the agents of such service. But because the surgeons' new general principles reaped benefits sooner than the internists', they were also the first to be haunted by the specter of Brooks's man whose only son had been sent off to fight in the South Pacific. Science taught about John Does and from that teaching much practical good had come. How was it though, asked Brooks, that good had come to be bound up with knowing more and more about less and less? Was it not possible that surgeons and other doctors had better ministered to the whole patient when they had known less of his parts? Brooks was not the only one to wonder, though most of the future complaint on that point would come from outside rather than inside the profession.

For his lifetime Barney Brooks tried his best to practice his profession both ways. He maintained the umbrella of general surgery over the blooming subspecialties for intellectual as well as political reasons, and he taught the old verities of diagnosis through careful history taking and physical examination and of sharpening one's old-fashioned powers of observation and thus one's clinical judgment. He believed in laying on the hands. Also, however, he worked in the laboratory and respected the facts. None of that made him unique, but it did make him representative of a synthesis that was dissolving fast. Later, after Barney Brooks had gone, a public tempted by the first good fruits and expectant of more of them also wants it both ways: both the remembered warmth and personalism of the old doctors and the scientific certainties of the new ones. Those two things were not self-exclusive, but as knowledge grew and science grew more demanding, the time and energy of the doctors stayed the same. The uneasiness that Brooks felt with his young surgeons foreshadowed problems that ever since would bedevil the relationship of science to all clinical medicine, surgery and otherwise. Science, it seemed, could serve too well, its good results driving up the demand for ever-better ones and the scientists ever scampering to meet it. But Brooks taught as he had been taught—that real scientists did not scamper; they plodded to the slow and measured beat of internal imperatives. How good for how long, he might fairly have asked of a future already then apparent, was a science so linked to service?

Science

9

From the meeting of science and medicine in the late nineteenth and early twentieth centuries came new institutions to solemnize and perpetuate that union. In it, the founders of the foundations—most notably the Rockefellers—saw wide field for lavish benevolence. Indeed, of the causes that ever captivated foundation philanthropy in the United States, scientific medicine ranks among the first and most enduring. Officered by men like Abraham Flexner, those foundations built and endowed other institutions—the medical schools—in whose reformed curricula, well-trained faculty, and select apprentices everyone placed high hopes. The new Vanderbilt Medical School of 1925 was only one of such places and was in no way unique as a shrine to the permanence of science in medicine and symbol of its beckoning future.

Flexner, Kirkland, and Robinson all liked to think of themselves as educators. True to that self-image, they built at Nashville with Rockefeller's money a working model of modern medical education. Robinson's first drawings pictured it. The deliberate coordination of the basic sciences with the clinical functions of a teaching hospital confirmed the unity of medical education and science that Flexner had preached since 1910, that Robinson had revered since Hopkins days, and that Kirkland too truly believed in. Robinson and his faculty busily set about filling in the operational details called for by such a broad outline. Borrowing from Osler, Halsted, and other early masters, they fixed the course descriptions and arranged the labs, clinics, and house officerships in a pattern that seemed to them ideal and that indeed changed little through the years. But if the forms of medical education so became fixed, the substance of the science it rested on was anything but fixed. In that, Burwell or Blalock, Goodpasture or Garrey surely found no surprise and surely felt no inconsistency. Neither did the foundation masters who saw their job not just as building and endowing the new medical institutions but as promoting the search for new knowledge that made them scientific.

Once, while wrangling with Kirkland in 1928 over the budget, Robinson had claimed that research justified red ink. As the educational program of the school finally was organized, he said, research activity had increased—and with it the frustration of scientists accustomed to better facilities and more ample funds for investigative work. Whether or not research justified deficits, it did in part account for them, which raised questions about how best to support it and why. Vanderbilt's medical endowment in 1925 stood at $2.45 million, all of it from the General Education Board, which during the first years of the school's operation also provided supplementary annual grants to help cover operating expenses. In 1929 the GEB capitalized those appropriations by adding $3.5 million to the endowment of the medical school and $4 million to the endowment of the hospital.[1] Operating budgets came from the income on that endowment, plus fees from students, patients, and any grants—most in the 1920s short term.[2] By 1929 the total GEB contribution to medical education at Vanderbilt for plant and endowment came to something more than $13 million. By the standards of the times that was a very large sum but one wholly in keeping with the general policy of the GEB since it had begun seriously to promote the reform of American medical schools. Through large grants for buildings and for permanent endowments, the board built and rebuilt institutions. By the late 1920s, however, just as the Vanderbilt project was at last getting started, changes at the Rockefeller boards foretold a different policy for the future.

As Flexner knew it at Johns Hopkins and as he had imagined it ever since, medical education and research were indistinguishable.[3] That was clear enough to Robinson and was reflected in the stable of young scientist-teachers he brought to Vanderbilt. The endowments provided to Vanderbilt and to other schools that were helped by the General Education Board were intended, along with fee income, to provide operating expenses and faculty salaries, and the board demanded no accounting of how much time faculty members spent on research and how much on teaching. But the endowment, as Flexner, Robinson, and Kirkland all knew, did not turn out to be large enough actually to do all that, even after it was increased in 1929. Faculty had to teach and tend patients or there would be no students or patients. Thus it was of research that they often complained—not of their responsibility to do it but of budgets that did not allow for the staff and equipment they needed. Though some found temporary relief in short-term grants from various foundations, none thereby secured the assurance of long-term commitment and continuity that their science often required. The effort to secure such commitment and thus to secure research at Vanderbilt succeeded in part in the early 1930s thanks again to Rockefeller philanthropy. Ironically, changes at the Rockefeller Foundation in the late 1920s seemed to help in solving that immediate problem, just as they signaled a departure from Flexner's precepts and the policies that had made the school a reality to begin with.

In 1928 a plan was adopted to refocus and streamline, so it was hoped, the functions of the four Rockefeller philanthropic foundations then active. The General Education Board, founded in 1902, had worked in reforming medical education, in uplifting primary education particularly in the South, and in some programs in the arts and humanities. The Rockefeller Foundation, set up just before the First World War, had concentrated on public health and medical education worldwide (the GEB's charter restricted its activities to the United States) and could count among its monuments the schools of public health at Harvard and Johns Hopkins, a modern medical school in Brussels, Belgium, and the Peking Union Medical College, which the foundation bought in 1915 and subsidized over the years through the China Medical Board with more than $44 million. In 1918 a memorial to the elder Rockefeller's wife was established; as its endowment grew, the Laura Spellman Rockefeller Memorial supported a broad range of research in the social sciences. Finally, the International Education Board had been created by John D. Rockefeller, Jr., in 1923 as a fiefdom for Wickliffe Rose, who had earned laurels as head of the Rockefeller Sanitary Commission in the fight against hookworm in the South. Under Rose the new board pursued a variety of research in agriculture and the physical and biological sciences.

Although they shared a general origin in the Rockefeller fortune and generally worked well together, each board was an independent corporation with its own trustees, its own resources, and its own officers. It was to sort out the inevitable overlapping of responsibilities and subsequent confusion that a committee of trustees representing all four boards recommended the reorganization that took place in 1928 and 1929. The aim was to concentrate in one agency all activities that had to do with what they called "the advance of human knowledge." As a result the Rockefeller Foundation, which was to be that one agency, emerged as the premier Rockefeller philanthropy.[4] Into it were moved research activities in the natural sciences, agriculture, and forestry from the International Education Board and the General Education Board; in the medical sciences, the arts, and humanities from the General Education Board; and in the social sciences from the Laura Spellman Rockefeller Memorial. Thus reconstituted, the foundation consisted of five divisions—the International Health Division (which had not been changed), and the divisions of Medical Sciences, Natural Sciences, Social Sciences, and the Humanities. That organizational change also signaled a substantive change in the direction of Rockefeller philanthropy away from institution building and sustaining, a role that had been so beneficial to Vanderbilt's medical school.

The foundation's official historian and its president from 1936 to 1948, Raymond B. Fosdick, ascribed the change to "the end of an era in philanthropy" brought on by two causes. By the end of the 1920s the boards had expended enormous sums "in the endowment of medicine, public health institutes, and programs in higher education." The General Education Board alone had disbursed $90 million for the building and endowment of American medical schools and, on a matching basis, $50 million to raise the endowment of colleges and universities. Giving on that scale obviously could not go on forever, particularly after the Great Depression drastically reduced both the earning power of the boards' own investments and the ability of other donors to match Rockefeller contributions. The times demanded prudence and some "new orientation of target, program, and technique." Research (or, as the trustees referred to it, the extension of knowledge), in contrast to more institution building, met those requirements; moreover, the newly built and endowed institutions of medical and higher education seemed to demand it. "The decision of the trustees to concentrate the work of the foundation on the extension of knowledge," Fosdick wrote, "was based on a growing conviction that the margin between what men know and what they use is much too thin. Psychiatric institutes can be created and medical schools strengthened, but as one professor [unnamed] expressed it, 'we haven't enough that we can confidently teach.' " So, the stockpile of knowledge that only research produced had constantly to be replenished. "There is a sense in which the practical applications of knowledge are the dividends which pure science declares from time to time," Fosdick wrote. "When pure science lags, or is interrupted by a cataclysm like war, then it is necessary to pay the dividends out of surplus; and obviously this process cannot long continue."[5]

It was hardly a new idea. Concern for research was always high with the Rockefeller boards and there was perhaps no grander monument to it than the Rockefeller Institute for Medical Research, founded in 1901 and headed by Simon Flexner. But among disciples of the faith that human progress depended in the long run on the extension of knowledge—and indeed flowed predictably from it—none among the Rockefeller men was a stronger advocate than Wickliffe Rose, who in 1923 had become head of both the General Education Board and the International Education Board and whose bold faith in science and the intrinsic interrelationship of all knowledge could be seen in the course of Rockefeller research strategy from then until long after he retired in 1928. "All important fields of activity, from the breeding of bees to the administration of empire," he declared, "call for an understanding of the spirit and technique of modern science. . . . Science is the method of knowledge. It is the key to such dominion as man may ever exercise over his physical environment. Appreciation of its spirit and technique, moreover, determines the mental attitudes of the people, affects the entire system of education, and carries with it the shaping of a civilization." And elsewhere: "Whether we will or no, civilization has become increasingly a matter of applied science. To be sure, science can be and is misapplied, but this is not to be laid at the door of science. Health, transportation, food, education— these are realms of activity that cannot be properly managed until more is known. The increase of knowledge upon which human welfare depends comes largely from the laboratories dealing in the most fundamental fashion with the physical and biological sciences. In cultivating these, universities make, therefore, a notable contribution not only to knowledge, as such, but to the art of living."[6] After Rose had gone, the presumption of the unity of science and progress lived on in the reorganized Rockefeller Foundation, whose first president, mathematical physicist and former University of Chicago president Max Mason, emphasized the structural unity of the foundation's five divisions that embraced essentially one program (as Fosdick put it): "the general problem of human behavior, with the aim of control through understanding."[7]

Abraham Flexner, who left the Rockefellers' service in 1928, saw rather differently the reorganization of the Rockefeller boards and their taking up the cause of research.[8] Neither the depression nor any intelligent understanding of the margin between what people know and what they use prompted the change in organization and orientation that to him was a colossal blunder. Flexner was never slow to criticize, but for the leadership of Rose, who restructured the General Education Board even before the larger 1928 changes, and for the masters of the "new" Rockefeller Foundation he reserved special derision. Under Wallace Buttrick, Rose's predecessor and Flexner's friend, the GEB had been virtually a small university, alive with ideas, its officers with contacts among the great scholars and scientists of the world, its policies guided by care for institutions as organic entities. Thus selectively the board had built and endowed; thus it had equipped others permanently to do good works. But under Rose, appreciation of colleges and universities as a whole disappeared. Looking around at the impressive work already done seemed only to have led him to conclude that the work of general endowment must be virtually finished. To Flexner, it was the GEB itself that was largely finished by the emasculation of its medical research activities (which incidentally Rose had opposed) in the 1928 reorganization, and the bedlam of misdirected granting that characterized the Rockefeller boards in the 1930s and 1940s to Flexner amply gave the lie to fatuous pronouncements about the unity and the utility of all knowledge produced by research. Scornfully, he cited the product of such scatter-gun philanthropy: $8,000 to Ohio State University for a scholarship in ceramic design applied to tableware; $2,500 to Cornell for photographic supplies "to be used in a study of eating behavior to be carried on in the Nursery School of the College of Home Economics"; $17,250 to the University of Virginia for three years to support an associate professor of rural economics and to strengthen the library; $2,500 to Harvard for study of crime and criminal justice in Greater Boston; $2,500 to the University of Munich's Institute of Physics for "the study of electrons and related problems"; $2,500 to the Royal Anthropological Institute of Great Britain and Ireland for its general budget; $750.33 to Harvard for "work in Oriental Art."[9]

Flexner's examples came from both the General Education Board and the Rockefeller Foundation in the 1930s and 1940s. Betrayed as he must have felt, he surely picked some of the more laughable examples of aid for specific projects. Not all grants were either so small or as seemingly inconsequential. Indeed, he also cited with praise large GEB gifts for endowment at Carleton College and at numerous institutions in Atlanta. But more important was the alarming trend away from the tradition of bold large-scale giving designed to build up whole institutions (giving that often entailed single grants of $1 to $5 million and of which he singled out Vanderbilt's medical school as a prime example) and toward the sort of small-scale, short-term projects that Frederick T. Gates had been accustomed to dismiss as "retail business." Of the GEB grant to Cornell for cameras to aid in the study of infant eating behavior, Flexner asked: "Who reads the books if written? Literally hundreds, perhaps thousands of such grants have been made. A few doubtless may be useful; but the method is wrong."[10]

Along with everyone else, Flexner knew that the flush times of the 1920s were over and that the holdings of the Rockefeller boards were not infinite. But in tightened circumstances he read another imperative from the one Fosdick said had moved the architects of the 1928 changes. They had looked at the substantial work already completed and at the shrinking power of their investments, and they had shied away from a sustained policy of further large-capital grants. Flexner the educator looked instead to the institutions where learning took place—the colleges and universities—and whose endowments in such times more than ever needed buttressing. True, the numbers needed were all the time getting bigger while the resources of the foundations were getting smaller. But if the foundations were to withdraw from the field and spread their grants to many specific short-term projects, some worthy and some not, then the endowed institutions of higher learning would be in for a "hard struggle." Their permanence mattered most, for under their auspices—not the foundations'—education and research took place.

It was the foundations' role to aid that good work by giving to a few of the most promising people at the most promising places the means to help assure their futures long after, for instance, the General Education Board had gone out of existence. Extinction of such boards seemed to Flexner inevitable if they were to remain faithful to the job of institution building that they had done so well while he was at the GEB—a job that was, he believed, what they could do best. Spend both principal and interest, he declared, and spend in large enough pieces and on worthy enough institutions that later generations too might profit. It would have required "educational statesmanship" of an order that Flexner did not believe the boards' leaders were then capable of so to invite liquidation, but what greater good would thereby have been served "if, say, two southern institutions already influential like Fisk and Vanderbilt had been liberally endowed: that would have set up models, and the remaining institutions would have fended for themselves." Though in time the General Education Board did liquidate (it closed its doors in 1960, the year after Flexner died), during the 1930s, when consistency might have consolidated earlier gains, its members and officers vacillated between some grants large and purposeful enough to be effective and the many more short-term commitments of which "it is impossible to make an estimate as to which have taken root and which are mere ripples on the surface." One thing was for sure: by so changing its mind "every few years," the board had the effect more and more of "reaching its long and clumsy arm into the policy-making machinery of the institution so 'favored.' "[11]

Even worse, to Flexner, was the fact that the new Rockefeller Foundation, with its much larger resources, also yearly dispensed millions for specific projects rather than for endowment for whole institutions while professing a shopworn faith in the unity of all knowledge and the beneficence of research—worse because it had more to squander. "The search for truth is, as it always has been, the noblest expression of the human spirit. Man's hunger for knowledge about himself, his environment and the forces by which he is surrounded gives human life its meaning and purpose, and clothes it with final dignity," wrote Mason's successor as president, Raymond Fosdick, in his review for 1946. It was language that befit an annual report, whose message was that if research was just subsidized then knowledge would be advanced and in the end all would be well. The common complaint that the foundation's support for research sometimes failed to "come to grips with human need" reflected only care about the execution of a philosophy and not about the philosophy itself in which research was held up as "an effective weapon" in what amounted to a moral contest with ignorance. Rather different were the voices that began to be heard in the gloom of the 1930s, some of them inside the Rockefeller boards themselves, that wondered "whether the civilization which we are building can utilize the knowledge which it has." The rise of totalitarianism abroad and persistent economic distress at home "gave pause to those who believed that the primary need of our age was more knowledge."[12]

Flexner's understanding of knowledge and its utility was less mechanistic than Rose's or Mason's. To him it made little sense to talk abstractly about knowledge and not about the institutions where knowledge supposedly was produced: the universities. Extending and transmitting knowledge was their purpose, which they accomplished through research and education. Flexner himself had officiated at the union of research and education in medicine specifically, and the result at the time were places like Vanderbilt. Their faculties worked deliberately at new knowledge and painstakingly transmitted knowledge to others. Gifts of money, which was what foundations had to offer, obviously could make such places more secure. But foundations could not substitute for them and should not substitute other purposes that might change their nature. The idea that research was a weapon just waiting to be pointed at the right enemies threatened through medicine to do just that. Medicine always needed more weapons to fight any number of widely agreed-upon enemies, and in research medicine found a wonderful problem-solving instrument to meet the challenge of rising expectations for useful service.

It is not difficult to see why in the eyes of patrons some forms of giving more than others seemed to suit the idea of research as an instrument. Specific short-term grants, whose focus could be changed quickly as first one then another topic promised best results, offered regular opportunity for intrusion and the power that comes with the ability to set trends and articulate fashions. Large grants for endowment offered fewer such gratifications. On the contrary, they demanded the patience to wait on capitalism at 5 percent, and of the patrons they demanded the faith to give up control of what they gave. The contrast was not always stated so starkly, however, and as real policies evolved it was commonly gentled by compromise. Rockefeller and other support for research at Vanderbilt in the 1930s reflected this fundamental confusion.

Flexner had always said that research and education were indivisible, and at the new Vanderbilt, organizationally at least, it appeared to be just so. There was no "research" faculty that did not also have its job to do in the school's daily round of teaching and learning. There were no full-time teachers not also expected to be found some of the time in the laboratory. Some of the volunteer clinicians, busy with outside practices, indeed often had small time and energy left for sustained investigation, while among the full-time staff there were those like Blalock who gravitated naturally toward research and became known chiefly for it. But no formal divisions segregated one from the other, and no patron, chancellor, or dean demanded accounting of precisely whose time was spent where and on what. Deriving only from endowment and fee income, departmental budgets for those years were small, in the early 1930s, for example, ranging roughly from $19,000 to $48,000 yearly, with medicine and surgery at the top and pediatrics, pharmacology, and preventive medicine–public health at the bottom.[13] They were also models of simplicity, itemizing only salaries (the lion's share) and modest sums for supplies and equipment. Research as a separate line item did not appear.

How research worked in those early years must in part be inferred from two seemingly contradictory pieces of evidence. Measured by their publications, Vanderbilt's researchers compared favorably with medical scientists elsewhere. But the litany of complaints raised by the school's first two deans, Canby Robinson and Waller Leathers, that research could not long be so supported raised the question of how it ever had been. Robinson had said at the beginning and until he left never tired of saying that Vanderbilt was not rich enough to do everything well for long. Leathers too, though a better financial manager than his predecessor, saw his scientists' need for other support. "The income of the Medical School is inadequate to supply the research needs" of the various departments, he reported to Kirkland in 1931, and as a result faculty were being compelled to seek grants from outside agencies to carry on their work.[14]

That year six Vanderbilt faculty members managed to attract such outside support but none of them for periods longer than a year or, with one exception, in amounts larger than $3,000. The exception was a grant from the International Health Division of the Rockefeller Foundation providing something over $20,000 a year to Paul Lamson, professor of pharmacology, for special investigation of anthelmintics in connection with public health work in the control of parasitic infection, a project begun while Lamson was still at Johns Hopkins and continued for a number of years after he moved to Vanderbilt. More typically, pathologist Ernest Goodpasture, even then an investigator of some reputation, received $1,250 from the Pouch Foundation, a grant discontinued on July 1, 1932. "I have been informed that Mr. Pouch died last year," noted Leathers to Alan Gregg of the Rockefeller Foundation, "and that this grant will no longer be provided." Goodpasture also obtained $250 from the National Research Council, which also gave $750 together to Sidney Burwell in medicine and Glenn Cullen in biochemistry, and $1,000 to anatomist R. Sidney Cunningham. Cunningham also received $3,000 from the National Tuberculosis Association and $2,000 from the Commonwealth Fund, which made him top grantsman.[15] Short terms and relatively small amounts characterized the other special grants that from the Mallinckrodt Foundation, the Carnegie Corporation, the Josiah Macy, Jr. Foundation, the John and Mary R. Markle Foundation, and the United States Public Health Service came to Vanderbilt's medical investigators throughout the 1930s. None satisfied.

The Rockefeller Foundation too, newly reorganized and newly dedicated to the advancement of knowledge, bestowed grants in like manner—to the consternation of Flexner and other critics who objected to putting the universities "on a diet of cracked ice." Those words belonged not to Flexner, who long held out for large capital grants to select important institutions, but to Alan Gregg,[16] who as director of the Rockefeller Foundation's Medical Sciences Division helped establish at Vanderbilt and elsewhere a scheme for research support that came down in between wholesale endowment building, which in straitened times no longer seemed possible, and the "cracked ice" of small yearly grants, which kept the researchers constantly hopping after the next hoped-for installment and gave the givers potentially too much power over what the researchers actually were doing. In 1931 Gregg and Leathers negotiated the details of a fluid research fund that both were confident would eliminate the uncertainty inherent in small yearly grants coming from a variety of sources and thus would give the scientists the assurance of continuity they needed to do good work. The fund also provided that the scientists would be judged by their own peers and not by nonscientist outsiders and thus would be protected from the interference and overzealous supervision not unknown to accompany large subsidy from a single source.

Judging from the research then in progress and contemplated, Leathers at first thought that a fund of $30,000 a year for each of five years would "be of inestimable value in supplementing the budgets already available for the ten departments in carrying on research."[17] The terms ultimately settled on were better than that, even though to get them the university had to agree, wearisomely enough, to raise matching funds on a sliding scale. The life of the fund technically was to run ten years, 1932–41, though the Rockefeller contribution to it of $250,000 was to be dispensed in outright grants of diminishing size over only the first eight years. The idea was to provide a constant research fund of $50,000 for each of ten years, consisting of the contributions of the foundation and of the university. In the first two years the foundation would provide the full $50,000; in the last two the university would. Over the intervening six years, the foundation's share was to fall on a fixed schedule as the university's rose on the same schedule. In the end a princely $500,000 was to go to research and research alone, an amount in excess of the regular operating budgets of the ten departments during those years.[18]

The condition that Vanderbilt match the Rockefeller gift with an equal amount made Leathers more than a little uneasy.[19] Toward that requirement he planned to count any grant obtained for specific research projects in the different departments; but, understandable as his plan was, it provided the contrary incentive for faculty to generate specific outside grants in order to enjoy the freedom and continuity that supposedly came only with a long-running constant research fund. Leathers also told Gregg that it was his understanding that the Rockefeller contribution to the fund would be paid without making it an absolute condition that Vanderbilt secure its equivalent sum for the ten-year period. It was enough, he thought, that if the fund was to be maintained at $50,000 a year then the university obviously had no choice but to secure the difference. The situation would only be made more unstable, and thus the purpose of the whole understanding subverted at the start, if the foundation for any reason threatened to withhold its share. It did not, though Gregg was clear enough about the foundation's expectations: "We shall watch with greatest interest the success of the fluid research fund not only as it may aid in the accomplishment of investigative work but as it may evoke interest from other sources of support in the research work of the staff of your school."[20]

The Rockefeller Foundation made payments of its share on a monthly basis and asked an annual statement covering expenditures of the sums provided by it and by Vanderbilt for research under the terms of the appropriation.[21] Beyond the general and obvious restriction that the funds be used only for research, the other additional limitation was that they not be used to add faculty-level personnel to any department. Rather they were to go for technicians, dieners, research assistants, equipment, and supplies, under the direction of the regular faculty, which was already securely supported by permanent endowment. Otherwise, the faculty controlled the fund. The procedural mechanism for that control Leathers settled with his department heads and with Kirkland early in 1932. A committee was formed to advise the dean on the funds' disbursement; clinicians Sidney Burwell and Barney Brooks and basic scientists Ernest Goodpasture, R. Sidney Cunningham, and Walter Garrey served. Requests for money might originate with anyone on the faculty but had to be channeled through the department heads. Requests were then referred to the dean's advisory committee, which in turn transmitted to the dean its opinion regarding the desirability of granting the request. Leathers wanted it understood that the committee should not be regarded as a regular faculty committee but rather as a group chosen from the executive faculty to advise the dean on the use of the fluid research fund. For its expenditure the dean was primarily responsible to the university board of trust, and requests for funds could be granted only with his and the chancellor's approval. Requests from department heads were to be accompanied by specific statements of purpose with the names of the individuals conducting the research and a tally of proposed expenditures for salaries, equipment, and supplies. If the request was for the continuation of an unfinished problem, a summary of work already completed was to be given. Later, each department head was to submit to the dean a final statement of expenses and results incidental to each grant made for work by the department's faculty.[22]

Carefully planned and administered, the fund worked well; at least it worked as its planners had hoped. Serious research was sustained at Vanderbilt at a level that Leathers had asserted was not possible on slim departmental budgets alone. As Gregg had hoped, other support specifically for research seemed to be stimulated, so that by 1940 the medical school had attracted slightly more money from other sources than was distributed by the fluid research fund. Including the fund, something over $560,000 went for research between 1932 and 1940.[23] Some of that outside support (the vast bulk of it from private sources: the International Health Division of the Rockefeller Foundation, the Josiah Macy, Jr. Foundation, the Mallinckrodt Foundation, the International Cancer Research Foundation, the Markle Foundation) may have been forthcoming anyway, but the endorsement implicit in a large research fund running for a number of years likely encouraged others to invest with confidence and high expectations in Vanderbilt's medical scientists. For the scientists themselves, the fund brought some assurance of regular sustenance and the possibility of planning their work according to scientific, not yearly budgetary, considerations. "The continuance of the grant from the Division of Medical Science of the Rockefeller Foundation," wrote pathologist Ernest Goodpasture, expressing a common sentiment, "has been the essential support from which all of the investigative work in the Department has depended. It serves to permit a planned continuity of research which is indispensable."[24]

On the average each of the school's ten departments received about $2,500 a year from the fund, though the actual yearly allocations and the departmental totals varied considerably. Anatomy received the most ($39,121), pharmacology the least ($12,570, though pharmacology also received larger outside support than other departments). In descending order in between, medicine ranked second and was followed by physiology, preventive medicine–public health, pathology, biochemistry, obstetrics and gynecology, pediatrics, and surgery. Out of $250,000 spent, in the end only $8,000 separated the totals for the five preclinical from the five clinical departments (the preclinical side got more), a happily even division between the school's two halves. Not infrequently researchers received more from the fund than they spent, and every department always came in under budget.[25]

However well the fund worked by such objective measures, it could never work well enough. Harder to measure but present certainly was the anxiety that attaches to the possession of something so good that it cannot possibly last. By the end of the 1930s Leathers had hopes that a separate and permanent research endowment of $500,000 could somehow be found to take the place of the Rockefeller fund, and he approached Gregg about the possibilities of such a Rockefeller gift.[26] But that was asking for the kind of large capital grant then out of fashion at the Rockefeller boards and his request was not greeted enthusiastically. Though the fund afforded to a degree "a planned continuity of research," just as Goodpasture said, and was marked a vast improvement over the "cracked ice of yearly grants" even then becoming more common, the fluid research funds at Vanderbilt and elsewhere reflected a confusion inherent in the Rockefeller Foundation's new dedication to the advancement of knowledge. If knowledge was something that could be bought and if the foundation saw itself as the purchaser, then the fund was a better means than most to that end. It paid, for the time, decently large sums of money; it promised to pay over the span of a full decade; and it respected the independence of the scientists who produced that knowledge. The patron was voluntarily insulated from the patronized: funds once granted were internally allocated and the scientists' work judged on site by fellow scientists. It stimulated (or so the record seemed to show) others who with money to spend were convinced that to spend it on the acquisition of knowledge in medicine promised high and certain returns.

If on the other hand knowledge was something that grew and if the university was the place where it grew best, then the fund was a half-way technique. A quarter of a million dollars was a lot of money, but who really could say whether that amount or ten times that amount assured new discoveries or whether it only raised the expectation of them? Other givers might swell even more research's coffers, but unless they gave for a long enough term they risked distracting scientists from their real work with constant worries over next year's funding. Thus compromised, truly genuine research might increasingly become something done only before someone gave money to support it. A term of ten years sounded in 1932 long and inviting, which it was, but it was still a fixed term during which one simple transaction took place: the foundation gave outright $250,000 to the university to be spent on research. It was normal for Leathers to hope for more as the end came in view. But could his or any other university where knowledge supposedly grew naturally, with a mere $250,000 and ten years, be changed into a hothouse where knowledge as if domesticated grew on demand? Or should it?

There are two kinds of hothouses. One provides conditions needed for the growth of things too delicate or too exotic to survive in the local natural or social environment. The other forces the growth of things that may or may not survive otherwise but for which there is on the outside heavy demand. As medicine, thanks to better knowledge, became an ever more desirable commodity, the research that produced the knowledge more and more required the second kind of hothouse. The money invested in research that resulted in new discoveries both true and lasting could be said to be well spent. The rest had to be accounted lost to the inefficiencies of science that not even the hottest hothouse removed. No amount of spending for the wages of laboratory assistants and the keep of experimental animals guaranteed useful results that made sense to foundation patrons. Naturally enough, they wanted to know that their support had served some urgent need or that from it some practical good had come. Giving was what they did, and by it they justified themselves. There was danger therefore in too much closeness between them and those they helped, especially if those they helped were researchers who produced a strange kind of commodity that could not always or even often be had for payment of more money alone. Universities did something else and at least in their rhetoric justified themselves differently. They advanced knowledge through research and transmitted it through education. They did not just pay to have research done; universities did research, whoever paid however much and whatever the results. More concretely, certain people in universities did research. The institutions themselves—their boards, bylaws, faculties, and endowments—stood in between those people and their philanthropic patrons. They helped insulate the serious scholars from nonscholarly worries; they had to look over their shoulders less often. That was good, and that was how the fluid research fund worked.

No foundation, though, gave forever to any one place for any one thing.

No matter how good the insulation between it and the researcher, both sides knew there were limits. In this particular case the limit was ten years and $250,000. Only figuratively then did the Rockefeller Foundation invest that amount in research at Vanderbilt; literally, the foundation spent it. It accepted acknowledgment in the publications of those it helped and in time moved on to other things at other places. True investment would have meant more boldly giving to Vanderbilt $4 or $5 million as a permanent research endowment, which would have amounted to a perpetual fluid research fund. Doing so at Vanderbilt and other worthy universities would have meant spending capital as well as income, but which was more important anyway, the Rockefeller Foundation or the universities? If in the long run knowledge mattered at all, the answer to a man like Abraham Flexner was self-evident.

The fluid research fund obviously fell short of Flexner's ideal of massive and largely unconditioned gifts for endowment that would make the Vanderbilts of the world finally secure. It was obvious too that not everyone shared a faith so absolute as Flexner's in the ever-beneficent union between research and universities. But with its fairly sizable appropriation of a quarter of a million dollars and its term of a full decade, the fund was considerably better than the "cracked ice" of yearly grants that Alan Gregg had warned against. Nor, bestowed on places like Vanderbilt whose record had proved their reliability, was it the sort of "retail business" sneered at by Frederick T. Gates. Far from it, for in the selective granting of research money to universities already committed to the advance of science and already staffed to do science was confirmation of the notion that in the concentration of resources for research lay the best hope of progress in medicine. A stern "to them that hath it shall be given" policy appealed intellectually and likely temperamentally as well to men like Gates and Flexner for whom crude equalitarianism held no charm. For Alan Gregg too, himself a doctor, and for other medical scientists it was also a policy based on merit alone.

Good results in research were always hard to get, even from the efforts of the most well-trained and zealous investigators. But for medical research, at least, what Harvard physiologist Walter Cannon called "the fertility of aggregates" seemed to improve the chances.[27] The new medicine invited, indeed required, free-ranging collaboration, not just among the various kinds of scientific doctors represented in the departments of a modern medical school, but with others—chemists, physicists, biologists, psychologists, and sociologists—that only a large university setting provided. From them all, not necessarily from formal collaboration but from the fertile presence of them all in one place, progress was more likely. Such essentially had been Canby Robinson's faith and the reason behind his compulsion first to see Vanderbilt's medical school adjoin the rest of the university and then to coordinate through the arrangement of physical space and through the choice of personnel the endeavors of the basic scientists and the clinicians among themselves and with each other.

Vanderbilt's "aggregate," though certainly not as large as some universities', was probably at least as fertile. From its medical scientists, much of whose work was supported by the fluid research fund, came in the 1930s a steady stream of articles reporting their investigations. With them everyone—the department heads, the dean, the chancellor, and the Rockefeller people— seemed satisfied that the advancement of knowledge was being well served. Likely it was, though as they all knew time alone would prove. Not all of the facts gathered and the inferences drawn could stand time's test; indeed not even from all the facts would any inferences be drawn at all, so cautious had these investigators learned to be. Not all of it was important or deserved especially to be remembered; not all of it has been. The single important advances that happened by chance to have been made at Vanderbilt rather than somewhere else tell, fifty years later as they did then, about their results, which was for many of the doers of medical research and for most of their patrons and spectators the chief value of it all. That is what many of their publications meticulously recorded.

Results and the therapeutic uses they were put to were the undisputed aim and product of science in medicine. Among the internists, surgeons, and other doctors on the clinical side, diagnosis and therapy—that is, service— defined the way every day they lived in the wards, clinics, and with their private patients. Knowledge, and the science from which it was supposed to spring, mattered most and mattered most immediately for the succor it could bring the sick people in their care. What, asked thousands of medical students and young doctors from that day to this, are the two or three facts about each of hundreds of maladies that most often will help most patients? For their living, they had chosen to live closer to the edge of things than did most people, and, unlike most intelligent and highly educated people in other professions, they could less well afford to dally in what might not matter. Even among clinicians, who in an academic setting such as Vanderbilt found in research much satisfaction and broad field for ample talents, experiments in the laboratory and projects in the field gravitated often as not toward the useful questions fairly close at hand. John Youmans's pioneering nutrition surveys first near home and later around the world documented the way to better health for millions of people, if but they or their masters would listen. Alfred Blalock's endless experiments to prove the nature of secondary shock vanquished one of the surgeon's most dreaded foes and, fortuitously, probably lowered considerably the cost in lives exacted by the Second World War. So it was supposed to work, and in that immediate hope at least most clinical researchers did their research. Some thereby no doubt hoped to relieve the lot of suffering humanity, others merely better to serve the few patients who were theirs. But whether modest or immodest, the researchers' motives at the bench as at the bedside were practical.

Indeed, to everyone who works for and then chooses to put the letters "M.D." after their names, practical things must matter. The profession since the beginning had existed to render service, and science had done nothing to change that. In many ways science only made better service possible and reinforced the old definition. There were, though, people on the preclinical side of the medical schools, most of them M.D.'s, whose immediate reference points were somewhat different. It was they—the anatomists, biochemists, pharmacologists, bacteriologists, physiologists, and pathologists—whom Flexner and Robinson aimed to cement into the structure of the new medical education and the new medicine. They too presumably were meant to serve. Many did; perhaps they all did. The topics of even the most esoteric investigations usually implied at least the possibility of ultimate application. In anatomy Karl Mason did important work on vitamin A; Jack M. Wolfe, though lacking the sophisticated tools available later, explored the physiology of the pituitary gland, the master gland of the endocrine system. Sam Clark and James A. Ward studied electrical effects on the cortex of experimental animals. Biochemist Morton Mason worked on renal function and hypertension, often in collaboration with clinicians Tinsley Harrison and Alfred Blalock. Studies in anesthetic agents and studies of barbiturates came from Paul Lamson's pharmacology department. Herbert Wells in physiology worked on serum proteins and osmotic pressure, and chairman Walter Garrey, an early student of auricular fibrillation, continued in studies of the transmission of impulses in the heart muscle.

Between research in the clinical fields and research in the basic sciences the Rockefeller men, whose fluid research fund paid for much of both, seemed to make no essential distinction. At least at the back of their minds surely lay the hope that all of it somehow, someday, would prove its worth in service. Not that application need be immediate: in science the advancement of knowledge was a sophisticated business that sometimes took years to pay off. But that it would pay off remained a faith among givers needing justification and among many getters who in the medical world saw service as their purpose. In medicine as in most other fields, the advancement of knowledge generally meant just what the foundation's unchanging motto said: "Service to Mankind."

Rare then were the basic medical scientists who did not hope that in the end their work would be useful, for with others who were medical doctors they shared the most determining of first things: four student years in a reformed medical school usually followed by years more of training in wards and laboratories. Add to that a lifetime spent in the realms of academic medicine (especially if those realms were coordinated as Robinson had co-ordinated them at Vanderbilt), and most of them knew one of the happiest of final things as well: the satisfaction of people whose technique helped them to take responsibility for others and so had enabled them to matter. But in between first and final things, the best of these basic scientists spent their days differently. One of the very best, pathologist Ernest W. Goodpasture, suggests how.

As the world judges people, Goodpasture was a great scientist and a famous man. Fame is by definition the world's to bestow. The world's understanding of "great scientists" is sometimes less competent, which with Goodpasture meant that fame was bestowed for the wrong reasons. His reputation illustrates how much the world claims to care for science and how little it understands the scientists, whose interest day to day is not to serve but to know. What this particular scientist wanted to know and spent his lifetime working at and the "discovery" that in the world's estimation made him great, though related, were different things. The discovery had great and immediate application and thus enabled medical science better to serve humankind. The problem, which led by chance to the discovery and remained a problem long after it, had less allure for the world though not for the scientist.

"America's Pasteur," the "Edison of Medicine," he was called,[28] thanks prosaically enough to what became known as "the egg." A pathologist interested in infectious diseases, particularly viruses, Goodpasture had the good fortune in the course of his investigations to hit upon a cheap and easy technique for cultivating in the laboratory uncontaminated viruses, which could then be used in the manufacture of vaccines to protect against infections. The idea—to use the living chicken embryo, simply a fertile hen's egg, as host for the virus—seemed inspired. As it was commonly related, the story of Goodpasture and the egg began with the need among virus researchers for a method to cultivate viruses in a way that would keep them pure and free from bacterial contamination. Only then would further study of them be possible and only then would there be any hope of obtaining virus in the quantities necessary to produce vaccines useful to medicine. Since the early 1920s, before coming to Vanderbilt, Goodpasture had worked with viruses, especially fowl pox, one of the numerous family of "pox" diseases and the one known to chicken farmers as "sore-head" after the eruptions it caused

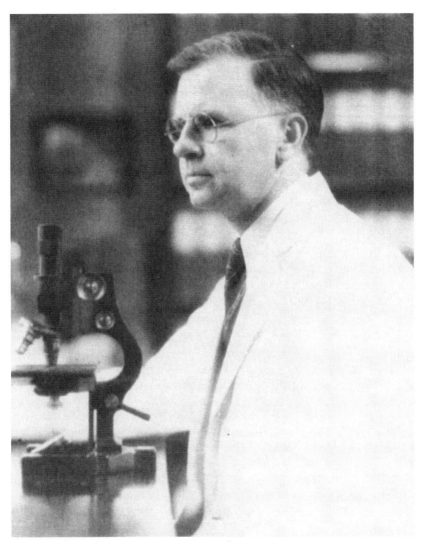

Science: pathologist Ernest W. Goodpasture

around a chicken's head and neck. For laboratory study it had certain advantages: microscopically some of its manifestations were easier to work with than other virus diseases; it was not contagious for humans, which made it safe for laboratory workers to handle; and chickens as experimental animals were cheap.

The egg had been used before in medical research, earliest and most obviously in the study of embryology but also as a medium for growing various disease-causing microorganisms. But it was Goodpasture, by now at Vanderbilt, who in 1931 thought of the egg—an abundant, essentially sterile, self-contained package of living matter—as a host for viral growth. With his laboratory assistant, Alice M. Woodruff, he cut a small window into the egg, inoculated the fowl pox virus onto the exposed chorioallantoic membrane, covered the hole with a glass cover slip sealed with paraffin, placed the egg in a small commercial incubator, and then settled down to wait. A few days later came the hoped-for result: the embryo showed a blotched appearance and other symptoms of the disease, the sign that said the virus was multiplying rapidly. Though reported in the *American Journal of Pathology* in May of that year, it aroused, reported one commentator, "no more national interest than an announcement two years earlier that [Alexander] Flemming in England had found a green mold which secreted a microbe-killing juice called penicillin."[29] Undaunted, Goodpasture moved on to see specifically what other viruses might also grow in the egg, and how they could be harvested, preserved, and transmitted through several generations. Smallpox was next: the egg proved nicely susceptible, so nicely that "a single egg produced enough vaccine to give lifelong protection to 1,000 children." Herpes simplex followed: "the modest little virus which causes cold sores, fever blisters. It thrived on an egg diet."[30] From there other scientists carried on, using the same technique to produce vaccines for yellow fever, typhus, Rocky Mountain spotted fever, influenza, and horse sleeping sickness.

It was of the practical preventive effects of it all, however, that most was heard. "This is a story of a Tennessee doctor who developed disease-fighting vaccines credited with saving more lives than any war has taken," reported a proud local writer of Goodpasture's accomplishment. "Thousands of soldiers in World War II and the Korean war survived long sieges in tropic swampland without a single case of yellow fever or typhus fever" thanks to his discoveries. So inexpensive had smallpox vaccine become "by his method of producing it inside an egg that whole nations have been vaccinated by it, in Europe, South America, Africa." The great influenza epidemics "that were the terror of World War I were no threat in World War II, because a vaccine made by his method was available to stop it."[31] Thanks to an egg-grown vaccine, horse sleeping sickness, which when it attacked humans killed 70 percent of those stricken, was virtually eradicated. There was hope even that some part of the egg might prove susceptible to the dreaded crippler, poliomyelitis. Even if that hope were not realized, "few events in research history have had any more significant results than Goodpasture's decision to try to grow fowl pox virus in fertile eggs." Simply: "soldiers abroad, civilians at home—millions of them—owe their lives to the medical magic of this modest Tennessee doctor."[32]

That story, correct in its general outlines and on most essential particulars, became a standard one in both lay and scientific circles by the 1940s. Those who told it and likely those who heard understood it as another installment in what might have been a newsreel on the forward march of science in the service of humankind. More, better, and cheaper vaccines save thousands of lives; that is, Goodpasture and the egg helped medicine better to serve. Always the story was related as the story of Goodpasture and the egg together, of the explorer and his discovery. The story's result was to link tightly the benevolence of the scientist with the usefulness of his science. Take away the egg and in the minds of most people Goodpasture, the savior of millions, would have faded to just another respected but rather mysterious research doctor who never saw patients but tinkered instead with things called viruses, so small they had never been seen.

This perception is sad—for the new medicine claimed much for its science, and in this respect the egg hides the scientist. Privately this particular scientist resented much of the acclaim and publicity that came to him because of the egg, and for what he really did it was of small account. No misanthrope, Goodpasture was pleased enough that the egg turned out to serve so well, but that discovery had not been the aim of his work before 1931, nor was it the great watershed afterward. He did not believe in "great discoveries" in the same way the newspaper writers seemed to. The egg helped him and others do some of their work better, but that was all. Probably if it had not occurred to him in 1931, it would soon have occurred to someone else. It was a small but very clear and very useful piece to the larger and more difficult puzzle on which he spent his life. Much of that puzzle is still unsolved twenty years after his death, something that would have been no surprise to him, so convinced was he of the complexity of what he was studying and of the time and work it would take to find the answers. It was no surprise, either, that his fame during his lifetime rested on one small clearly useful piece of a puzzle, a piece that represented more technique than science.

Science and medicine had come of age just a generation or so before Goodpasture did, and he later confessed to have been attracted and stimulated as a student of medicine by the aura of what he recalled as the "romantic period of medical research." It had shone all across Europe, especially Germany, France, and the Low Countries, in the second half of the nineteenth century, and by the turn of the century it brightly illuminated North American shores as well. Matthias Schleiden, Theodor Schwann, and Rudolph Virchow had firmly established cell theory, while under the tutelage of Louis Pasteur and Robert Koch and their protégés the germ theory of disease had spawned the new science of bacteriology. To sanitary science, which empirically had already saved thousands of lives, now came the understanding of immunology. Old concepts of vital activity and the spontaneous generation of living matter had wilted before Antoine Lavoisier's chemical interpretation of respiration and Friedrich Wohler's synthesis of urea. The optimistic predictions of great advances for experimental medicine through scientific physiology made by Claude Bernard, who himself so firmly laid its chemical foundations, seemed to be coming true. The impressive strides of scientific research in medicine justified again the idea of progress, which in the nineteenth century general peace and rising prosperity had already made the spirit of the age. The happy conclusion of Herbert Spencer's version of evolutionary theory applied to human history, that progress through knowledge and adaption was not just possible but necessary, seemed borne out by scientific research that promised and produced the cures that stopped disease and made life better.[33] The scientists themselves may have been tempted to wonder if all physiological functions and biological phenomena generally could not "be brought to the experimental test."[34]

The allure of that exalted romance in the beginning was the same for Goodspasture as it was for a good many others who wanted to be doctors in the early twentieth century. No matter that, later, he went down different, more mysterious paths from his practicing colleagues, his entry and early years in the exciting world of scientific medicine saw the simple success and unambiguous achievement befitting the great promise of his chosen profession. He was one of the only two of Robinson's original new men with local roots in Tennessee and at Vanderbilt, and to many of his friends and admirers his stature was enhanced when later in life, an eminent man with opportunity to go elsewhere, he clung to those roots.[35]

Goodpasture was born on a farm in Montgomery County, Tennessee, and was raised there and in Nashville, where at Vanderbilt he earned his bachelor's degree in 1907. After a term as a college teacher in West Virginia, he went to Hopkins a year later to learn medicine with the class of 1912. He knew then that pathology would be his field and upon graduation he pursued it with alacrity. A Rockefeller Foundation fellowship supported him at Hopkins his first year out of school, and in 1913 he formally joined the pathology department there as an instructor and acting resident pathologist in the Johns Hopkins Hospital, working under William Welch and George Whipple. In 1915 he stepped up to become resident pathologist in the Peter Bent Brigham

Hospital and instructor at Harvard under William T. Councilman. For 1918 he was on his own, as assistant professor at Harvard, as pathologist in uniform at the Chelsea Naval Hospital in Boston, and as professor at the medical school of the University of the Philippines in Manila.

He was thirty-six in 1922 when the next opportunity came, and between then and 1960, when he died, he held three more posts, all offering ample scope to do the things he wanted. For two years, 1922 to 1924, he first experienced what it was like to run his own laboratory, as director of the William H. Singer Memorial Research Laboratory in Pittsburgh. Such laboratories being still small-scale, it was his chance less to administer than to investigate problems that interested him, at the head of a group of other talented scientists. With one of them in particular, Oscar Teague (who was also a Vanderbilt graduate), Goodpasture began to concentrate on the problems that would become his life's work. With that good start to his credit, Canby Robinson offered him the post of professor of pathology at the new Vanderbilt Medical School and chief pathologist in the Vanderbilt Hospital. He accepted in 1924 and remained there until his retirement from academic medicine thirty-one years later. That long tenure was interrupted by only two detours, the first actually a preface to the new job, and the second a responsibility pressed upon him and not one of his greater successes. In the academic year 1924–25 he went abroad (as did most of Vanderbilt's new men), at the expense of the General Education Board, as a visiting scholar at the Institute for General and Experimental Pathology of the University of Vienna. And from 1945 to 1950, in addition to his regular work as head of pathology he served as dean of Vanderbilt's medical school. In 1955, at age sixty-nine, he retired from Vanderbilt and became scientific director of pathology at the Armed Forces Institute of Pathology in Washington, D.C., a post he held until 1959.

At all those places the things Goodpasture wanted to do related to the study of infectious diseases. In that, he viewed his work as a continuation of a large and memorable epoch in the history of medicine reached in the last decades of the nineteenth century, when from the work of Pasteur and Koch sprung the twin fields of bacteriology and immunology. Illustrating for him the importance of that turning point, Goodpasture recounted (third-hand at least) an episode at the International Congress of Medicine in London in 1881 at which Lister, Koch, Pasteur, and other luminaries had gathered to hear the latest advances. Pasteur, who had not before met Koch, witnessed his demonstration of the growth of bacterial cultures on solid media and was duly impressed—but not Englishman Charlton Bastian, a staunch heterogenist who would not be moved from his belief in spontaneous generation.

Exasperated and appalled, Pasteur reportedly threw up his hands and cried: "My God, my God, do you still believe that? My God, it just can't be possible!"[36] Of course, it was not possible, at least not for many for much longer. The new microbe hunters soon established a new doctrine that in time became an old orthodoxy: that specific infectious diseases were caused by specific microorganisms and by nothing else. With that doctrine of the specific microbial etiology of infectious disease, nature yielded up numerous useful secrets, many of which translated fairly directly into better practical medicine. Logically it might have seemed that the doctrine itself should embrace all infectious diseases, but there were some that did not yield to the specific methods of Koch and Pasteur. The job of investigating them, which Goodpasture said might once have been "relegated to the mopping up operation of the twentieth century," in fact became in the twentieth century "a vast terrain of rich potentialities for those who went in," Goodpasture among them. "It was the Lilliputian land of the viruses, the rickettsiae and sundry recalcitrant obligate and facultative intracellular parasites."[37]

By the time he began his work in earnest in the 1920s, others over the previous two or three decades had made significant explorations in that Lilliputian land. As established by the early bacteriologists, the biological nature of the specific parasite of a disease was in the main determined by growing the causative microorganisms on a suitable artificial medium outside the body of the infected host or by investigating the infecting organism still inside the tissues of the host. The bacillus of typhoid fever, for example, had grown successfully on an artificial medium; the plasmodium of malarial fever was studied microscopically within the host. But for the purposes of establishing specific causes, there were some diseases, apparently infectious, whose causative agents could neither be grown on lifeless media nor be visually identified with certainty under the microscope. Their nature, therefore, could not be discerned by experimenting with them in pure culture (something very difficult to obtain before the egg), nor could it be simply apprehended by sight. Such agents were detectable for sure only by their effect on the host organism (which might range from a single bacteria to a human being), typically often by specific changes wrought within certain of the host's cells.[38] Those changes appeared in diseased tissue under the microscope in the form of inclusion bodies in the nucleus or in the surrounding cytoplasm of a cell, which were not normally a part of the cell's constituents. In all viral diseases the presence of such inclusion bodies had not in the 1920s been demonstrated, among them poliomyelitis, Rous's chicken sarcoma and fowl leukemia, and D'Herelle's bacteria-attacking bacteriophage (which was, incidentally, the chief scientific interest of Martin Arrowsmith in Sinclair Lewis's 1925 novel).

But it was this feature in many of them that Goodpasture believed held the best promise in the search for fundamental insights into their structure and behavior.

There were other distinguishing characteristics of the organisms causing viral diseases, among them their apparently minute size, which enabled them to pass through, for example, the earthenware and porcelain filters that caught ordinary bacteria. From this feature came the general label for the group: "filterable viruses."[39] Viruses characteristically also could be preserved in glycerine and some of them were known to be very resistant to drying. They seemed to thrive only on specific tissues of the host; that is, they were tissue specific. The poxes, for example, appeared only on the skin, while polio and rabies were manifested only in the nervous system. No viruses had been cultivated with certainty on lifeless media; living matter seemed necessary for their reproduction. The viruses generally had the capacity for biological variation; like the living cells where they grew they could undergo mutation. And relatively avirulent strains of some of them could be used to induce immunity through vaccination, as with smallpox and rabies. Recovery from virus diseases was usually associated with immunity to them in the future. Various investigators had offered several interpretations of the identity of these active agents, describing them as animal parasites, plant parasites, bacteria, toxic substances, or perhaps enzymes.[40]

But it was with the demonstration and interpretation of the specific intracellular inclusion bodies present in many viral diseases that Goodpasture and others chiefly concerned their investigations into cause. In some diseases—smallpox, vaccinia, and paravaccinia—inclusion bodies appeared in both the cytoplasm and the nucleus of the cells for which the virus had a special affinity. In herpes simplex, herpes zoster, varicella, foot and mouth disease, and (more exotically) polyhedral disease of caterpillars, they were observed only in the nucleus; in trachoma, rabies, sheep pox, and fowl pox only in the cytoplasm.[41] Even before methods of filtration were instituted that could free virus from other microbial contaminants and thus establish filterability as a criterion for assignment of diseases to the virus group, intracellular inclusions had been discovered in the hosts of diseases whose causative agents later proved to be filterable. The existence of inclusion bodies in the disease mollusculum contagiosum had been known since the early 1840s. Otto Bollinger demonstrated those in fowl pox in 1873. Seven years later Alphonse Laveran's discovery of the malarial plasmodium spurred the search for inclusion bodies in diseases of unknown cause. During the 1890s it seemed likely to some investigators (Guiseppe Guarnieri and T. von Was-ielewski) working with variola and vaccinia virus that the intracellular inclusions represented a protozoan or animal parasite. In 1898, however, a German commission to investigate foot and mouth disease announced that the virus, which could be neither cultivated nor seen, could be filtered free of bacterial contaminants and therefore must be too small to be seen with the optical microscopes then available. It was then plausible to infer that other disease-causing agents that had baffled the methods of the bacteriologists might also be so filtered and thus placed in the same group of ultramicroscopic organisms.[42]

That raised a problem for those who had thought that the visible cellular inclusions typical of some of the diseases were some sort of protozoan parasite, inasmuch as the observed size of those inclusions was hardly compatible with their passage through the finest of filters. It was still possible, however, that somewhere in its complex life cycle the parasite existed in such a minute (and filterable) form that it could be imagined not to constitute but to inhabit the inclusion bodies themselves. That possibility seemed more probable when in 1904, experimenting with smears from fowl pox virus, Borrel observed enormous numbers of extremely minute particles, uniform in structure, whose size and profusion could account both for the filterability of the virus and for its evidently high concentration in the cells of the susceptible tissue. Discovery of analogous structures in mollusculum contagiosum, vaccinia, variola, and trachoma followed, leading to the theory (advanced by Stanislaus von Prowazek and B. Lipschutz in 1907 and 1919) that the tiny particles, in fowl pox since known as "Borrel bodies," "are individual living agents, which divide by constriction, invade cells, and multiplying within them cause the cells to react to the invasion by forming substances which envelop the microorganisms, thus segregating them and grouping them into an intracellular mass." Accordingly, the inclusion bodies, too large to be filtered, ceased to represent the parasite and became products of the host cell's reaction to a much smaller particle. Whether that particle was protozoan or something else, whether it was the virus or still another representation of it, was still uncertain. But it was around such tiny evidence that the search increasingly circled.[43]

For the study specifically of the relationship between such particles and the cell they supposedly affect, fowl pox was a good disease because cellular inclusions and the granules within them were one of its prominent features. With it Goodpasture and his assistants worked in the late 1920s, steadily tracking the virus or its shadow across that Lilliputian land. With C. Eugene Woodruff he demonstrated that fowl pox inclusion bodies at least were something more than nonliving products of cellular degeneration, which was a theory advanced after the single protozoan parasite theory and quite its opposite. He showed how, by a laboratory process of chemical digestion, the inclusion bodies, themselves resistant to the action of the chemical trypsin, could be freed from the surrounding skin cells of the lesion that the trypsin quickly destroyed. Thus liberated, the inclusion bodies were washed in a sterile saline solution to assure that the fluid surrounding them was innocuous, and then they were inoculated into the feather follicle of a healthy chicken. The characteristic fowl pox lesion resulted, which demonstrated that the isolated inclusion bodies were—or were vessels for—the infective agents of the disease.[44]

That was important largely for the question it then raised, the question of which parts of those inclusion bodies were actually responsible for transmitting the disease. The shape of the isolated inclusions seemed to change with the fluid that surrounded them. In saline solution they were compact hyaline structures, but after washing and immersion in distilled water they swelled and developed vacuoles, or small cavities, in which "dancing about in rapid Brownian motion," tiny granules were visible. Goodpasture then crushed an inclusion body on a slide to view the Borrel bodies, which were, he concluded in comparing the two, the granules seen in the vacuoles of the bloated inclusion. The inclusion body then appeared to be composed of Borrel bodies embedded in some kind of semi-permeable ground substance, possibly a lipoprotein.[45]

When immersed in water the inclusion bodies swelled in their linear dimensions by one-third to one-half, which indicated a doubling or tripling of their volume. While handling them during that process, Goodpasture and his assistants happened on one of those events that in experimental science sometimes reward the diligent observer. If the swollen inclusion bodies were allowed to dry, they promptly exploded. That seemed attributable to increased surface tension and no reduction in volume, but what really mattered was that as the drying inclusion bodies tore themselves apart, the Borrel bodies inside were set free. And they were what Goodpasture was now after. Painstakingly, using a capillary pipette and Chambers microdissection apparatus (he was working with particles no larger than .25 micron, 6,000 to 20,000 of which he conservatively estimated were contained in each inclusion body), he prepared slides smeared with Borrel bodies and with the sharp tip of a glass rod scraped across them to harvest a small portion of the smear. The tip of the rod, with, he hoped, its cargo of numerous Borrel bodies, was then inserted into the feather follicle of a healthy chicken (just as before the entire inclusion body had been introduced) and broken off to be left there, glass and all. That procedure was repeated with smears from 17 different inclusion bodies and 17 chickens, all of the scratch inoculations from a given inclusion body made into the follicles of a single bird. As controls, 118 inoculations were made in an identical manner except that the glass points were run through the pools of distilled water used to wash the inclusion bodies before their "explosion." All proved negative, indicating both that the fluid was noninfectious and that the glass itself had not produced a foreign body reaction suggestive of a fowl-pox lesion. From the 135 genuine inoculations, 52 did produce the disease.[46]

Ever cautious, Goodpasture hesitated to conclude from the experiment that one specific part of the inclusion body smear—the Borrel bodies—had caused the successful inoculation, but that was in fact what he had shown. Here was how he put it: "These facts [that the lipoid component of the inclusion bodies was shown to be noninfective, and that no other component within the inclusion bodies had been isolated other than the Borrel bodies], together with the enormous number of Borrel bodies in a single inclusion and their perfect uniformity in size and shape, lead us to think that in our various experiments the Borrel bodies represent the important part of the inoculum—the actual virus of fowl-pox."[47] The operative word was "represent," for he did not say that the Borrel bodies actually were the virus. But they were the smallest representation of the virus ever shown, and he had fairly clearly demonstrated that they were the causative agents of fowl pox. He had tracked the virus one more step, and that knowledge, he hoped, would aid in theoretical and experimental interpretation of other virus diseases.

From such experiments Goodpasture was moving constantly toward the idea of the relationship between the virus and its host cell as the key concept and moving away from the cruder notion of filterability, which unfortunately had given the group its name. The activity of the virus in relation to the cells of the host, what was meant by the term "cytotropism," promised to be of major biological importance. It had been shown that different viruses had special affinities for different kinds of cells: rabies, herpes, poliomyelitis were attracted only to nervous tissue and thus were neurotropic; variola-vaccinia and the poxes were attracted only to the skin and thus were epidermotropic. All were cytotropic: they thrived, reproduced, and did their mischief only from within the cells of the host organism. Viruses were known to increase in quantity at the sight of the specific changes they effected (the fowl-pox lesion, for example), and—in the phrase that appeared ever more frequently in Goodpasture's work—in "intimate relation" with the cells they altered. So little was then known about the physical conditions that exist and the chemical changes that take place within the walls of a cell that Goodpasture feared that study of the dynamics of that relationship was bound to be slow. He was also convinced that it was the place to look.[48]

It would take much more work to resolve the two divergent views then current on the nature of viruses: one, that they were extremely small living parasites that grew within and in intimate relationship with the cells of a host, or that they were nonliving toxic agents that caused the cell itself to reproduce the same agent and thus account for the continuous regeneration of the poison. Goodpasture's evidence was pointing toward the first hypothesis: that viruses were living parasites, though in the late 1920s he still remained tentative. Viruses clearly had some of the characteristics associated with living matter, among them the ability to reproduce themselves in series. Yet they still eluded cultivation on nonliving media, which would have provided the ultimate proof of their vitality. Unquestionably, they were intracellular, which meant that work more strictly to define their nature would necessarily take investigators farther and farther into the living cell. A clearer picture of that tiny landscape would await techniques that Goodpasture did not then have available (electron microscopy specifically).

But neither then nor later was his immediate aim (nor was it his nature to expect) definitive answers. The more significant the problem a scientist worked on, it seemed, the less likely that the problem could ever be brought to a true conclusion. And the problem of the viruses, Goodpasture knew, was a very significant problem. The question of whether viruses were living or nonliving matter, though the immediate experimental question, was not in truth the real one. Suppose, on the basis of solid though imperfect laboratory evidence, that they were shown to be living parasites as Goodpasture even then was coming to believe. Having thus reduced an idea of living matter to its most elemental manifestation, the scientist logically asked not just about the nature of that particle but about the nature of life itself. That was as much a metaphysical as a scientific question, and whether or not the ultimate truth would ever be known was a puzzle that, with thoughtful nonscientists, many of these sound and sensible people, who were trained to put things to the experimental test and to respect the facts, surely wrestled with at quiet times and in private places.

Just as difficult was that the truth that clearly was the scientists to know, the truth about the physical world that came with the advancement of their knowledge through research, changed. As they tested and retested their and their fellows' theories, as they constantly brought to new problems fresh ideas and fresh prejudices, new facts proliferated. But the prospects for their permanence shrank as the search for them accelerated. Thus Goodpasture expected no definitive answers and settled in his science for the fun of the search alone. The best searches had as much to thank to luck and good hunches and the sense to see where to go next as to new hardware and better techniques—whether the electron microscope or the egg.

The egg, which was a triumph of technique if ever there was one, came after Goodpasture's most fundamental work: his tracking of the as yet invisible virus to the constituent particles of the inclusion bodies of fowl pox and his demonstration that those particles were the infectious agents of the disease. Later, the egg served as means for investigating the nature of other (though certainly not all) known viruses and some other infectious diseases. The chorioallantoic membrane of the chick embyro was not susceptible, for example, to the growth of some viruses, that of mumps, for one, cultivation of which in monkeys won Goodpasture almost as much popular acclaim as the egg itself.[49] Polio too, a more dreaded scourge by far, Goodpasture found especially troublesome and left its solution to others.[50] But with or without the egg (whose practical promise for producing better and cheaper vaccines he also left largely to others), he worked quietly to know better the biological nature of these intracellular parasites. He did not underestimate the difficulties of understanding the cell-parasite relationships—the framework for it all. The ability of parasites to inhabit the interior spaces of living cells might be an assurance, he once said in part playfully, "that nature left alone to its own evolutionary maneuvers is designing us to be more efficient hosts, just as the insects have become for some of their parasites; and thereupon would be removed naturally and automatically the stigmata of our present infectious diseases. If we were not so impetuous, a few millenia of progress would doubtless resolve for us more problems than these that presently beset and trouble us."[51]

Both he and the doctors who heard him (he was delivering the Alvarenga Prize Lecture for 1941 before the College of Physicians of Philadelphia) knew, however, that it was the business of medical science to deny such orderly processes of nature. And for what his colleagues understood as Goodpasture's large contributions to medical science, they enobled him as they did only a few. They called on him for twenty-five special lectureships (including the DeLamar Lecture at Johns Hopkins and the Harvey Lecture at the New York Academy of Medicine, both in 1929; the Loeb Lecture at Washington University in 1938; and the Shattuck Lecture at the Massachusetts Medical Society in 1940), awarded him seven prize medals (including the Kober Medal of the Association of American Physicians for 1943 and the Kovalenko Medal of the National Academy of Sciences for 1958), and bestowed on him four honorary degrees (Yale, 1939; University of Chicago, 1941; Washington University, 1950; and Tulane, 1957). Among special appointments, he served as a member of the Board of Scientific Directors of the International Health Division of the Rockefeller Foundation (1938–40; 1942–44). Among societies, he was member of the National Academy of Sciences and (more rare for a medical man) the American Philosophical Society. From his seniors in science came personal praise for his work and requests for counsel with theirs. Shortly after "the egg" was published, E. Paschen in Hamburg, discoverer of the "Paschen bodies" in variola-vaccinia (analogous to the Borrel bodies in fowl pox), wrote to Goodpasture. He was eager for more details on happenings in Vanderbilt's pathology laboratory, and he enclosed photographs of his own inoculated eggs.[52] Simon Flexner in 1924 sent congratulations for the series of papers on herpes that Goodpasture had published with Oscar Teague the year before: "They are a model." And in 1937 Abraham Flexner offered his best wishes on Goodpasture's election to the National Academy of Sciences.[53]

Goodpasture was not unappreciative. He had after all fairly earned it, and praise warmed him as it does most people. But he must have suspected that some of it at least, though offered in generous spirit, was wrong in its understanding. Like the public who in newspaper and magazine stories saw pictures of the white-coated man with microscope and eggs and read about Goodpasture whose idea had saved thousands of lives, "the antibiotic-happy general practitioner" (Goodpasture's words) and many clinicians in academic medicine did not know him either. They viewed research from the perspective of their business, which was useful service. On a linear scale, they linked it forward to therapy, whose needs inevitably shaped what they did in the laboratory. "The procedure of research is much the same irrespective of purpose or problem," Goodpasture wrote, "but the attitudes of investigators differ." Goodpasture's attitudes were not those of many of his clinical colleagues. Almost every researcher in the academy (whether devoted to experimentation or to the clinic), including Goodpasture, mouthed the usual homilies about the importance of an atmosphere where the intuition and curiosity of the investigator had free play. Goodpasture, on the topic of viruses, also wrote: "The significance of the relationships that exist between obligate intracellular infective agents and the cells they inhabit has hardly begun to be explored, although in those relationships lie some of the most fundamental phenomena of biology."[54] He did not say that in those phenomena lay the promise of lifting from the shoulders of humanity the burden of infectious disease. That promise was there, as he well knew, and he welcomed it. But in research, which was how he spent his days, it did not govern.

On the same linear scale, Goodpasture linked research not forward to potential therapies but back toward fundamental principles of biology whose implications might be larger than all of medicine and which had after all preceded it. In the Lilliputian land of the viruses he had come upon disease-causing, apparently living particles, in size and shape (he wrote in 1950) "overlapping with bacteria at one end and with protein molecules at the other." In the twenty-five years since he had begun his own work with viruses, some nuance had been added to the old debate over whether viruses were living or nonliving matter. By then they were thought either to be retrograde forms of probably extinct but once free-living microorganisms, or to consist of large molecules of nucleoprotein primarily derived from the cells of the host. The former idea had for Goodpasture the advantage of beginning with an entity, probably a bacteria, that was endowed with the attributes of life. Yet he also thought that the latter, for the purposes of biological speculation, at least offered an evolutionary and not a devolutionary phenomenon and raised from the dust, strange as it seemed, the old problem of spontaneous generation of living matter that Pasteur thought he had disposed of decades before. Not that such theories were necessarily mutually exclusive: both assumed a virus to consist of a single molecule, and the factual basis of both theories suggested a molecule capable of reproduction and mutation, both important characteristics of living things.[55] Either way, Goodpasture was probing backward, looking for a source or a cause as the beginning point from which to ask how things happened since.

It was a search that to Goodpasture throughout his life illustrated the basic problem (and there were other examples besides viruses) of a subject that opened onto "the ancient and perpetual problem of life processes" but which held perhaps small immediate promise of utility—and perhaps no promise at all. How well such subjects were being tended, especially in the United States, concerned him over the length of his career as a scientist. When he came to Vanderbilt in 1925 neither the department of pathology nor any other preclinical or clinical department had a separate budget for research. The costs in time and materials of experimental and clinical investigation could be met, it was hoped, from the school's regular resources: income from endowment and fees. They could not for long. To the rescue, the Rockefeller Foundation, newly committed to the advancement of knowledge, offered what to almost everyone except purist institution builders like Flexner was a fairly ideal solution. The fluid research fund was for the time remarkably generous and accompanied by essentially no strings: an assured $250,000 over an eight-year period for whose allocation the faculty alone was responsible. It was a rare thing: money without a master. Including the two final years when the foundation's contribution fell to zero and Vanderbilt supplied the full sum, the fund ended its life in 1942—a time that, as later events showed, was not unfitting.

An era in the history of medical research at this particular university and in the country generally was then about to end. The nation was fighting its greatest war by panel and committee and it bequeathed to its postwar history the habits learned in crisis. As they were enlisted first in war and later in peace, medical research and the university medical schools, which since the beginning of the century had wonderfully produced so many useful things, followed larger national patterns. Of a major shift in those patterns, there was in research no clearer symptom than the shift in the relative importance of the comparatively long-term unsupervised subsidies of a fluid research fund and the term grant-in-aid phenomenon so familiar ever since. In the implications that this shift carried for a rather different approach to science, Goodpasture saw for the basic sciences special danger. The pursuit of knowledge to enrich understanding of fundamental principles could not be hurried: "it cannot be measured in time because it has no end." Besides, the best exploratory science was wasteful, and unless patrons, public or private, accepted the inefficiencies inherent in work whose very substance were things only poorly understood, then that kind of science could not function. Patrons of science, who made grants-in-aid for "projects," and scientists did not speak from the same intellectual vocabulary. "A project is an entity; it is something concrete; it can be described, defined, budgeted and evaluated by a remote committee; it can be time-limited to a year or so; it has the crispness of a contractual relation, a *quid pro quo;* it has the fiscal address of a good business proposition."[56] It was not Goodpasture's science.

By the time Goodpasture served as dean, from 1945 to 1950, most of his own research was behind him. It was a troubled time at Vanderbilt and elsewhere that did not suit his temperament or his history. There is about him (and some of the other of Robinson's original new men whose careers stretched beyond the war) something of a yearning for the world that they and Robinson had, so they thought, designed for permanence years before. But boldness is individual and, though surely present in many scientists in more recent years, it would become less apparent as their numbers increased and the institutional arrangements for their support changed. Masters multiplied as expectations rose. While the techniques of science ever improved, its purpose diffused. Basic scientists like Goodpasture felt, perhaps, such anxieties first and most intently, but, generalized as those anxieties quickly became, others in academic medicine and in practicing medicine would know them too. Habituated to believe that what they did—medicine—rightly ran to largely internal scientific or at least professional rhythms, they found more and more of their attention and energies consumed by challenges from the outside.

PART FOUR

Challenge and Response

Dependence 10

The techniques of doing medicine and science practiced at Vanderbilt in the late 1920s and 1930s were products of a special kind of freedom. Goodpasture's doubts in the 1950s about the fate of science and thus about the future of medicine rose from the fear of freedom lost. With foundation support Vanderbilt's medical school had bought independence from the community. Under one roof it had built its own self-contained physical plant. Endowment enabled it to pay new full-time teachers and to subsidize medical students and the hospital patients on whom they learned. A fluid research fund assured investigators of the continuity of support they needed to do good work. Neither the power of government at the federal, state, or local levels nor the demands of the private marketplace intruded greatly upon it. Designed for permanence and for a while functioning just as designed, Vanderbilt Medical School was a true "institution" after Flexner's own heart.

That did not mean, though, that Vanderbilt's values were therefore foreign or somehow hostile to the values of the community. In a pool of shared community values probably deeper then than now, the claims of science in medicine were to the layman already self-evident, even if not all people yet had opportunity to sample the product. But independence did mean that medical education and science as they were done at Vanderbilt were not directly accountable to the community. Both Flexner the educator and Kirkland the university builder would agree that it was an enviable position for an educational institution dedicated to learning. From where Kirkland stood at his retirement in 1937, the medical school (which was already famous and was then adding another large wing, thanks again to the General Education

Board) was a conspicuous success and one of the greater accomplishments of his fruitful career. It still was two years later when he died on the shores of his and Flexner's Canadian lake.

It was a good time to go, for what followed marked the steady erosion of that independence Kirkland so cherished. No one deliberately planned it that way, and some, like Goodpasture, fought to stay the tide. They failed. Had it been otherwise, theirs would have been a dubious success, however. They might have made the independent medical school of the future into precisely the kind of foreign body in the community that it had not been in the beginning, when the values of the community had been more agreeable. Independence would have been purchased at the price of isolation, something the school could ill-afford in a community that expected increasingly to be consulted about medical education and research and that increasingly was asked in one form or another to pay for it.

In the 1940s and later, the kind of freedom that Vanderbilt had enjoyed in glorious early days became socially less admissible and economically no longer possible. Even as scientific medicine grew more esoteric in its knowledge, which in a sense might have seemed to dictate greater isolation, it was being pulled back into the community. It was not just the local community, which was what had mattered to the old proprietary Vanderbilt of pre-Robinson days, but rather the community at large, which through various agents was making modern medicine a proprietary interest. Vanderbilt's story henceforth is the story of response and adaption to that community. Some of the original intellectual architecture endures and is a fitting testament to the skill of its builders; science still flourishes at Vanderbilt. But the loss of freedom required much new growth and remodeling. The disruptions of World War II, which Vanderbilt's medical staff prayed were "for the duration only," foretold it.

Wartime on the home front saw the methodical mobilization of the nation's productive capacity toward the single goal of victory. The requirements of victory brought many prewar institutional patterns into sharp relief and reconfirmed them in such broad areas of American life as industry, agriculture, and in much of education. Government fought the war by recruiting the talents of its citizens, and in the proven skills of the nation's industrial captains and their allies in banking and finance it summoned the ingredients of victory. Not just patriotism alone, but hard cash and public subsidy in various other forms moved them. Capitalists, whose old-fashioned homilies about free enterprise, individualism, and the American way had been decidedly out of fashion in government circles during Roosevelt's New Deal, answered the call, eager to do the work and to reap the glory. With their energies and the government's money, the nation lifted itself from depression to perform the prodigies of production that won total victory. Reform wilted, and an older capitalism, now allied with and elaborately financed by the state, took the new shape that it would keep after the peace. The substance, however, which since the 1920s at least had defined American life in the grammar of size and abundance, was not new and did not change. To "mass employment, mass production, mass advertising, mass distribution and mass ownership of the products of industry" the *Saturday Evening Post* ascribed the strength of the nation at war and at once said much of prewar experience and postwar developments.[1]

But size and abundance had decidedly not been the dominant themes in medical research and education at Vanderbilt before the war. Thus as medicine there was enlisted in the war effort and was forced to the national pattern, it was hastened down paths where it had not been before. At Vanderbilt the war experience itself was not particularly decisive in the loss of independence, but there were signs generally suggestive of the shape of things to come. In both education and research it felt the intrusion of the larger community that was at war. The intrusion therefore was blatant; Vanderbilt could not resist it and did not really want to. But both in the daily round of teaching and learning and in the conduct of science the tight, tidy, and self-regulated world of Robinson's new men was, with so much else, reshaped for victory.

In the training of doctors, the medical school found itself forced to do more and more with less and less. The year 1942 saw the institution at Vanderbilt of the national accelerated program of physician education whereby new first-year classes were admitted every nine months (June 1942, March 1943, December 1943, September 1944, and June 1945), the school operating on a year-round basis. Four years of work were covered in three calendar years, with another class of seniors graduating every nine months. All male medical students not physically disqualified had to join army or navy reserve units in order to complete their education without being drafted; thus Vanderbilt's student population became overnight predominantly military. Admission standards were not lowered (at least not formally), and not until 1945 did Vanderbilt admit students selected by the army and the navy rather than by its own admissions committee. At the graduate level of house staff training in the university hospital, there was more improvisation to try to balance manpower needs in the armed services with the need to maintain educational standards in the medical schools and their teaching hospitals. Under the "9-9-9 Plan" worked out between the schools and the Procurement and Assignment Service for Physicians of the War Manpower Commission, young M.D.'s served three nine-month terms as interns and as junior and then senior residents. Essentially a loan by the surgeon general of military personnel to civilian institutions, the plan helped maintain the house staffs whose members, as commissioned officers, would otherwise have been called to active duty after only one year of internship.

An inadequate house staff quota was one of the most frequent complaints of faculty, who found their own ranks sorely depleted just as the accelerated program made teaching loads heavier. Although the Procurement and Assignment Service froze a supposedly adequate core of faculty on the essential teaching list, many others enlisted to serve the cause more directly. Hugh Morgan, head of medicine, departed at the outset to head the Medical Consultants Division of the Office of the Surgeon General; John Youmans, his replacement, went two years later to become director of its Nutrition Division. Others joined the Vanderbilt 300th General Hospital unit and saw service in North Africa and Italy. For those who stayed behind less glamorously to mind the home fires, the desperate job of turning out more doctors with fewer teachers put everyone to the test.[2] More than usual the school relied on the volunteer services of its part-time clinical faculty, whose private practices were already overfilled because of the wartime doctor shortage. Everyone served long, hard hours for the usual low pay and in deteriorating conditions, and it was no surprise that as the war dragged on some were attracted by offers from other institutions.[3]

Yet it was a national emergency, and there is about those individuals—who taught the parade of students, who supervised the house staffs, and who traveled to countless committee meetings of countless agencies concerning the national defense—a certain stoutness typical of the home front generally, where most soldiers and civilians were determined to see the thing through, often as not with a smile. Even the stiffest of upper lips quavered, however, and the morale that springs from seeing everyone doing much more than their part sagged as strains mounted. On top of already slimmed-down and inexperienced house staffs, a nationwide shortage of nurses, anesthetists, and orderlies made operation of the hospital doubly difficult. Perhaps no kind of building gets harder use than a teaching hospital, and, at Vanderbilt's, maintenance postponed or ignored for lack of money, material, or labor piled up quickly to compound postwar problems.[4] And most frightening, that thing on which Vanderbilt probably most prided itself—high-quality undergraduate medical education for the select few—was falling, a casualty to wartime necessities. Biochemist C. S. Robinson complained that the class entering in 1944 needed not merely to review certain fundamentals but to learn them to begin with. The quality of those beginning the year the war ended "has continued to deteriorate to establish a new low."[5] Goodpasture, who reluctantly assumed the deanship on Leathers's retirement in 1945, surveyed the sad effects of wartime dislocation: "The results of maturity, inadequate preparation, faulty selection, accelerated tempo of studies and many unfavorable psychological factors were beginning to appear in the increasing number of students who failed in medical subjects, and in a generally lower scholastic attainment. Contributing to this result also were the depleted faculty and staffs and the excessive and continuous character of the teaching load."[6] Goodpasture was as proud of Vanderbilt as he was honest about what had become of it, and writing those words likely hurt.

Thus the community at war intruded upon education at Vanderbilt. Unambiguously it demanded, through the federal government, more doctors quickly. It mandated an accelerated program to get them. The medical school did what it was told, to the accompaniment of much stress, turnover, and shortages of every kind. The intrusion was made in the name of patriotic duty and was made fairly enough. Intrusion into research was justified similarly. It was directed by an agency of the federal government whose purpose was to marshal through research the new knowledge needed for victory. Though through the 1930s the idea of federal research grants to universities had generally seemed inappropriate,[7] the probability that the United States would soon be drawn into the war in Europe led Roosevelt in 1941 to establish the Office of Scientific Research and Development (OSRD). It was inspired and headed by mathematician and electrical engineer Vannevar Bush, a former vice-president of the Massachusetts Institute of Technology and a leading figure in American science. Over the course of the war, OSRD contracts worth millions of dollars went to universities and corporations for work on everything from proximity fuses to penicillin, from flame throwers to the atomic bomb.[8] The results were impressive and demonstrated that even scientists, long viewed by many as impractical idea-men, could be mobilized in the work that really mattered. As a wartime agency, the OSRD understandably was concerned less about the long-range effects of its subsidies than it was about winning the war. Its purpose was not to build up institutions to do research but rather to get research done. It was natural therefore for it to turn most frequently to those large institutions and companies already best staffed and equipped to do the job. OSRD work was concentrated at places like Dupont and General Electric and, in the academic world, at Harvard, Columbia, the California Institute of Technology, and MIT (the latter alone by the middle of 1945 held contracts worth $117 million).[9]

Vanderbilt, which was then neither large, wealthy, nor widely renowned for its work in science and technology, shared in this assignment but modestly.

The medical school received eight OSRD contracts through the war, totaling approximately $172,000. The medical staff who did the work saw them clearly for what they were: contracts for "to-order" research with a specific practical aim in mind. It was hardly the kind of research they at least professed to believe in. On the other hand, they saw in the contracts simple subsidy for research, and research was one of the things they did. Even if the aims of that research were for the moment dictated by wartime needs, mere subsidy was better than no subsidy at all. And who knew, perhaps in more normal times the terms of subsidy, if it continued, might be more congenial to their scientists' scruples. Administered by the OSRD's Committee on Medical Research, contracts first came to the medical school in late 1941 and early 1942, just as the ten-year term of the fluid research fund was running out. But only crudely could the OSRD subsidies be said to have filled the void left by the end of the older kind of support. The terms of the fluid research fund had been loose to say the least; those of the wartime government contracts were categorical in the extreme. They aimed to do different things. What the OSRD aimed to do was increase the store of useful knowledge of specific medical problems and conditions relevant to the conduct of the war. It wanted the scientists who worked at that knowledge to feel that they too had contributed to the war effort.

One of them was Cobb Pilcher, the brilliant young neurosurgeon who as head of the Section on Neurosurgery of the OSRD's Committee on Medical Research supervised some fifty war research projects across the country. When not on a plane or a train, he worked with colleagues back at Vanderbilt under two OSRD contracts on problems of chemotherapy in craniocerebral wounds. He studied the use of the sulfanomide drugs, then in early stages of development, in experimental infections of the brain and its covering, and he explored the effects of penicillin in the treatment of infections of the central nervous system. In brain surgery itself, he conducted experimental and clinical studies in the use of two new hemostatic agents, fibrin foam and the gelatin sponge, for the control of bleeding during surgery.[10]

Pharmacologist Paul Lamson, who at Alfred Blalock's invitation had joined in the summer of 1940 the subcommittee on shock of the National Research Council, gathered a small group at Vanderbilt under an OSRD contract to investigate the effect of anesthesia in shock. He carried out work to find a way of overcoming the reduced respiration that attended use of certain intravenous anesthetics then being introduced, and in related work he showed that the sulfanomides did not seriously affect the anesthetic action of intravenous anesthetic agents. Making a chemical attack on the problem of shock, the Vanderbilt group showed the extent to which the metabolic processes of the body were upset by shock, perhaps the most striking of which was the breakdown of coenzymes by the asphyxia produced in shock from hemorrhage.[11] In anatomy, Sam Clark and James A. Ward studied concussions and the effects of blast injuries, something the world was seeing much of just then, while in medicine Rudolph H. Kampmeier studied the use of penicillin in the acute stages of that hardy camp follower, syphilis.[12]

Other schools' files hold contracts for similar kinds of war work. Their depleted faculties probably undertook it as dutifully as did Vanderbilt's, and when it was all over they were praised in letters of commendation like the one sent in July 1946 to Vanderbilt's dean from the chairman of the Committee on Medical Research: "The new knowledge gained through the efforts of these investigators and their professional and technical colleagues not only strengthened our war potential and increased our national security but has provided additions of permanent value to the theory and practice of medicine, surgery, and related fields of medical science. You may be justly proud of the record of accomplishment of these members of your faculty."[13] The OSRD also provided more individualized tokens of the nation's gratitude, distributing engraved certificates of merit to everyone who had been engaged satisfactorily under an OSRD contract for at least six months. Decorated with a fierce-looking American eagle and Vannevar Bush's signature, they found their way onto thousands of study walls beside the diplomas, certifying solemnly that the holder had "participated in the work of the Office of Scientific Research and Development contributing to the successful prosecution of the Second World War."[14]

But war is hard on science, and it is not for scientific substance that the work done under OSRD contracts at Vanderbilt holds significance. Rather it is important as it represents a shift in the equation of power and dependence that determined how research got done and a shift in the nature of the relationship between those who did research and their patrons. Vanderbilt's medical scientists did the work out of genuine patriotism but also because the government paid, and research, as was acknowledged even by the late 1920s, invariably required some kind of special subsidy. The government paid, however, only on certain terms and according to procedures that carefully spelled things out. For example, the specific purpose and details of Vanderbilt's first OSRD project (the study of drug therapy in head wounds) were agreed upon ahead of time by Cobb Pilcher and the Committee on Medical Research. The contract itself defined how the books would be kept. Pilcher's work was to cost not more than $35,000 over a period of twenty months beginning December 1, 1941; the figure included a sum equivalent to 50 percent of the salary items to compensate Vanderbilt for the increase in general expenses such as utilities, maintenance, library, and incidental clerical costs attributable to work under the contract. Reimbursement was to be on an "actual cost" basis, upon receipt of vouchers classified according to the provisions of the contract. "Actual cost" meant expenditures by the contractor (Vanderbilt) for salaries and wages of employees directly engaged under the contract (plus Social Security taxes payable by the employer), and for supplies and equipment needed to do the work, for telegrams, long distance telephone and postage, and for traveling expenses not to exceed subsistence of $5.00 per person per day, standard Pullman lower berth fare, and five cents a mile by private car. There were standard procedures for the disposition of nonexpended materials. The government retained sole power, in the event of patentable discoveries, to determine whether or not application would be filed and over the title to any patent that might result. The results of work done under contracts were not to be made public without the written consent of the OSRD's contracting officer, and the university was to be vigilant of the dangers of sabotage. Finally, if progress seemed unsatisfactory, the government could on thirty days notice terminate the agreement.[15]

The mail from Washington showered Vanderbilt's OSRD investigators with "administrative circulars" that governed various aspects of war work and that, while taxing already harried investigators, seemed the unavoidable price of subsidy. In closing out one of Paul Lamson's projects, university treasurer Andrew B. Benedict chafed at running into "a tremendous amount of red tape." He sent to each head of an OSRD project the agency's five-page memo on "Accountability for Property at the Termination of a Contract," with the weary comment that "there seem to be a good many of details in connection with these matters but as they are requirements placed upon us which the OSRD is not willing to waive, we shall have to comply with them."[16] The contract dealing with anesthetics and shock was classified restricted, with the notation that anyone revealing its contents was subject to prosecution under the Espionage Act. Only persons investigated and cleared by the army, navy, and the FBI were to have access to confidential information and the files themselves when not in use were to be kept in a locked filing cabinet or safe. At Vanderbilt the need for secrecy in science in wartime was not then much debated, even though it sometimes entailed bothersome things like fingerprinting. Wrote Cobb Pilcher, whose contracts were not classified but who had received the OSRD's fingerprinting circular anyway: "I assume therefore that the recent communication regarding fingerprinting does not pertain to my contract. If it does, although obviously a waste of time on a non-secret matter, I see no particular objection to our conforming rather than raising an objection which would lead to endless correspondence and confusion."[17] Such were the daily, nonscientific trials of scientists in wartime.

What seemed only nuisances signified more than that. War research was indeed to one degree or another important, and in it many scientists were able to say they had done their duty. But it was also distracting and, if their complaints are to be believed, inimical to a tradition that, while not old at Vanderbilt, was already revered. In focused intensive work on shock or concussion, medical research was made into another instrumentality of victory. It served well: American troops suffered less than they might have and more came home again to pick up peacetime lives than otherwise would have. War showed just how well science could serve. Science in medicine served especially well and so justified itself anew. Total war and final victory demanded nothing less. Those demands left little time for reflection. Researchers scrambling to meet wartime needs as reflected in the subjects of OSRD contracts frequently did their greatest practical good in perfecting the application of general principles others had worked out earlier. It was in World War II, recall, that Alfred Blalock's insights into the nature of secondary shock received a grand application. It was then that Goodpasture's "egg" saved thousands.

It was then too that further fundamental work declined. Some private grants continued as they had before the war, when money from foundations and drug and chemical companies had matched the fluid research fund. But even with money, time and energy during the war were limited and assigned to other things. Heavy teaching loads made laboratory time scarce; what there was went to war work. "There has been carried only a restricted amount of fundamental research which I dare say has been interfered with to a considerable degree," wrote Leathers three weeks before D Day. "It is noticeable that the spirit of research has in a considerable measure disappeared under war conditions. The work of this kind has been greatly limited."[18] On that point all the "certificates of merit" were mute. Their good words spoke of service, not knowledge. But the best research done at Vanderbilt before the war had put knowledge first and service second. As the war neared its end, there were some who, as they slowly emerged from underneath government contracts and twelve-month teaching schedules, hoped it could be that way again.

The "spirit of research" whose passing Leathers lamented during the war owed much to the independence purchased in the 1930s by foundation philanthropy and by the fluid research fund in particular. Then investigators had done what they wanted, securely subsidized for a decade and insulated through the university from those who would harry them for results. As fate would have it, when that all ended the war both replaced the foundation with the government as the source of subsidy and altered the expectations placed on the research thus paid for. During the war the government, fixed on victory, expected to get what it paid for, and its contracts clearly defined the things it was after. Even though new and useful scientific knowledge about medicine could not be requisitioned in quite the same way one might requisition tanks or submarines, it could nonetheless be purchased. And in that transaction the scientists-turned-"contractors" ceased to enjoy a freedom that had earlier been viewed as a prerequisite for doing good science. They were also just then losing freedom as educators too, by mandate greatly accelerating the course by which they made doctors out of college students. Both losses, most Vanderbilt leaders assumed quite rightly, were sacrifices temporarily to be endured during a national emergency; when peace came their old freedoms would surely be restored. For the most part they were. To survive as scientists, Vanderbilt's doctors needed both freedom and funds. In the past they had had those things, and it is not surprising that in 1945 as they anticipated an end to the war's dislocations they looked to the future filled with hope.

The fluid research fund had made an enormous impression at Vanderbilt and was regularly held up as a model of how research could best be stimulated and stabilized. The wartime experience with OSRD, however, led many to anticipate that the federal government and not the foundations would become research's chief patron in years ahead. Measured in useful service, government-sponsored war research had after all resulted in an array of good things: the development of penicillin and the sulfa drugs, the use of plasma and blood substitutes for transfusions, the discovery of potent insecticides and vaccines to fight typhus and yellow fever. Vanderbilt was a small school and had participated in that work only modestly but enough at least to claim some of the spoils and to hope the future might hold more. Vanderbilt's medical scientists might complain bitterly about the dispiriting effects of "for-hire" research; they also could not help but be impressed by the sheer scope of government support for research during the war—and wonder, as Leathers did, whether "the momentum which has been given medical research, because of the war, [would] be continued or must we see a dwindling of the funds and opportunities with the result of failure to make continued progress in medical education and the results of new knowledge the treatment and control of disease?" It seemed probable that financial aid in the shape of federal grants-in-aid would sustain "the momentum." "It is exceedingly important," Leathers wrote early in 1945, "that Vanderbilt University avail itself of the trends in this matter in the postwar program."[19]

There were by then plans afoot. With Roosevelt's backing, OSRD director Bush appointed four committees to prepare recommendations on the future of government support for scientific research after the war. By spring 1945 the Medical Advisory Committee was circulating to medical deans a memorandum on the ways federal funds might be utilized in promoting research. Leathers (who would shortly be succeeded as dean by Ernest Goodpasture, who was a member of the Medical Advisory Committee) went to New York to confer with the committee and saw in its proposal promise of the kind of help Vanderbilt had not had since the days of the fluid research fund.[20] It tentatively outlined a "National Foundation for Medical Research" to be established as an independent agency of the federal government. To be administered by an executive council and an advisory board appointed by the president on recommendation of the National Academy of Sciences, the foundation would provide financial aid to medical research in three ways. It was the committee's opinion "that the broadest needs of medical research can best be met by locally administered, unrestricted funds," and to that end it proposed to grant to medical schools lump sums whose allocation would fall to a research committee of faculty specifically set up for that purpose. Long-term grants would be favored, and "the needs and promise of development in the applicant institutions" would be considered in making recommendations. Unrestricted research funds so distributed would, as the committee put it, ensure that "limitation in available information or lack of foresight on the part of the Advisory Board or Executive Council will not blight investigators or investigations of a tentative nature, or prevent development of fields which at the moment have no general recognition or appeal." Also envisaged was the use of unrestricted funds to establish junior fellowships for students in medicine and medically related fields to permit more specialized study of medical research techniques than was possible in the regular curriculum. Junior fellowships were not, however, to be used or viewed as general scholarships defraying the cost of medical education. Most medical schools produced practitioners; junior fellows were supposed to become scientists.[21]

The foundation's support for research would also take the form of another kind of fellowship, to be awarded those who already held the M.D. or the Ph.D. degrees. Renewable for up to six years and carrying stipends commensurate with university salaries, these fellowships were intended to enable talented young scholars contemplating research careers and with a potential for leadership in medicine to broaden their research experience either at their own or at other institutions. Fellows should engage in research training and in actual research but were not to exclude such activities in teaching and the clinical care of patients as sound research training might require. But as with the junior fellowships, which were not to be used as general scholarships, these fellowships were not to be used primarily to meet the needs of practice, either to obtain postgraduate degrees or to qualify for certification by the specialty boards. Finally, there would be a program to award categorical grants-in-aid to universities, medical schools, and other nonprofit scientific institutions for the support of specific projects or investigators. "Where circumstances warrant," long-term grants would be favored.[22]

Vanderbilt's researchers who had thrived on foundation subsidy in the 1930s could hardly themselves have put it better. The proposed granting of unrestricted research funds to be allocated by the faculties themselves was the perfect reincarnation of the fluid research fund, though this time the funds were to be drawn from an even fatter exchequer and not improbably for a longer period of time. Such support would be granted with an eye to strengthening whole institutions whose commitment to research clearly merited it. And it promised to decentralize the control of research monies through numerous universities and medical school administrations, thus safely insulating scientist from patron. The fellowship programs provided the enticements needed to assure a steady stream of new recruits for medicine's laboratories. Specialized grants meanwhile still allowed for the deliberate attacking of problems of great public urgency, which was essentially what the OSRD had done during the war and whose example was powerful among postwar planners.

It was a balanced proposal, for all parts of which there was sound practical precedent. Only the underlying general principle that "the health of the nation is a matter of public concern and merits public support" was new, though hardly revolutionary. The United States Public Health Service already had a long history (Vanderbilt's first federal money for research came in 1937 through the Public Health Service's program to fight syphilis), and during the war the generally superior medical care rendered to the country's armed forces had proven the worth, at least for an emergency, of what was basically state medicine. As the postwar era dawned, it was apparent that many shibboleths about the danger of interference implicit in public subsidy were breaking down, and it was on precisely that point that the Committee on Medical Research went to some pains to allay lingering suspicions. Actions of the proposed public research agency were to be couched as recommendations and invitations only and were never to be construed as binding upon any investigator. "Thus the National Foundation for Research would come to share in the leadership of medical investigation without challenging the priority of individual initiative or freedom of research, and with a minimal danger of coercion and regimentation, which lead not only to mediocre work but to disastrous destruction of the research spirit. Community of interests, independent scientific curiosity, and regard for the common weal must in peace replace as a cohesive force the patriotism of war."[23]

Thus all of the old verities would be honored by a new master, in whose service the scientists would find perfect freedom. The proposal for the new public agency did not say how much of its resources would be apportioned to unrestricted support to institutions and how much to fellowships and categorical grants to individuals, or what might be the criteria for making those divisions. It was on the amount going to unrestricted institutional support, after the manner of the fluid research fund, however, that hinged the credibility of the new foundation as guardian of true research in the old sense. But as a proposal only, some vagueness was expected. Its authors were guilty of no special disingenuousness or naiveté for tentatively seeking to combine things that were not always or even often perfectly compatible: in this case, an understanding of science in medicine as an instrument of public progress, with the veneration of science more abstractly as the key to knowledge whether or not it was useful. Not all of the committee's proposal ever saw the legislative light of day, and the shape that public support for medical research took after the war, in the vastly expanded National Institutes of Health, reflected more the realities of public policy making where the expenditure of tax revenues was accompanied by the political necessity of real and regular accountability to the people's representatives.[24] At Vanderbilt the trial balloon elicited generally enthusiastic response. Only the irascible Barney Brooks replied that he could not "possibly understand how any one with any respect for scientific accuracy could submit even an estimate of funds which could be usefully employed in the indefinite future, with even more indefinite knowledge of the conditions which will exist." His colleagues, less constrained, replied hungrily with wish lists for research that had yearly price tags ranging from $3,000 (anatomy) to $70,000 (pharmacology).[25]

Brooks may simply have been out of sorts that day, although his concern for the amount of money that actually could be applied productively to research then or in the indefinite future was also a concern of the authors of the proposal for the new foundation. They were scientists themselves and knew that the path from subsidy to discovery was seldom a straight one. Perhaps fearful that supply would outrun demand and thus help create it, they urged that federal subsidies for research be "modestly initiated" and "conservatively increased only with the demonstrated capacity of the country to utilize them." However instrumental science in medicine had shown itself to be, they did not want to throw money at it just because money was there. Moreover, they did not want the proposed research foundation to get into the broader business of supporting institutions that could not support themselves. That was something that would have been considerably more radical than any plan merely to subsidize research alone and was something they professed to want to avoid. They were proposing federal support for medical research and not for medical education, though as Flexner had said years before one could not really be had without the other. The urgent need of medical schools generally, the places where both research and education primarily took place, was not in 1945, they said, for public underwriting but rather for a more solid permanent financial base. To that end, they urged "that every consideration be given to methods of increasing medical school endowment, *pari passu* with the addition of special funds for research purposes."[26] That proved hard to do.

In the early postwar years it quickly became apparent that "special funds for research purposes" were considerably easier to get than new money to bolster old endowments. Because much of the special research money came from the federal government and, as it turned out, in the form of term categorical grants to individuals and not as the unrestricted sums to institutions that the Committee on Medical Research had favored, research tended within the medical schools to self-segregate in terms of budgets and personnel. Mainly federal research grants constituted by 1955 a third of the income of American medical schools, which were becoming, even the technically "private" ones, dependent on NIH for survival. Though enrollments grew slowly, faculties mushroomed until by the end of the 1960s there averaged more than one full-time faculty member for every two medical students. Most, thanks to NIH, were not primarily teachers, however, but rather were researchers, nearly half of whom were supported in part from federal funds.[27]

Such massive support for research was both a blessing and a distraction. Indeed, the sum of medical knowledge grew enormously, but as it did Flexner's old dictum that research and education were inseparable (a dictum to which Vanderbilt's new leaders all had subscribed) came finally unstuck, even though catalog rhetoric would not let it peacefully die. It came unstuck at Vanderbilt because the school no longer found itself of its own resources able to support the things it was called upon to do and the things its architects felt it should do. Hospital and medical school endowment had never yielded enough to subsidize students, patients, and research, but in the 1930s the fluid research fund fortuitously had brought outside help on the select terms that made real unity possible. Beginning in the 1940s, research was subsidized from the outside largely on other terms that made unity ever less real. It was also in the 1940s that endowment ceased adequately even to subsidize students and patients, thus reducing even further the old freedom and driving the school more and more into the community.

The wartime experience shook severely the little world Robinson, Flexner, and Kirkland had called into being only twenty years before. The curriculum was hurried to the point where good faculty members complained of teaching poorly. Students with things on their minds other than becoming doctors sometimes performed poorly. House staff and nurses were too few and too much worked. In the laboratories and wards up and down the long corridors, researchers investigated to government requisition. Though all did their duty, for no one could normalcy return fast enough. To most people "normalcy" meant the way things had been before the war. It did to Waller Leathers, the dean then, who had tried to defend his faculty from raids by the military and other universities, to produce decent doctors, and to turn out creditable research. But Leathers, who retired in 1945 and died a year later, was spared revelation of how unlike the early days things henceforth would be. Goodpasture the quiet scientist succeeded him, to preside for five troubled years over matters far from his mind's desire in the laboratory and over events he could not control.

At medical schools like Vanderbilt, which on the strength of the foundations' money and their own faculties' talent were reared up in so short a time to such magnificence, it is strange that fear so quickly overtook them. It was likely part of a larger national pattern of postwar uncertainty that left many people in many walks of life worried over what would come next. Having fought to total victory on all fronts, the nation found thrust upon it burdens of active world leadership that took continued exertion and much getting used to. Thousands of servicemen returning from Europe and the Pacific knew for sure only that they wanted to get home. They did not know whether home was going to be the proverbial land fit for heroes to live in or, fresh in the memory of many of them, another depression-ridden disappointment brought back by the end of war production and their own return to the labor market. Those who had stayed home to run the factories around the clock shared their fear. Everyone wanted the war to be over, but no one wanted things the way they had been in the late 1930s when the shadow of low production and high unemployment still stretched long across the land. From all that the new world of academic medicine had been insulated, though not perfectly. Medical schools too in the 1930s saw the value of their endowments shrink and patrons grow more cautious. Some of their best human talent was sacrificed to the necessities of retrenchment: such was Canby Robinson's fate at Cornell. But medical schools also prospered, at least relatively. Salaried full-time teachers, though never paid munificently, found themselves more secure than some of their practicing colleagues who lived by the market; indeed, secure academics at well-endowed universities might actually see their standard of living rise as the cost of living fell. Vanderbilt's medical school in the 1930s prospered well enough, actually adding both to its endowment and to its buildings.

Thus if Vanderbilt's doctors were uncertain after the war, along with other

Americans, they understandably thought more in terms of a simple restoration of the recent past than did the factory workers, many of whom had not known peacetime prosperity since the 1920s. All of a sudden, however, Vanderbilt's prewar world seemed rapidly slipping away, to the accompaniment of not a few anguished cries that it should all go for naught. Declining return on investments, small expectation of enlarged endowment, diminishing reserves, higher operating costs everywhere, and augmented demands for service of various kinds spelled critical times and not just for Vanderbilt. Deans and other leaders of medical education filled the professional press with warnings and prescriptions, and in 1947 the presidents of nineteen leading universities (among them Vanderbilt's new chancellor, Harvie Branscomb) issued a joint public statement on medical education that indicated just how close to the edge they thought things had come.[28]

As educators they claimed naturally enough that the future of medical care and public health depended on medical education and not on the new hospitals and clinics, the new drugs, medical insurance plans, and state subsidies that so impressed the public. A continuing supply of well-trained physicians had to be secured for the future, a job that the country's forty-three private and twenty-seven tax-supported medical schools were not then prepared to do. Medical education, they explained, was the most expensive kind of professional training, and only by large increases in endowment, or long-term gifts, or both could its costs be met, particularly in the private schools that typically had "set the pace." The war had been hard on all medical schools, stripping their faculties and commandeering their laboratories, and until they fully recovered, which would take time, talk of new schools to meet the growing need for doctors was foolish. Grants for research, they said, seldom eased daily operating costs, while aid from foundations though once munificent promised just then not to exceed $4 million a year, which was a fraction of total operating costs. Several leading schools were predicting that in the near future they would need twice their current income just to maintain current levels of operation, and more would be needed if new areas were to be explored as science and the times demanded.

Other areas of higher education too, said the nineteen university presidents, would need expanded support in years to come, but the claims of medical education are "obvious and paramount to the actual health and well-being of every citizen, and we speak for it here with special emphasis." That must have pleased their medical deans, though what exactly they had in mind beyond that is not clear. They did not publicly anticipate or ask for federal subsidy for education, though whether they really believed that the people would choose to pay for that education privately rather than collectively is a moot question. They claimed to, confidently: "We believe that if this situation is clearly understood by our fellow citizens, they will rally to the support of medical education. Through private support American medical schools have set a standard for the world. Private support should not now abandon them through ignorance of the facts, temporary uncertainties, or absence of mind." Clearly the statement was not prescriptive except in the most general way. Rather it was educational and political. The presidents would set the facts straight and shake up the absent-minded. And they would go on record that private support was the key to the future just as it had been in the past and that the hour was already late and the need extreme.

The presidents' general perception of the rising value Americans would place on their physical health was right. Though they would not always do so privately, the people would pay and pay willingly. Medical education, more broadly defined as the years went by, did move ahead. By most measures, it prospered enormously. But the fears that time later proved illusory just then filled the days of sober and clearheaded people. How fragile was a place like Vanderbilt, Goodpasture soon discovered to his own great despair. When he became dean in 1945 everything seemed wrong. The quality of the medical students was not what it should be and their performance was down.[29] War research was one thing, but the lack of unrestricted funds for basic research had resulted in "a drastic reduction in the extent and depth of original inquiry."[30] But it was the university hospital that was cause for the most immediate crisis and that brought into sharp relief the school's failing ability to sustain its old independence.

The problem with the hospital, which in Robinson's plans had been so closely integrated with the medical school, was this. In its clinics and wards Vanderbilt's medical students learned their clinical medicine. It was an educational tool of the medical school and, as originally conceived, only secondarily a service institution to the community. To function properly as an educational tool it required both a certain quantity and a certain quality of patients—or in the medical vernacular, "clinical material." There had to be enough beds to supply classes of fifty students ample opportunity first-hand to see and to begin to treat disease. As first constructed, the Vanderbilt Hospital barely had enough, and in some areas like surgery it fell considerably short. The construction of the new wing in the 1930s kept it adequate only for a time. But just as important, those beds had to be filled with the right kinds of patients. Not just any sick people would do, but only those who illustrated the variety of pathological conditions that students needed to see. Constantly to achieve that educational goal, the hospital staff who were also teachers maintained tight control over who was admitted and who was not.

To do that day in and day out required purchasing patients from among the community's indigent sick. The hospital bought them with free care made possible by endowment and low costs.

It was an ideal arrangement but stable only as long as costs rose no faster than the endowment income available to meet them. At Vanderbilt, where it worked well for not much more than a decade, hospital deficits had already by the late 1930s led to the imposition of limits on free care. After the war, deficits grew apace of rapidly inflating operating costs, and by the end of 1948 losses resulting from care of indigents were averaging close to $300,000 a year. As the hospital's reserve funds were expended, medical school endowment was shifted to balance the budgets, which resulted in the loss of those funds for strictly educational purposes, and in 1947 and 1948 the income on $6 million of university endowment was used to defray the hospital deficit. Clearly, the need for income was wrecking the old dogma that only those patients be admitted who in the eyes of the staff were useful for teaching purposes, regardless of whether or of how much they could pay. Going outside, Chancellor Branscomb tried without success to persuade the governments of Nashville and Davidson County to pay $8.50 per patient per day for local poor treated at the university hospital. Finally, on May 1, 1948, free care of indigents was completely eliminated when all patients were required to pay the minimum daily charge of $8.50, either from their own funds or from some supporting agency.[31]

The conflict between the need to fill the hospital with paying patients and thus raise income and the need to fill wards and clinics with the most useful teaching cases was not resolved until well into the 1950s and then only by reliance on third parties. But in the first postwar years that prospect was not at all clear, and how realistically to balance Vanderbilt's responsibilities against its very limited means was subject for some considerable debate, none of it academic. Late in the war the medical school had commissioned an outside study of the Vanderbilt Hospital and its relation to medical care and education. The first of several to appear over the next three decades proffering analysis of present problems and advice on how to meet the future, it appeared in 1946 under the name of the chief consultant, Basil C. MacLean of the Strong Memorial Hospital at the University of Rochester.[32] Like the reports that followed it, this one (which made fifty recommendations ranging from major changes in executive organization and financial procedures to the need to contract with an exterminator to keep down the cockroaches) did not read the future perfectly, but it did parade all at once the host of problems that measured the school's and the hospital's limits against what likely would be expected of them.

It saw those expectations not only in terms of a concept whose triumph in the 1960s and 1970s congeries of public and professional forces had assured but also in terms that already in the 1940s seemed to some self-evident. Though Vanderbilt was not especially quick to acknowledge it, the concept of medical schools as part of large medical service centers, with ever-expanding responsibilities in the medical or (as it would increasingly be called) the "health" field, was something that in time would render ever more remote the austere world of Robinson's courts and corridors. If the consultants in 1946 were to be believed, Vanderbilt needed to become a medical center, or at least to take the lead in forming such a center in Nashville. In a number of cities there had already developed close geographical and organizational ties between medical schools and university and municipal hospitals, bringing, ambitiously, "to all classes of patients all types of medical service under the highest standards of professional supervision."[33] Nashville and Vanderbilt needed to move in the same direction.

Their ability to do so, the report said, would in part be determined by local economic conditions, which was to say again that the age of glorious isolation was over. When compared with ten cities of about the same size, Nashville in 1940 ranked tenth in per capita income and its surrounding counties well below the rural level of living index for the country as a whole. For Nashville and an area within a radius of approximately fifty miles that its hospitals served, there were 2.45 beds per 1,000 population, considerably below the 4.5 to 5 beds per thousand then thought to be a desirable minimum. It seemed evident, therefore, that needs could not be adequately met without more beds and better utilization of beds already there. Vanderbilt (with 340 beds—more than any other Nashville hospital), ever wary of who was admitted, in 1945 had an average occupancy rate of only 64 percent, something obviously intolerable financially for the hospital and because it set poorly with "the service aspect of the institution,"[34] which would increasingly define and legitimate the medical center of the future.

Vanderbilt needed to do better and to appear to do better. It is "an unusual condition," the report said charitably, that at such an important institution "emergency facilities are almost non-existent." Students learned much from them, and the public rightly expected them. Rightly or wrongly, the public partly judged things by their appearance, and by the end of the war Vanderbilt made a poor showcase. Though part of its general dinginess was due to wartime shortages and inefficiencies, there was "little evidence of imagination, supervision or inspection. The visitor, on entering the main lobby of the hospital, finds himself in an atmosphere suggestive of a third-rate hotel, Spartan-like in its barrenness and discomfort." Outpatients commonly used it as a waiting room and on one occasion a member of the resident staff was seen using the lobby for a nose and throat examination. "The loud instructions of the house officer were accompanied by guttaral sounds from the patient in a performance which could hardly add dignity to the foyer of a university hospital." The lobby of the medical school (which Robinson also had handsomely done up with oak paneling) was worse, suggesting "a combination of a bus station, a five and ten store and Coney Island. It lacks only a juke box."[35]

Doing better—more and better-utilized beds, up-to-date equipment, better nursing, clean and modern facilities, all the things that made for public service—required, for the first time and with great urgency, a more realistic relationship between charges and costs, something up to then as foreign in academic medicine as in university life generally. The consultants in 1946 predicted that with payment being made less by individuals and more by insured groups, both public and private, truly cost-related charges would be socially acceptable. More and more, hospital care was being viewed as a necessary commodity, to be paid for, most often collectively, by those who used it or who might use it. The "tincup era" of hospital finance was about at an end,[36] and as it ended so was diminished the old philanthropic character of the university hospitals and clinics. As the people determinedly mobilized their resources, first through private and later through government insurers, to buy the medical care that in their judgment had joined food, shelter, and schooling as a requirement of the good life, the university medical center dispensed its services more and more for fees charged to someone on the outside. Too poor to go it alone, they had small choice.

In time, Vanderbilt like most others made the choice. There was, however, another way, which while taken neither then nor later, retains more than historical interest. Goodpasture, in 1948 and 1949 a very frustrated dean, proposed it. It is important not because Goodpasture was the dean or because his views were widely shared (which they were not) but because it represents in "pure culture" (as he would have said in the laboratory) the dualism of science and service in medicine, just as the great era of service was getting under way. The dualism would not again at Vanderbilt be stated so starkly; compromises and generally easier times inevitably gentled it. Still, to see it now is to be reminded not merely of one particular crisis at one particular school but of two fundamentally different (though not necessarily incompatible) ways of regarding what medical schools like Vanderbilt were supposedly about. Goodpasture did not get his way and probably never expected to. What he did get, forced to it as he was by crisis, was the pleasure of an analytical exercise. As a scientist he was good at that, and as if he were working on his viruses he carefully broke the problem down and asked how things happened.

He proposed to discontinue at the earliest possible date the undergraduate curriculum of the medical school and, utilizing all present facilities and resources, to create in its place a scientific institute devoted to medical research and education at the graduate and postgraduate levels.[37] Though bold, the proposal was a radical departure from the past in practice only. In principle, it confirmed the past, specifically Vanderbilt's history since 1925. As then reorganized, he argued, the medical school and others like it symbolized the rapid development of scientific knowledge applied to medicine during the first quarter of the twentieth century. That in turn rested directly upon the preceding quarter-century of scientific discovery, made possible by the application of the experimental method to basic problems of biology. The work of Pasteur, Koch, and Bernard were typical of that luminous era. The rapid accumulation of scientific knowledge useful to medicine, Goodpasture said, thereafter "captivated the imagination of leaders in medical education and directly the philanthropy of American wealth toward an integration of this new science into our American educational institutions." Integration meant the essential unity of research and education, and because medical teachers henceforth could not divorce themselves from research, it became necessary to train a new breed of teacher-investigators. New medical schools had to be created and old ones renovated to accommodate the new science and prepare its future leaders. Hopkins led the way, and Vanderbilt, though among the last to follow, embodied the new ideal of scientific medicine more comprehensively than any other. Its experience since its fresh new beginning in 1925 proved the wisdom of that revolutionary undertaking. Marching hand in had, research advanced knowledge and training applied it.

That experience also showed how general education lagged behind the forefront of scientific knowledge. When the new school opened it was without question necessary to concentrate as it did great expense and effort on undergraduate medical education aimed at supplying a higher level of practitioner and at discovering new talent for research. Not a little of the knowledge so transmitted and most of the inspiration for it sprung from medical science's first heyday in the late nineteenth and early twentieth centuries. In the meantime, the public had grown to appreciate the beneficent effect the new education was having on its own welfare. And, Goodpasture wrote, "this public has at last determined that it will have in full measure the fruit of discoveries and the services of the profession trained to administer them." The public did not, however, often appreciate the increasingly complicated techniques in research and training upon which all hope of better service rested. "We therefore witness at the present time a great avalanche of funds for research along particular lines that have a public appeal, coupled with an inordinate and unprecedented demand for services, with what seems to be a complete absence of comprehension, even on the part of potent influences, of the underlying essential element of adequate support for the structure from which both research and application must always depend; namely our institutions of higher learning." The foundation had been laid less than a century before but already was crumbling. "Because the public wants medical service, it will have it, and we can see the handwriting distinctly on the wall": the American Medical Association was idolizing the general practitioner; the military, the public health service, and social reformers were crying for more doctors; proposals in Congress were giving precedence to the number of medical graduates rather than their quality. "In this rapid reorientation of emphasis upon service at current levels, educational and research potentials are becoming dissipated and weakened except perhaps in a few temporarily fortunate institutions."[38]

Vanderbilt was not one of them. In the midst of such demand it found itself bankrupt financially and with slim prospect of the resources needed to set things right. The local government would not support indigent patients; faculty and staff were being dissipated to the city hospital and the veterans hospital. Through financial necessity the Vanderbilt Hospital had been converted into an essentially private service institution of little value to teaching or research. Too many personnel were underpaid, too many departments understaffed and administered in a skeleton form only. Already there had been too much patching and filling, some of it no doubt a hangover from wartime habits of muddling through. But further absence of a true policy promised to bring the house down. Offering one, Goodpasture appealed to what had been the purpose, policy, and program of the school in its first twenty-five years: the fostering of research and medical education at the highest level. He hoped it would continue to prevail.

Medical education at Vanderbilt in the 1950s and after did not need to take the same form it had in the 1930s. Indeed if it did, it would no longer be education at the highest level. Anyone with one ear to the ground could not doubt that the nation would support undergraduate medical education, in both state and private schools, and at a level of standards attained during the past twenty-five years. "Existing undergraduate schools will be enlarged and others will be built," Goodpasture said. "Public demand and governmental support will effectively see to this." What worried him were the prospects for sustaining at a higher level the combination of research and education that provided the creative talent and leadership needed "if we are to go forward rather than to sink to the low level of service distribution for which the demand is so compelling today."[39]

The program Goodpasture envisaged would instead lead the school to a new high ground in research and the advanced training of select medical scientists. The undergraduate curriculum would be abandoned, along with the department of preventive medicine and public health. The remaining preclinical departments, in close relationship with the science departments of the college, would offer graduate students the master's and the Ph.D. degrees. In the past, great need had been experienced for research laboratories designed specifically for clinical investigation, something then accomplished in a number of small isolated facilities throughout the school (for example: the Rh laboratory in pediatrics, the EKG laboratory in medicine, the EEG laboratory in anatomy). Under the new scheme, several large division laboratories would be set up for the conduct of significant clinical research. The division of nutrition, already established under William Darby and intermediate between medicine and biochemistry and transcending many departmental barriers, was a good example of what should be done also with parasitism and immunity, endocrinology and metabolism, cellular growth and cancer, cardiovascular physiology and radiobiology. The clinical departments themselves would, where competent leaders were available, be broken up into individual specialties each headed by a chief: neurosurgery, gynecology, orthopedics, and so forth would become separate units whose continuation depended on their filling an assigned number of beds in the reorganized hospital.

The university hospital would, in Goodpasture's plan, be converted into a teaching and research institution for postgraduate training in the several advanced clinical specialties. Even in the clinical fields the primary emphasis would be on research, and hospital admissions policy would be governed by the availability of the appropriate staffs. Postgraduate students did not require the great variety of patients so important to undergraduates, which was one of the great problems of the hospital as then operated. Under the new system, patients (all of whom would be teaching patients) would be highly selected to match the particular competence and facilities of a particular service. The staff of each specialty would operate in both teaching and research only within a carefully specified area. Under such conditions Goodpasture believed the hospital could adequately fill its beds either with private or with subsidized patients; however, it could be stipulated realistically that the hospital must operate at cost, a demand that could not be made given the teaching conditions needed for the instruction of undergraduates. Specifically, there was on hand already the professional ability to develop specialties too long neglected, among them psychiatry, ophthalmology (for which he cited the Wilmer

Ophthalmological Institute at Johns Hopkins as a good example), neurosurgery and chest surgery, nutrition, and endocrinology. Dermatology was one of the most sorely neglected specialties in the country. Work in radiobiology and active isotope therapy was just beginning. Orthopedics, urology, otolaryngology, and plastic surgery all held much promise. There was broad field for work in tuberculosis and cardiovascular disease. Gynecology needed to become a specialty under its own leadership, while pediatrics, which was becoming a hospital within a hospital, could fill beds in any number of special areas.

On it all would be spent the entire income from the school's and the hospital's $14 million endowment: then about $560,000 a year. The preclinical departments would get $150,000, the divisional laboratories $100,000. Each specialty on the clinical side would be as self-supporting as possible: patients would pay, and staff would collect fees for service rendered and would themselves pay office rent. One hundred thousand dollars from the school would cover laboratory space and research facilities. Overhead was figured at $170,000, while $40,000 remained unallocated, possibly to go to fellowships.[40] Tuition and special grant funds would be extras. Best of all, government aid could better be accepted by such a research institute "without the dread and apprehension that overshadow government subsidy of education."[41]

It was a stunning proposal that in some respects foreshadowed some of what was in fact to be: the divisional laboratories and the breakdown of the clinical departments, for example. On the main points, however, it had the effect of a star shell, which momentarily shows things in stark and eerie relief and then returns them to murky darkness. The choice to Goodpasture was simple enough: continue educating medical undergraduates, which with existing resources would mean compromising on the old Vanderbilt standards; or, set sights on advanced specialized research and teaching, which with the same resources would mean important contributions to the true scientific substance of medicine of which still precious little was known. The first would be a pathetic comedown for a school that overnight had risen to eminence. There was no justification, he wrote, "for a Vanderbilt Medical School whose objective is only the graduation of its complement of physicians to serve the health requirements [of the nation]." The second alternative, though, promised to preserve in new form the old spirit of science since the early days of its union with medicine. "There is and always will be need and a great need for advancement of knowledge and superior training. Our modern civilization, not its medical aspects alone, must be supported by the best minds of the Nation, trained in the most advanced technical boundaries of science if we are to go forward intellectually."[42]

The second choice (on which, incidentally, Goodpasture staked his job as dean) was also, at the exalted level of whole institutions, analogue for his own private convictions about how scientists justified their work. He pictured Vanderbilt's medical school as a school of science whose special field was medicine, not as a school of medicine more broadly conceived but whose tools and techniques came from science. Knowledge about how human biology worked, not service to meet rising demand for medical care, defined what it really did or should do. That more knowledge historically had made for better service and the probability that it would continue to should not be allowed to confuse things and make the linkage appear more direct than it actually was. Better service was fine, and such as it was, it rested on better science. But better science never led necessarily to more and better service, which failure detracted not a bit from its worth as science.

The plan presumed more boldness than can commonly be summoned in large committee-governed institutions. The last time the school had so radically changed course (then in principle as well as in practice, back in 1919 when Kirkland and the General Education Board struck their deal), it had been enticed by the power both of great subsidy and of irresistibly superior ideas. In 1949 Goodpasture had no GEB, and what he proposed could be too easily construed as the betrayal of a golden past built on those ideas. His argument that only by changing practice could principle be preserved was subtle and not fitted to convince people for whom much pride and prestige were at stake. Besides, Goodpasture had probably worked out more clearly for himself the proper relation of science and service than had many of his less analytical colleagues. Most of them shrank from the thought of apparent retreat and were unpersuaded that somehow ways and means could not be found to enable the school to go on doing and doing well the things it always had. Even his close friend and confidant, anatomist Sam Clark, who saw the plan before anyone else and said he believed in it, could not bring himself to desert the basic undergraduate curriculum, especially "in the face of the great need for doctors."[43] Pharmacologist Paul Lamson (like Goodpasture one of the original new men) argued that what Vanderbilt had been for twenty years it could with effort be again: neither a "super-science institution" nor a "mass production medical school" but above all a school peopled by students and talented scientist-teachers "obligated to no one."[44] Psychiatrist Frank Luton likewise found abandonment hard to contemplate, and neurosurgeon Cobb Pilcher, though finding the plan for a great center of postgraduate instruction "one of the strongest and most inspiring proposals in my experience," felt that it would "best be based upon the firm foundation of an undergraduate medical school," providing it was returned to its old standards of quality in teaching and research.[45]

There were other more cautious ideas, which more closely approximated actual developments. A special committee was appointed to advise the dean on ways out of the financial crisis. Consisting of Amos Christie (pediatrics), John Burch (gynecology), Henry Clark (director of the hospital), Hugh Morgan, and Cobb Pilcher, it judged that efforts should first and foremost be directed to the survival of the undergraduate medical school. Admitting that if research died education would languish, they saw education that produced new research workers as the greater imperative: "Medical schools must foster and nourish medical research, but in order to do so they must survive as schools." Vanderbilt's ability to survive, they said, was crippled by lack of community support, which it had never cultivated, and the inability of the hospital to utilize satisfactorily the indigent sick. There was not even a limited private practice plan whereby professional fees were partly returned to the school to help finance it. As a solution, they proposed a community-university hospital plan to help square the rights and interests of the local profession with the interests of the university. Such a plan might include construction of a new city hospital to be operated by the university but providing an open, nonteaching service to local practitioners. The present university hospital then could either be closed or used for special purposes such as cancer research or possibly even as rentable office space. New sources of support needed to be discovered and the community had to be compelled to assume the financial burden of indigent care. On this point in particular Pilcher felt so strongly that he said the university should announce publicly that the hospital would close its doors on July 1, 1949, unless completely relieved of operating costs by the community, and he said, "I should not be in favor of its being a bluff."[46]

Chancellor Harvie Branscomb, who like his predecessors spent much time and energy on medical tangles, also had looked for closer relations between Vanderbilt and the community as a way out of current tangles. Hospital beds had to be filled and paid for, and paying patients from the community would help to do that. Meanwhile neither he nor the university's board of trust relished the possibility of giving up the medical school, no matter how impressive a research institute was to replace it. Branscomb presented Goodpasture's plan with the recommendation that it not be accepted, and though the difficulties hardly ended there, the board's rejection of it meant that in the future things would somehow have to be worked out short of divestiture.[47] They were, slowly and with much wringing of hands—but not with Goodpasture in charge. He did not leave the deanship in a huff, but he was serious about not wanting to preside on terms other than those he had outlined.[48] Quitting the business of educating M.D.'s was something never seriously discussed at Vanderbilt again, as Goodpasture's successor, John Youmans, and his successors went about the harried work of tending to that job and the many others thrust upon medical schools in recent times. Goodpasture's analysis of science, service, and expectations in medicine, however, only gained in relevance.

John Youmans was the last of the original new men to preside. His tenure saw key departments pass into younger hands, and it saw the new leaders become old. He was a more successful dean than Goodpasture: he had more training, for one thing, already a veteran of the deanship at the University of Illinois. He also had an administrator's shyness for apocalyptic thinking and institutional changes (like Goodpasture's proposal) that hinted betrayal of past glories. Though Goodpasture's analysis of current trends in science and medicine was correct in the abstract, his proposal judged incorrectly the degree to which universities through their boards, chancellors, and deans commonly crave institutional completeness. The completeness that included medical schools had been sanctified long ago by Flexner, and at Vanderbilt it was an article of faith and nonnegotiable. With such thoughts safely put behind it, the school continued in the 1950s to turn a few college students into doctors (classes still hovered around fifty) and, also faithful to Flexner, to build up medicine as a distinct discipline of science. Increasingly that meant breaking medicine down into subspecialties. At the same time, demands for service and growing public subsidy reduced even more Vanderbilt's old independence. Alan Gregg once described medical research's beginnings as a private matter and its evolution into a public one as part of a natural history of inventions, whose power to affect the lives of large numbers of people eventually compels the people to assert their own control if not their proprietorship over the invention.[49] It turned out to be not greatly different at Vanderbilt in medical education and medical service, where the growing allocation of public resources showed clearly what the public valued.

During the first disrupted years after the war, the fear, implicit for a moment at least, that the public would not pay and that the whole grand edifice of modern medical education might disintegrate as costs rapidly outstripped the traditional means of meeting them, proved unfounded. Goodpasture had known that when he said that if the people want more doctors and more medical care they will surely have them one way or another. Youmans and the others knew it too. The things that Vanderbilt's medical school produced every year would enjoy ever-greater demand, happily for its graduates for whom jobs were never a problem and for their mentors who basked secure in the community's esteem. But for private schools like Vanderbilt, boom times in medicine also threatened to and did change their nature. As the school stepped gingerly through the 1950s, at once cleaving to memory of Robinson's perfectly designed world and keeping alive some of its substance and all the while piling up a hefty array of NIH grants-in-aid for research, it became apparent that events were running ahead of policy.

Research presented the fewest difficulties. Unambiguously it had been ordained during the old order and abundantly it would be supported in the new one from the beginning. In this, both the practicing profession as organized in the AMA and the medical schools were of one mind. Money for research was in keeping with the Flexnerian prescription for advancing medicine as science, which inevitably added to the skill and power of practitioners. Research made possible excellence, a word increasingly used during the 1950s. It did not, however, threaten in any direct way the sacred realm of private practice. The stick of higher standards and better quality through science could still be used convincingly to beat down demands for a higher quantity of service as well. For Vanderbilt's doctors and scientists, the coming of public monies for research shored up and in time greatly expanded the scientific function of the medical school as it had originally been conceived. That function clearly needed some shoring up. To a significant degree the school's strength and reputation rested on its record of producing a relatively large amount of high-quality research; on that foundation the school had risen to an eminence out of proportion with its age. In this respect especially, Robinson and his new staff had built well.

But by the late 1940s their old level of activity and productivity was lacking, and it disturbed Youmans. Reduced numbers of Vanderbilt's faculty prominent in learned societies, reduced major publications, and fewer high-level research projects all said something new was needed. The faculty had not yet recovered from the war's depredations, which was surely part of the problem, along with, as ever, money. Needed, said Youmans in 1950, "is a faculty of real students and investigators who are adequately supported on a continuous basis permitting them to exercise their talents in the most effective fashion." It could not be done, said Youmans, bravely expressing an old conviction, "solely or even for the most part on the basis of recurring grants-in-aid from outside sources, governmental or otherwise. Our task is to provide from continuing University sources, adequate salaries and reasonable budgets to which these additional funds can be added."[50] What Youmans and his faculty wanted for research was different from what they got, though they quickly enough settled, as did their colleagues at most of the medical schools, for subsidy that met hardly any of the old conditions once so nicely embodied in the fluid research fund.

As Goodpasture had said, the independent medical schools—even one so small as Vanderbilt with its respectable $14 million endowment—relatively speaking were desperately poor. And Vanderbilt became even poorer. From poverty and persistent high demand for what it produced came dependence. In research, government grants-in-aid for specific projects was the price of dependence. Goodpasture had serious doubts, as did pharmacologist Paul Lamson, who on the general crisis of the school and hospital wrote: "Grants without strings are of course splendid. I was on a committee of the National Institutes of Health where money was given with strings. . . . This group controls our work. We lose our freedom. We have to tell what we intend to do—which one cannot do in true research, and if they do not approve of what is to be done we get no money, and if we stick to our program no further funds are granted. We now face the situation of having to give up the rich man's enviable position of freedom from economic want to grub as 99 per cent of mankind does for money to keep up alive."[51] But most of the doctors, if they felt any, kept their philosophical agony to themselves. Even though "grubbing for money to stay alive" seemed hardly to befit the activities of so dignified a profession, there was little choice to do anything else.

Throughout the 1950s government grants for research increased steadily as did, on a different scale, grants from private sources. Whatever the source, most ran for specific terms and covered specific projects. Together, such soft money for research grew faster than the regular budgets, and before the middle of the decade they were fully half as large as those budgets.[52] With $130,000 from the National Cancer Institute (matched by $70,000 from the university) a new science laboratory went up across the north court of the medical school to help accommodate the new activity, which by 1955 had in Youmans judgment again reached a desirable maximum given current facilities and personnel.[53]

Research thus nicely rebounded, so nicely in fact that it raised a question about the intentions of its new patrons with regard to both the researchers who did the work and the medical schools where the work got done. A revitalized national fascination with science (or more precisely with the good material things that could come from research) was one of the legacies of the war, which had been fought and won in part by the wizards of science. In a dangerous postwar world really only half at peace and where the United States found itself in the unaccustomed role of leader, science more than ever was summoned to the nation's service. Research and development became sacrosanct articles of a faith that said through science the republic could be made both prosperous and secure. In medicine the claims of research in perilous times were about as obvious as those of research in nuclear physics.

A strong argument can be made that, through its growing subsidies for medical research, the public through their government was simply trying to buy something whose value to it seemed clear. Money changed hands with the expectation that a specific product would be had for it. With subsidy also went some direction, perhaps not as heavy-handed as Lamson had said, but direction just the same. It is a view supported by the fact that at Vanderbilt research grants with few exceptions went to the individual scientists or at most to the departments but not to the school as a whole. Patrons who had in mind to assist medical schools as institutions to carry on their own research functions would have distributed their money differently: witness the old fluid research fund. But aid to institutions of medical education to carry on research, unlike aid to scientists themselves to carry on research, would have required at some point close examination of the medical school research function in relation with its other functions in education and increasingly in service. At that point (not yet reached in the 1950s) the possibility of government interference with education and service destroyed the consensus that once had united the practicing profession and the medical schools behind public support for research.[54]

As it was at Vanderbilt, the effect of research subsidies that singled out "principle investigators" for aid rather than the whole school was to put a premium on a certain brand of entrepreneurship among faculty, who to do their research were forced to compete for favors beyond the university's power to dispense. Whether that talent had any relation to an individual's talent to do good research is another problem; usually it was probably irrelevant. Not irrelevant for such people, however, many of whom did very good work, was the problem of tending two masters: the one in whose laboratories they worked, and the one who paid for the work. Cleavages of two sorts resulted, both of which began to erode parts of Flexner's old ideal. Between the university and its various schools power traditionally ran along a dean-to-chancellor axis. In the medical school, however, that began to change to an axis between the chancellor and powerful department chairmen or the leading researchers who controlled the federally supported scientific enclaves within the medical school. Feelings of attachment and loyalty decentralized, which hardly served to advance the unity of university and medical school. Within the medical school, meanwhile, the new means of patronage pried research away from education and service. At least the existence of research enclaves within the school and not really governed by it emphasized research's separate status and mocked the integrated design of courts and corridors, which became finally an artifact unrelated to the way things really functioned. Though few wanted to admit it, a pattern had been established in which the medical scientists sometimes appeared to be the de facto wards of the state and the medical schools they worked in appeared to be branches of the NIH.

No one really intended such a pattern. No one cravenly bartered away his or Vanderbilt's independence for mere money. But as but one small part of a large national trend, Vanderbilt, which was not independently rich and with no prospect of becoming rich, could either align itself with that pattern or invite a period of genteel and likely fatal decline. It chose the former, not quite in absence of mind but, during Youmans's tenure, not really by conscious policy either. If its now aging first new leaders saw in the pattern the sad end of a kind of freedom and unity they had known years before, there were many more younger people, just as good scientists as they had once been, whose survival as scientists outside that pattern was hard to imagine. Theirs was the strength of youth and of numbers. But it was not even that the veterans resisted what then, as in their own youth, was touted as another step in the advance of medical science. Moreover, medicine, first in research, then in education and service, was only following as it had before the larger culture.

In the 1950s and after, that culture reflected the people's increased desire to purchase collectively things they once had provided for as individuals or had gone without. Medicine, like an old-age pension, was one of those things. Sometimes the agency of that collective purchase was private, as with Blue Cross and Blue Shield and other third-party insurers against the cost of a hospital stay. Sometimes it was public, as with the research subsidies of NIH and later with federal aid to medical education and with Medicare. The public purchase of medical research, less controversial than the purchase of education and service, came first. And despite the repeated assertions of people like John Youmans about the superiority of unrestricted internally allocated research funds (which remained rare), such purchase did work. Science, at least as it was evolving in medicine, may have been more resilient than Goodpasture in his gloomier moments suspected. The younger medical researchers, who had never known what it was like to work under a fluid research fund, obviously adjusted to the new forms. They did very good work. How much different it might have been had the National Research Foundation ever been constituted as its first planners wished we can only guess.

In its service function, still expressed in the 1950s chiefly through its hospital, the medical school found no patron comparable to NIH. Makeshifts resulted as the managers of the medical school and the university tried desperately to resolve the conflict between the need for income from patients and the need for the proper kinds of teaching cases to conduct an undergraduate medical school. Branscomb and Youmans, who got on well,[55] knew that balance sheets could be improved by the admission of more private patients who paid; and under a new hospital director, Richard Cannon, the numbers did improve. They knew too that private patients whose admission, diagnosis, treatment, and follow-up were not controlled by the hospital staff reduced the hospital's effectiveness as a laboratory for teaching, which supposedly was its purpose to begin with. Thus, in the early 1950s, they went outside, not for money, which for subsidy of hospital patients was not then there, but for more patients. Goodpasture and the 1946 consultants had proposed that the city build a new hospital adjacent to Vanderbilt where indigents could be cared for at community expense and used to teach medical students, a plan that did not materialize.

The next best thing was for Vanderbilt to go to where the city's patients then were: Nashville General Hospital. After long and difficult negotiations, the city and the university entered into a contract effective August 1, 1952, whereby Vanderbilt would take over the professional operation of Nashville General, the cost of operation (then about $750,000) to be paid by the city. Eight to ten additional staff members were provided for the outpatient department, and full-time heads of medicine and surgery were appointed. Certain clinics were transferred to Vanderbilt for better service, and arrangements were made to move patients back and forth between Nashville General and Vanderbilt so as to augment the cases available for undergraduate teaching.[56] Unfortunately, the financial results were less happy, as deficits accumulated from unpaid patient accounts, the same problem that beleaguered so many teaching or charity hospitals, Vanderbilt's own included. Even though the contract was renegotiated on more favorable terms, the relationship did not last. Fearing that the hospital would be closed, nonprofessional employees put pressure on the city council to end Vanderbilt's encroachment.

For Vanderbilt's part, Branscomb expressed dissatisfaction with the degree to which Nashville General had actually been utilized to assist Vanderbilt's medical program. A better arrangement, he thought, would be for Vanderbilt to contract to care for indigents at Vanderbilt itself, thus enabling the city to close its outdated and ramshackle facility and enabling Vanderbilt to fill 100 of its beds with city-subsidized indigent patients. Not everyone agreed, among them some Vanderbilt faculty who said the result would be an endless parade of drunks and runny noses and constant interference from local politicians over what services were to be rendered and for what cost.[57] Some relief was had by utilizing for undergraduate teaching the wards of the Thayer Veterans Administration Hospital, but poor availability of teaching patients at Vanderbilt was a continuing complaint among faculty as well as the hospital managers who stared constantly at stubborn deficits. There was even talk of moving the third and fourth clinical years of the school to another city (Chattanooga was mentioned and the possibilities were explored), which would have meant a dismemberment quite as radical as the one Goodpasture had contemplated.[58]

There is sometimes virtue in a policy of muddling through, if what truly matters or what truly needs doing cannot just then be accomplished. Preserving the medical school in the same basic form (the four-year undergraduate curriculum) and with the same function it had had for years (the education of M.D.'s) was uppermost in the minds of individuals like Youmans and Branscomb, and their efforts to hold things together a year at a time ultimately had their reward. Like Kirkland (another fierce institutional loyalist) before them, they guessed the future rightly and determined to keep Vanderbilt somehow in its path. When medical insurance at last assured filled and paid-for hospital beds, thus lifting the old burden of having to rely on indigents, the hospital was still there to be filled, and the third- and fourth-year students were still there to serve out their clerkships in the old Oslerian tradition.

The education of those students at Vanderbilt proved more resistant to outside intrusion than either research or service in the decade after the war, and the daily rounds of teachers and students gave the impression of business much as usual. The faces, though, of some of the key teachers were new. When Youmans became dean in 1950 there was already need to seek five new department heads (preventive medicine–public health, physiology, surgery, obstetrics and gynecology, and experimental medicine), and soon there would be others. Youmans saw filling the vacancies as the greatest opportunity since 1925 to infuse the school with fresh spirit and to restore its momentum. In a sense it was; the senior faculty as it was reconstituted represented, like its predecessor, much talent and energy. Further comparison is unfair, because what it no longer shared with its predecessor was a free and open field. In their role as educators the faculty members professed many of the same ideals cherished by Robinson, yet, obedient to the steady advance of medical knowledge, they made specialism the order of the day and so helped fracture old unities. Hugh Morgan came back from the army powerfully impressed with the organization of medical care along specialized lines and gradually the department of medicine blossomed into subdivisions for allergies, pulmonary and cardiovascular diseases, infectious diseases, nutrition, clinical physiology and experimental medicine, endocrinology, gastroenterology, and neurology. Surgery, free after 1951 of the tight rein of Barney Brooks, went down the same road with specialist enclaves that clearly reflected the way in which science was breaking down the body: neurological, ear, nose and throat, thoracic, urological, and orthopedic surgery. Plus there were plastic, pediatric, and experimental surgery and surgical pathology. Since the war ophthalmology, psychiatry, radiology, and anesthesiology were established as independent departments, and a division of hearing and speech sciences was organized.

The growth of medical knowledge was reflected more in the growing number of courses than in any radical changes in the structure of the undergraduate curriculum. There was some tinkering with various scheduling formulas—semesters, trimesters, and quarters—and beginning in 1952 a summer quarter was added to provide more clinical experience for third- and fourth-year students. It was required for juniors but optional for seniors, only four of whom signed up in 1953. To Youmans's disappointment, the faculty backed off a year later and substituted an extension at the end of the second year to introduce the clinical clerkship. The basic outline was retained: study of medical sciences during the first two years, work with patients in the final two years, though in surgery and gynecology fourth-year students worked the wards and not the clinics, reversing the old pattern.[59] The students themselves were largely the same: many had attended Vanderbilt's undergraduate college, most were southern, male, and upper middle class. Their numbers were few.

In education there still was much substance to the old image of independence, less so in the laboratories and the hospital. With only 200 or so students working toward their M.D.'s, Vanderbilt was one of the smallest of the nation's medical schools. It still owned its own hospital (however troubling that ownership might be), and its students and teachers still spent most of their days inside Robinson's original building, which by then was showing its age. It took ten years, but by the mid-1950s the worst of the postwar trials seemed to be over. Youmans managed well and with his colleagues breathed a sigh of relief at improving budgets and a rebuilt faculty busily tending research and teaching. Youmans and the others also knew that any such periods of relative stability henceforth would be brief. Science in medicine, more richly patronized than ever, was speeding things up, and no one, it seemed, in academic medicine or elsewhere, anymore planned or built for permanence in quite the way that Robinson had.

"In respect to the physical plant of the Medical School–Hospital building, extensive rehabilitation, additions and modernization are needed," wrote Youmans in 1955. "Without any increase in the size of classes, the continuing need for additional activities, requiring additional space for equipment and personnel, made necessary by the continuing march of medical science, must be met. Increasing change in the nature of illness, and the type of patients and the form and pattern of medical care will call not only for certain kinds of change in the hospital and outpatient facilities (for teaching) but also in personnel and in administrative organization."[60] Youmans worried about complacency. If new brick and mortar (during Youmans's tenure new laboratory buildings were added for the basic sciences and for experimental surgery, as well as a new office building adjacent to the hospital for clinical faculty) and if planning and self-study were any sign, he need not have been concerned. If much of the brick and mortar from those days later seems to lack pattern (wings were added and courtyards filled in a jumble of styles), it may be because the planning for the future that Youmans counseled was undertaken not for purely academic or scientific reasons. Rather, the future had to be read so as to assure a hand in shaping it, lest someone else shape it first. Planning increasingly entailed not just articulating policies that to one degree or another embodied ideas; it was guessing at someone else's intentions. As medicine's domain greatly expanded during the 1960s and 1970s and as those with claims upon it multiplied accordingly, planning to keep up with "the march of science" more and more became planning somehow to keep control over what one did. The future that Youmans was looking at would afford no more grand designs like Robinson's. Strangely, as the knowledge and power of medicine grew, the circle in which medicine's people had freedom to think and act seemed to diminish.

Vanderbilt's loss of independence, brought on most immediately by rising costs but ultimately by the very success of what it did, meant that more time and energy would go to managing the relationship with those by whose grants and appropriations it lived. As the university was driven back into the community in order to survive, it confronted there expectations once irrelevant to what went on in Robinson's austere wards and laboratories. A generation of academic doctors, who had been raised in a private world that was essentially self-regulated and self-sufficient, found themselves in middle age to have become essentially public servants. On everything that they did— the research that advanced medical science, the teaching that made others into healers, the care of sick people—others acting collectively had made compelling claims. In a moral sense, Vanderbilt rightly always had been a "public service institution"; it produced the doctors the people of its region needed. So Flexner had said it should. But as it was called upon to produce more doctors and more services in return for public subsidy, it became a public service institution literally as well. Over the last twenty years it has adjusted to that necessity with a certain caution. With demand for the services of medicine ever escalating, just as Goodpasture had said, it cannot escape the community. Nor, it seems, will it forsake its other older nature, which was fixed in its origins: to establish medicine as a discipline of science.

Service and Science

11

On the things that the Vanderbilt Medical School had produced so reliably since 1925—exceptionally well-trained young physicians and research into the scientific basis of disease—concern in the early 1960s focused sharply. Times were good, national self-esteem and confidence were high. Appetites were growing, though not, it seemed, any faster than means available to satisfy them. With such striving many thousands were at once proud and comfortable. The names that their leaders gave to those years—the New Frontier and the Great Society—were well suited to mobilize anew popular idealism and to confirm older national meanings. The peculiarly American ambition to do all things well for all people all of the time boldly asserted itself. Medicine, which in previous decades had so well proven its promise, was an early and easy target. It remained one long after the Kennedy and Johnson years were a memory.

Symptom of the country's growing appetite was a growing confusion between the words "medicine" and "health." Vanderbilt Medical School had always been precisely what its name said: a place where people taught, learned, and practiced essentially curative medicine based on science. To learn enough about how specific disease processes worked in order to cure or possibly even prevent their occurrence was its aim. When knowledge was imperfect, as very often it was, its physicians and surgeons treated symptoms and hoped for the best. One of the legacies of the union of science and medicine was thus to think specifically in terms of disease-causing agents that in one way or another made people sick. Figure them out and you solved the problem. "Health" was something else, altogether more comprehensive. Social, eco-

276

nomic, environmental, and spiritual factors determined it, along with the biological ones that more clearly were the domain of scientific medicine. But more and more during the 1960s and the 1970s, the traditional providers of medicine were looked to for health as well. Rightly or wrongly, more was asked of them than before. Among the nation's front line of medical providers, the practicing profession generally, the reaction was mixed. Some condemned what they saw as an unwarranted rise in public expectations for what they could do. Others variously aligned themselves with the rhetoric and the substance of what seemed the fashion of the future: "health care delivery," an omnibus phrase that somehow was supposed to subsume knowledge and the techniques of scientific medicine with care for matters of distribution, access, and consumer satisfaction. Although science and research-oriented medical schools like Vanderbilt were hardly in the front line, they too felt the stresses of the nation's changing tastes.

Its independence already well-eroded but with a fixed idea of what it should and should not be about, Vanderbilt responded ambivalently. It found itself in the 1960s and 1970s operating in a secularized consumer culture that put a high premium on physical health. Nationally, insistent demands for more and better health care (as medicine had come to be called) were manifest in certain predictable ways. Most familiar and least threatening to a school like Vanderbilt, the national consensus remained essentially unshaken that research into the biochemical mechanisms of disease must go forward. Indeed, through the middle 1960s enthusiasm for research, measured by the support of its greatest patron, the National Institutes of Health, reached new highs. More recently, a troubled economy has made for less spaciousness, and a changing ideological climate has cast doubt over the proper role of government in health matters generally. But public support for research in medicine will likely be with us for a long time yet and, compared with support in other academic disciplines, at still fairly bounteous levels. Another national consensus, growing steadily since the end of World War II, centered on the need to produce more doctors. Though that need was more self-evident to some than to others, even the American Medical Association eventually acknowledged it. By crude numbers alone, the jump in population growth rate occasioned by the postwar baby boom pointed to very real shortages, added to which the proportionally greater number of M.D's made necessary by the spread of specialization, and the rising popular expectations placed on the profession, led to considerable hue and cry to expand and speed up production. A part of the Flexner era thus ended, as medical school classes were expanded and more medical schools were built. The service that more doctors and better science rightly should render constituted the third persistent concern of these years. The debate over how to achieve the proper mix of doctors (how many of which kinds of specialists and how many generalists), over their even distribution to all areas and populations and over the optimum means of health care delivery generally, was often strident and raised questions about basic purpose that could be deeply troubling at a school like Vanderbilt.

Vanderbilt reacted to these things differently, but the common effect of them all was markedly to increase the school's size and its functional and administrative complexity. In 1958, the year John Youmans retired, the school and hospital were still housed in the original 1925 building, to which there had been only three additions: the hospital wing built in the late 1930s, a modest basic science laboratory (shared with the university science departments), and a surgical research laboratory. By 1980, the once massive core of Robinson's old structure had been swamped by its appendages. The A. B. Learned Laboratory had risen to seven stories. New hospital space protruded to the west, capped by a circular wing. On Twenty-first Avenue, where originally a porte cochere and curved drive had announced the entrance to the Vanderbilt Hospital, the Joe and Howard Werthan Building and new library and laboratory space had crept virtually to the city sidewalk. Courtyards had been filled in. Finally, as if it would bear no more, the grid gave up its unifying function. A massive education building, Rudolph A. Light Hall, appeared on the other side of Garland Avenue and next door was built an even more massive new hospital whose three towers and twelve floors housed nearly all of Vanderbilt's 545 beds.

In the 1950s, the phrase "Vanderbilt Medical School" still signified the totality of Robinson's first design. By 1980, the phrase "Vanderbilt Medical Center" had replaced it, signifying a much larger totality and something of a different design. The medical school (which Robinson had not liked to think about as separate from the hospital, the laboratories, and whatever else there once was under that large first roof) had become one unit of what, among medical administrators, was an "academic health center" or an "academic medical center." As things grew, they also differentiated and at the top required special managerial talent. John Youmans first carried on and off the title of director of medical affairs, a designation increasingly common in American medical schools by the 1950s. But the school was still relatively small then, and Youmans was essentially a dean. His successors, first John Patterson and then Randolph Batson, played twin roles as both dean and director or vice-chancellor for medical affairs. In the mid 1970s the jobs were separated when Vernon E. Wilson became vice-president for medical affairs with several associate and assistant vice-presidents under him. John Chapman became dean of the medical school with his own assorted associate and assistant deans. Robinson (a part-time dean and full-time professor) and Leathers had gotten along essentially with one assistant (Beverly Douglas, also an active faculty member) and a secretary or two. Their present-day counterparts have more substantial staffs—and less time to teach and see patients.

Such growth measures a kind of prosperity. The American people individually, but increasingly collectively, had decided to buy more of medicine's goods and services. Vanderbilt was one beneficiary of their decision. The quality of its response, however, is not fully evident from the numbers alone. Expansion was also accompanied by a modest amount of self-renewal, nowhere more deliberate than in the area of its very oldest activity, undergraduate physician education. For the first time since 1925 the faculty reformed the curriculum. Curriculum reform was not a little in the air in the 1960s in medical and in other kinds of higher education, and Vanderbilt moved in the assuring company of some other very good schools, among them Case Western Reserve, Stanford, Northwestern, and Johns Hopkins. Common to such changes was a clear trend to relax the rigid, lock-step type of program in which every student studied the same things in more or less the same prescribed pattern, and to allow more flexibility and more opportunity for elective work. Related was the move to provide a more continuous medical education by correlating more closely medical and premedical, clinical and preclinical programs. Further, better integration of course material would, it was hoped, eliminate needless duplication of material covered at different levels. And in some places, effort was made to shorten the overall time needed to educate doctors, thereby helping more quickly to increase the supply. Though far from the boldest, Vanderbilt's changes savored of that same spirit.[1]

Credit for the initial pushing and shoving belonged to John Patterson from Stanford, the first dean chosen from outside Vanderbilt circles since Robinson himself was picked in 1920. But not until 1964, two years after Patterson had left Vanderbilt, was a reformed curriculum actually implemented. Long in the gestation, it worked well. The assumption was that Vanderbilt's responsibility was to produce individual physicians and surgeons with widely divergent skills and talents but who shared the basic core of information needed for them to function as doctors. Thus the new curriculum (which was new only in part) was divided into basic required material to be taken by everyone and numerous elective courses to be selected by individuals to complete their programs. The electives were taken for credit and were to be taken seriously. To help in course selection, each student was assigned a faculty adviser. The medical school even switched to a semester schedule so its students might elect offerings in other departments of the university. How it worked in the department of medicine, still quite as much the keystone department as in Robinson's and Burwell's day, suggests its effect.

The second-year introductory course on clinical medicine became a new required offering, "Methods in Clinical Science," an interdepartmental course designed to acquaint students with the basic laboratory techniques and principles employed in clinical medicine. Weekly meetings consisted of lectures introducing the theory and clinical indications for laboratory methods, followed by laboratory periods for small groups, stressing the practical application and demonstration of lecture material. Laboratory procedures that lacked reality in present-day medicine were dropped, more demonstration sessions were introduced, and greater emphasis was placed on metabolism, basic biochemistry, and physiology in laboratory procedures. Anatomists, pathologists, radiologists, physiologists, biochemists, as well as clinicians, did the teaching, thus giving new life to Robinson's old ideal of integrated co-operative medical education. The instruction of second-year students in the methods of physical diagnosis and history taking ran in tandem with the work on laboratory procedures, and it completed the students' preparation for the third-year clinical clerkship. Strengthened by the elimination of a number of required lecture hours that formerly were given by other departments during the same period and that conflicted with students' ward responsibilities, the third-year clerkship remained the backbone of the undergraduate's clinical experience. It was an old but sturdy orthodoxy that medical students learned most rapidly and most responsibly from intimate participation in the work-up, diagnosis, and management of patients. And in the teaching wards of the Vanderbilt Hospital and the Veterans Administration Hospital (built just across Garland Avenue in the early 1960s) the students worked under the close supervision of house and teaching staff. They presented cases for criticism, made rounds, and attended a growing number of teaching subspecialty conferences. The fourth-year curriculum was altered to allow assignment of every student to one morning clinic period a week in the outpatient clinic department. It was hoped thereby to give students a better continuing responsibility for a selected group of ambulatory patients over a long period and to improve their understanding of the complexities of medical care as contrasted with the problems of the diagnosis of disease. In an atmosphere providing consultation from many branches of medicine, they acquired greater understanding of the specialized ancillary services available for the care and rehabilitation especially of patients with chronic illnesses. In the meantime, they further refined their skills at history taking and physical examination.[2]

It was with a broad range of electives, however, that students after 1964 could tailor their medical education to their own interests in ways their predecessors had not enjoyed. Electives multiplied and were available to students at all levels. In addition to the formal offerings, wrote David Rogers, head of the department of medicine when the changes were implemented, "virtually any kind of investigative or clinical program can be worked out on an individual basis through consultation with the faculty member who will assume responsibilities for supervision and guidance of the student." The department's initial twenty-six offerings multiplied many times and included formal course work, medical specialty clinics, clinical clerkships, and clinical research electives. At various times students might look at science-oriented subjects like medical genetics and cytogenetics, clinical biochemistry, disorders of fluid and electrolyte metabolism, clinical endocrinology, or renal pathophysiology. Or they might cast broader nets and come up with the problems facing the prospective intern, medical philosophy, the psychosocial aspects of life-threatening illness, or death and dying. Fourth-year students might do special clinics on allergies, dermatology, diabetes, endocrinology, gastroenterology, hematology, rheumatology, and the chest. Elective research programs were available in such specialty areas as infectious diseases, nuclear medicine, ischemic heart disease, and biomedical engineering.[3]

It was the same throughout the school. On the four-year calendar that plotted out the way medical students spent their time, the blocks given over to elective time grew more numerous. In the first two years, Wednesday was reserved for electives. The third year was filled largely with ward rotations, but the fourth became essentially fully elective, the seniors serving as clinical clerks in electives on the outpatient service or in a variety of positions as inpatient clerks or as research fellows at Vanderbilt or other institutions. Indeed, it was possible for fourth-year students (beginning in the summer of their junior year) to lead lives as peripatetic as some of their mentors. As the catalog rhetoric said, the idea was to give the students maximum opportunity for individual development. To make that possible, parts of the required core curriculum were trimmed (anatomy, for example) but never so much that the fundamental structure in 1980 would not have been recognizable to the new school's first reformers back in the 1920s. But the growing number of electives and their variety clearly did say that there was more and more to teach. Not all electives proved permanent, but it was in the nature of a system that responded both to the students' choices and to changes in science that self-renovation came naturally.

Such reform was probably necessary; it was also lasting. Reform, innovation, and catering to individual development characterized higher education generally in those years, including medical schools. Compared with some other places (Harvard, for instance, which for awhile denuded its basic science departments), Vanderbilt moved cautiously. It retained the old fundamental structure for educating doctors: two years spent mastering at least the basics of the medical sciences, followed by two more years spent beginning to apply that knowledge in a clinical setting. Years more of apprenticeship followed that. Vanderbilt did not, like some, experiment with shortening the time it took to get an M.D. degree. Vanderbilt did not train doctors in three years just to help ease what in the 1960s and early 1970s was widely proclaimed as a critical national shortage of health manpower.

Vanderbilt did not, however, leave that problem wholly to others. Indeed, with its old freedom gone, it could not. During the 1960s and the early 1970s probably no one theme dominated medicine and medical education more than the public's perception of the need for more physicians. It was a perception manifest in government action targeted on the nation's medical schools, which had sole responsibility in the United States for training doctors. By the end of 1967 there were more than forty federal laws on the books that had direct or indirect effect on medical schools, usually providing some kind of financial assistance. That number was swelled by a steady stream of health professions educational assistance acts and amendments, nurse training acts, allied health personnel training acts, and heart disease, cancer, and stroke amendments, which poured forth from Congresses ever more preoccupied with health.[4] And though the idea of health was coming to be interpreted ever more broadly, it was on the supply of physicians—the traditional keepers of medical knowledge and the traditional purveyors of medicine—specifically that most attention was fixed. More physicians, it seemed, meant better health.

Conferences, studies, and special reports sponsored by government agencies, private foundations, and professional organizations focused public and professional concern.[5] In 1966 the problems took on the appearance of special urgency with President Johnson's creation of the National Advisory Commission on Health Manpower, charged to attack with a number of task forces what the president termed a "critical shortage" in health manpower. That urgency was reflected by the creation in January 1967, within the Department of Health, Education, and Welfare, of the Bureau of Health Manpower with separate divisions of physician manpower, allied health manpower, health manpower educational services, nursing, and dental health. Such professional organizations as the American Hospital Association, the Association of American Medical Colleges, the American Academy of Pediatrics, the American Nursing Association, and the American Public Health Association issued reports and generally agreed that large numbers of additional health personnel were needed to meet present and future requirements. The American Medical Association too, the voice of the practicing profession and long wary of threats to overcrowd it, aligned itself with this particular sign of the times in medicine. In June 1966 it established its own committee on health manpower to investigate the national situation; a year later the committee confirmed "the critical need for more physicians, for a better distribution of physician resources, and for allied health personnel in all categories." Conclusively, the AMA board of directors declared in favor of "an immediate and unprecedented increase in physician output" and said that "the most rapid way to obtain this aim without reduction in the quality of education is by expansion of existing medical schools although new institutions will be required as well. . . . Those schools whose enrollment has remained relatively static for years need to review their policies regarding the number of admissions in light of national demand."[6]

Vanderbilt's was among the most static. Indeed, of the changes that affected its educational responsibilities over the last fifteen years, the change in class size is most apparent. Though but one aspect of the growth in the size of the entire institution in these years, larger number of medical students broke sharply with old tradition and put new strains on Robinson's old buildings, hastening their replacement. Since the reorganization of 1925, only fifty-two carefully chosen students had been admitted to any entering class. The school physically was built to accommodate that many and no more; the small teaching hospital was designed to accommodate just enough patients to teach that many and no more. The number of hospital beds had expanded somewhat, but the number of spaces at many laboratory benches had not. (It was a standing joke, during the years when classes began to expand and before space had expanded, that students' admission would be decided on intellectual and educational merits and by the width of their bottoms, which literally determined whether they would fit in at Vanderbilt.) But besides the limitation of space, it was institutional habit that kept classes small. The faculty, itself not large until the growth of the late 1950s and 1960s, liked it that way and with good reason. Vanderbilt had one of the highest student application/acceptance ratios in the country—and not unrelated, one of the lowest average attrition rates—about 4 percent, against the national average, in the mid-sixties before the expansion came, of about 10 percent.[7] With students who were overwhelmingly male and white it was a closely knit old-fashioned southern school that did the best by a few. It had the pick of the region's best-prepared young men (and a few women), and it made of them some of the country's finest doctors. The vast majority of its graduates, after vigorous residencies at Vanderbilt or elsewhere, went into specialty practice, and Vanderbilt ranked high with the schools among whose graduates a select few chose careers in academic medicine.

Its graduates in 1980 chose much the same kinds of careers. Vanderbilt did not become a mill to produce average doctors to meet high popular demand, as Goodpasture once feared it might. An M.D. degree from Vanderbilt still meant something out of the ordinary, but there were more of them. Beginning in 1967 more students were admitted, until by 1977 the class size (though still among the smallest in the country) doubled to 103. It was done, as elsewhere, largely at public—that is, at federal—behest, and it entailed, in addition to physical squeezing and shoving and the urgent planning of new buildings, some adjustment of self-image as well. For it was here, in the realm of education in the 1960s and 1970s, that Vanderbilt suffered another blow to its independence, much as it had earlier in another realm, when research had become dependent on NIH. Vanderbilt was but one of many schools in a broad national trend. Increases in class size were in part a general result of the growing public consensus that the nation, to be healthier, needed more doctors, and that the medical schools, as public service institutions, were morally bound to provide them. The increases were also the result of specific federal actions to entice and coerce the medical schools to do more of what they had always done.

The incentive was federal aid to medical education, which finally became reality with the Health Professions Educational Assistance Act of 1963. It authorized federal matching grants for construction and improvement of medical school facilities plus a six-year program of loans to students in medicine, dentistry, and osteopathy. Amendments later set up a scholarship program, and basic and specific improvement grants were designed to increase both the quantity and the quality of medical education. The forgiveness principle for student loans was introduced in 1966, which allowed cancellation of up to 100 percent of principal and interest if the physician practiced in a poor rural area designated by the secretary of health, education, and welfare. Vanderbilt students first received loans under the act in 1965, and while funds under the act did not keep up with financial needs, the assumption thus existed that financial aid for medical education was available and that costs therefore need no longer deter qualified students from training for a medical career.[8]

Though the people, acting through the federal government, could not, either practically or constitutionally, simply decree the creation of more doctors, they could buy them, which was the end effect of public aid to medical education. The medical schools (or at least their deans, as reflected

in the actions of the Association of American Medical Colleges) were eminently agreeable to the prospect of federal money for educational purposes,
after having experienced in the 1950s an unbalancing of the educational
process caused by massive federal funding for research alone.[9] They were
agreeable, that is, assuming that federal support for education would cover
the true costs of the expanded job they were expected to do. On that point,
however, the gap between initial promise and later performance widened
disappointingly as the years went by.

Nowhere was the gap more evident than in connection with the Comprehensive Health Manpower Training Act of 1971, whose stated purpose was
to increase the number of the nation's "health professionals" and one of whose
provisions was the introduction of the so-called capitation grants to medical
schools that met certain legislative requirements. It provided a certain number
of dollars for each student enrolled and required of every school receiving
such aid that it enroll more students. Unlike the basic institutional grants and
specific projects grants that had been and still were available, capitation
brought with it the principle that federal financing was "necessary for the
regular operational support of schools of medicine."[10] It was also the first
time that federal support had been made contingent on the fulfillment of
certain qualitative program requirements within the schools that accepted
aid. Of nine kinds of activities, schools had to present a plan to carry out
projects in at least three. They included, in addition to increasing enrollment,
such things as shortening the length of medical training; establishing interdisciplinary programs and promoting the team approach to health care;
training new types of health personnel including physician assistants; increasing the enrollment of disadvantaged students; undertaking the training of
primary-care health personnel; offering innovative programs in the organization, provision, financing, and evaluation of health care; establishing programs in clinical pharmacology and drug abuse and in the science of nutrition.[11] It was a fair catalog of the nation's health concerns in the 1970s and a
measure too of how those concerns were changing and broadening the
meaning of medicine in America—of how "medicine" was coming to mean
"health." Vanderbilt conformed, as it had to. Most of all it educated more
students.

In return, it did not get what it had bargained for. Capitation monies
proved notoriously flexible, never amounting to more than $2,300 per student
in any year. Within ten years of the program's beginning, with medical
enrollment at record levels and thus assuring abundant future supply (some
predicted a doctor glut by the 1990s), it appeared that capitation would likely
be abandoned. Such public aid to medical education at Vanderbilt produced

results not all of which are yet apparent. More clear and something tied directly to its history, Vanderbilt's basic product and the quality of that product—well-trained M.D.'s—seem to have been fairly indifferent to the source of the funds that paid for it all. Public funds for medical education did not, of course, pay for nearly all of it. The true cost of educating doctors is notoriously complicated to figure and is commonly borne by resources other than those tagged strictly educationally. Vanderbilt's graduates continued to rank near the top of national medical board examinations and to win residencies at leading institutions across the country. Few of those graduates themselves thought much about whether public assistance for medical education had added to or detracted from their own education. They were simply the happy beneficiaries of the national demand for more doctors. Capitation marked the high point of that demand.

They were not, however, the only students getting an education at Vanderbilt's medical school even though physician education remained its central purpose. As more was learned about health and disease and as the public became more insistent about health care delivery, a modest array of other kinds of students tramped up and down Vanderbilt's corridors. The spectrum of health-related education was broadening rapidly. In addition to student nurses[12] and hospital house staff, who had long been a part of Vanderbilt, there were educational programs in the university hospital for nursing technicians and practical nurses, radiological technicians, dietary interns, physical therapy interns, and inhalation therapists. "We should no longer consider the Medical Center as being a school only for the training of medical students," wrote dean Randolph Batson in 1964. "Indeed one might justifiably consider our role as being that of a health related university."[13] So it has remained. By 1980 the number of nursing students approached 600 (579), while under the umbrella of the "allied health professions" smaller numbers of students studied to become dietetic interns, medical technologists, radiation therapists, technologists in nuclear medicine, and specialists in blood bank technology. Graduate students working for master's or Ph.D. degrees in basic science departments increased steadily in the 1960s in response to abundant federal training support (46 in 1963–64; 141 in 1968–69), and though there was a leveling off in the leaner years that followed, predoctoral graduate education remained a part of the school's educational mission (there were 116 degree candidates in 1979–80, most in biochemistry, pharmacology, microbiology, and pathology). The preclinical departments also offered nondegree work to a number of fellows and postdoctoral students (86 in 1979–80), mostly in biochemistry, pharmacology, and physiology. Continuing medical education courses greatly multiplied, largely in the clinical departments, which provided opportunity for practicing doctors to come to Vanderbilt for short periods to refresh and keep current on a wide range of subjects. In 1979–80 there were eighty-four separate offerings, attracting over 4,000 registrants.[14]

In its education function alone, the school became a very busy place. The demands on its faculty rose, as did their number. In 1958, the year John Youmans retired, there were 355 faculty members, 128 of them full time; in 1964 there were 555 and 271 respectively.[15] Later, as the medical student body was expanded, faculty grew too, by 1980 to 966, 457 of whom were full time (316 in the clinical subjects, 141 in the basic sciences).[16] Such growth meant that from the late 1950s to the late 1970s the ratio of students to faculty steadily fell from 1.3 students to every faculty member in 1957–58 to .8 in 1977–78 (the national average for those years was 2.9 and 1.3, respectively).[17] Though not all of those faculty members were regular teachers (some indeed seldom saw students at all), growth in the numbers of faculty more than kept pace with growth in the number of students and sustained a relationship on which the school had long prided itself, even as things unquestionably got more crowded.

The expansion of physical space to meet expanded education responsibilities long lagged behind, which made the Vanderbilt Medical School in the middle 1970s a sad example of an old building, which, though once masterfully conceived, no longer worked. Over the previous twenty years there was no litany more universal among the faculty than the cry for more space. In research, square footage was one secret to attracting and holding good scientists, and it was for research that some expansion had come in the 1950s (the A. B. Learned Laboratory and the S. R. Light Laboratory for Surgical Research). Obviously, education occurred in those places, just as it did in the various extensions that were added to the old hospital. But it was not until 1977, with the completion of Rudolph A. Light Hall, that Vanderbilt got its first completely new (since 1925) building dedicated to medical education. That building broke—literally—away from the school's integrated design, rising on the other side of Garland Avenue from the rest of the school and hospital, though it was attached to the hospital's west wing through an underground tunnel. Built for about $12 million—from gifts to the university by Rudolph A. Light and from federal funds—it brought to the school the first hint of luxury since Canby Robinson had the original hospital and medical school lobbies fitted out with handsome oak paneling. "Collegiate Gothic" was long gone at Vanderbilt, and the new building rose in a modern modular style, having in common with its parent across the street only its red brick veneer. Its 209,000 square feet contained large lecture halls and commodious student lounges, up-to-date laboratory equipment and electronic teaching tools, and the Howard Hughes Medical Institute. There was all the hardware for computer-assisted instruction (basic science examinations were commonly taken at computer consoles) and even a television studio allowing the taping and replay for instructional purposes of complicated medical and surgical procedures. Students loved it, and the departments of biochemistry and physiology, which took up residence there, found in its ampler spaces compensation for removal from Robinson's old grid.

Medical education at Vanderbilt thus changed in quantity. It is not quite fair, however, to say that it did not change in quality as well. It was not that the general quality did not remain as high as ever, which it did, or that its graduates did not continue to become specialists, which they did. Rather, the substance of much of what they learned was new and there was more of it— to which burgeoning electives partly testified. For that, Vanderbilt students and medical students elsewhere had research to thank. Since the school's new beginning in 1925, research had been the coequal of education in defining Vanderbilt's purpose and mission. Flexner had said research and education were one, and Robinson's new leaders—talented teachers and investigators together—made them one at Vanderbilt. It was a durable dogma that made most sense when the sources of support for research and education were the same. For the researchers and educators, one master was easier to serve than two, especially when that master was relatively far removed from the daily life of the school and was willing that the judgments about science and education and the allocation of resources be made internally. So things had worked at Vanderbilt in the 1930s.

The dogma made less sense when in the 1950s and 1960s large federal support for research—but not yet for education—forced things to a new pattern. In no small part because Vanderbilt had been good at science before the war and because in the first decade afterward it had wisely recruited a second generation of investigator-doctors in keeping with that tradition, it stood in good position to reap the harvest of research dollars that poured forth, especially from an expanding NIH. Beginning in the late 1950s, NIH expanded significantly, and for a few halcyon years the trough of public dollars for biomedical research seemed bottomless.[18]

How much the supply of research dollars created a demand for them is hard to say. But by the early 1960s the fashion of research was such that the *Journal of the American Medical Association* felt safe in saying that "it is generally recognized today that every good medical teacher should participate in some type of research activity, since his powers of critical observation are thereby sharpened and his perspective in his special field of interest is improved, especially with regard to his appreciation of new specific discoveries."[19] Obviously, not all good medical teachers in the United States could do good research, even if they "should." Some of the research turned out under those conditions was less than first-rate, and the temptation unquestionably did exist for people who were not true investigators to undertake research because the money was there. Although the mechanism of passing on applications—the peer review system of the NIH study sections—was always technically competitive, it was inevitably less competitive the fuller the trough seemed to be.

Vanderbilt's investigators received generous support, but unlike some schools that built research programs only in response to the coming of large public subsidy, Vanderbilt built on habits already long established. The research activities of individual faculty members at a complex, integrated medical school where many people do many things are hard to measure. Some people clearly did little else. Some were clearly leaders around whom lesser lights gathered to do some of the work and so to justify themselves in the thing that at Vanderbilt mattered so much. Everyone at Vanderbilt claimed reverence for research. Probably more people than at most medical schools actually lived that very special life, not that that number was large, however. Some happily balanced research with other kinds of work that to them as doctors also mattered much. The aggregate is easier to see. The publications of the faculty rose more than commensurately with its numbers, and their expertise was widely sought at home and abroad. Many sat on NIH study sections and participated regularly in the programs of national scientific and professional organizations. If Vanderbilt once had had the appearance of a tight and provincial little medical school, its faculty in the 1960s and 1970s became one of the most itinerant in the country, thanks largely to their research prowess. Their interests ranged widely over basic and clinical fields. Biochemists worked on the metabolism of amino acids, carbohydrates, lipids, and vitamins, and they advanced understanding of membrane biochemistry, the structure of proteins, and the function of enzymes. Molecular endocrinology, however, was probably source of the department's greatest renown. In microbiology, research centered on two types of large biological molecules: the nucleic acids and the proteins. In studies of synthesis and translation the nucleic acids, bacteriophage (bacteria killing bacteria), and herpes virus (with which Goodpasture once had worked) were used to analyze the process of replication of viral DNA. The connection between the structure of viral RNA and the degeneration of normal cells to malignant ones was also investigated, while protein analysis was pursued through investigation of several toxins and enzymes. Pathologists of Goodpasture's old department focused on the molecular structure of proteins and cell membranes and on the mechanisms of the immune response. The department of physiology's program of basic research in the field of hormone action and metabolic regulation probed how hormones and other chemicals reacted with living cells. Cyclic AMP and GMP, special compounds found in minute amounts in most of the cells of the body, were subject of studies of some of the enzymes involved in their action. On the clinical side, pediatrics research dealt with disordered endocrine metabolism, such as was evident in the juvenile onset of diabetes, and worked toward prevention, not just the treatment, of such infectious diseases of childhood as meningitis and pneumonia. Problems associated with intercranial hemorrhage and with respiration, common pathological processes that threatened the prospect for normal childhood, were also investigated. Medicine, the largest department in the school, was especially recognized for its work in endocrinology and diabetes and for its study of the effects of hormones that regulate glucose metabolism. There were also studies on the metabolism of drugs in various disease states, genetic studies on chromosomal abnormalities, and studies on all aspects of inchemic heart disease. Blood platelets, cyclic AMP, and the prostaglandins received attention, as did clinical problems like liver failure and the body's immune response to malignant tumors.[20]

Long tradition and continuing success kept research at the very top of the faculty's priorities. Though the faculty was still not enormous, it had in many areas grown with its subject enough to provide the critical mass needed to do good science. Moreover, it had the proper mix of different kinds of scientists to make interdisciplinary collaboration on complicated biological problems a matter of course. In its numerous research centers,[21] M.D.'s and Ph.D.'s from many departments dealt with a number of biomedical phenomena and disease processes, which called for a large component of the classic practical and problem-oriented activity of medicine as well as the abstract and principle-oriented approach of science. The faculty's reward system reflected its members' values. There was but one track to tenure at Vanderbilt—a straight academic one that demanded distinction in research in the clinic or in the laboratory. And when one faculty member received in 1971 the highest honor of the Nobel Prize (physiologist Earl Sutherland for the discovery of cyclic AMP), it was almost as if Vanderbilt itself was being honored, not just for the work of one man, but for its whole long and sustained research endeavor.

But no matter how dedicated and how good they were, much of the faculty's enterprise still rested on the uncertain ground of public subsidy. The best scientists believed that the need of individuals to compete for that subsidy was healthy for science; it assured quality. They had learned to like being

judged by their peers on the outside rather than by their colleagues on the inside. For a time, the bounty was munificent and the demands for accountability minimal. Even though NIH grants usually ran for periods of only three to five years and sometimes seven, the researchers kept their freedom (in contrast to Paul Lamson's complaints of the late 1940s), and as long as there were appropriations enough to go around, few complained about the arrangement's structural weakness. The country got much of what it paid for—productive biomedical research—from the medical school–based scientists only too happy to oblige. Budgets and faculty at Vanderbilt rose impressively and the laboratories hummed. But it was not an activity that brought to it or to private medical schools generally any measure of institutional stability. Most of Vanderbilt's basic scientists lived literally by their wits, which was bracing. It could also be risky.

For a while (the middle 1950s through the late 1960s) the union of science and medicine symbolized in biomedical research commanded largely unquestioned respect and great power to secure public support. Science since the war, and science in medicine particularly, decisively had put forward its claims in the political marketplace. Its unparalleled success could be measured by the growth of the university-based research establishment, sustained by the state but governed largely by the scientists themselves.[22] Research's mandate, however, was eroded by the continuing evolution of expectation that in the beginning had sanctioned it. Research paid for by public money in the United States was supposed to produce tangible results: a better national defense, a higher standard of living, or, in medicine, healthier people. It did all of those things. But in medicine, research had had some fabulous successes long before large public subsidies came along, which plausibly fueled expectations that money—from anywhere—could buy useful results. It could not always, or quickly.

The greatest successes of research in medicine had probably come in the field of infectious diseases, beginning in the public eye in the 1930s with the development of penicillin and in the 1940s and 1950s of other chemotherapeutic agents that attacked the specific microbial agents known to be fundamental mechanisms of disease. The discernibility of such fundamental causative mechanisms was key, and in infectious diseases it had not come overnight in the 1930s. Rather, it was the product of half a century of arduous experimental work that established the reality of such things as microbes to begin with. The work of Pasteur, Koch, Behring, Metchnikoff, Erhlich, and others, which associated certain kinds of microbes with certain infectious diseases, opened the door to many medical wonders, but at first the practical payoff was small. Gradually, by the turn of the century, the phenomenon of immunity was being developed, and the existence of antibodies and specific immunizations for diphtheria, tetanus, and other infectious agents was demonstrated. In the 1920s the basic work of Heideberger, Cole, Gobel, and Oswald Avery (whose brother Roy was a pathologist at Vanderbilt) opened up the field of immunochemistry. Numerous types of streptococcus bacteria were identified, and in the early 1930s the link between streptococcus infection and rheumatic fever became clear. But for the anxious physician waiting for things that would be useful in practice, there was for years little to show. It was really only in the late 1940s and in the 1950s that an applied science of infectious diseases widely proved the practical worth of all the basic work. Pneumonia, tuberculosis, syphilis, polio, typhoid, and numerous bacterial infections—once largely untreatable—came under medicine's effective control. The viruses, as Goodpasture well knew, were more difficult and are still elusive, though promising work proceeds.

There are two points. First, the great success of scientific medicine in the field of infectious disease was the fruit of much fundamental research that took years and whose practical usefulness was for many people hardly apparent. But the work went ahead, and it is good for us that it did. Second, medicine's success in dealing with infectious diseases rested on the known existence of special microbial entities that could be proven to be the causative agents of specific diseases. Thus the scientists had a target, which they could subject to various kinds of experimentation from which in turn effective therapies and preventive measures have risen. For many of the maladies that remain to plague humankind, however, there is as yet no such insight into, no such grasp of, the key inner mechanisms that actually explain how such diseases work. Though there is progress, we do not yet know the mechanisms of cancer, heart disease, hypertension, and stroke. We have some ways to mitigate some of their harmful effects, ways that, though wonderful by past standards, are essentially halfway techniques and often very expensive ones. We do not yet understand primary cause. Until we do, the measures to prevent or decisively terminate these kinds of illnesses will remain mysteries.

Such, however, are the kinds of problems that increasingly occupied the NIH-subsidized medical researchers from the 1950s onward. It is not that the challenge of infectious disease ended, but successes there did turn scientists to the remaining more difficult puzzles of the great chronic afflictions. And there, they had to begin just where Pasteur and Koch had begun. They had to search experimentally (that is, slowly and often inefficiently) for causative agents. Only then, only after they were sure, could they begin to think about applying their new knowledge. In the natural history of a scientific process, what the basic researchers were doing in the chronic diseases was a very early event. How fast that history would unfold is an unanswered question. Perhaps with luck it would run faster than it had with the infectious diseases (about seventy-five years from the early basic discoveries to their full blossoming in therapeutic usefulness), but there was no guarantee either that it might not run even slower. For a research enterprise that had become the proprietary interest of the public, that possibility was fraught with peril.

The very fact that the American public had rushed so eagerly to subsidize science in medicine measured their high hopes and expectations for it. That was certainly understandable, considering the very real and seemingly sudden successes of science in infectious diseases during the great antibiotic era. Unfortunately, it was too easy to forget what those successes had cost in time, trial, and error. In money, they had cost probably less than the people, through their government, would choose to spend on cancer, stroke, and heart disease. Whether more money in the 1920s and 1930s could have speeded up the scientific process is unknown. That the expenditure of large sums of money more recently against the chronic diseases can speed up the scientific process seems a clear hope. It may. If it does not, the question is one of how much time, trial, and error then will seem acceptable.

Signs of impatience were evident soon enough. Research in the 1970s indeed produced much new knowledge, some of it useful. It did not produce the decisive therapeutic breakthroughs in the chronic diseases that had been witnessed in the 1940s and 1950s in the infectious diseases and that—quite wrongly—many had viewed as sudden developments. NIH, though by the 1960s a firmly established public institution, ceased to enjoy the acclaim it once knew and came under closer congressional and executive scrutiny. Moreover, its growth was curbed as public attention drew away from research to other more gratifying ways of spending the nation's health dollars.[23] It was a volatile business. Between 1955 and 1960 Vanderbilt's revenue from grants and other sponsored programs, most of them for research and most of them federal, rose from about 30 to 75 percent of the school's total income. By the mid-1960s it neared 80 percent. In dollars, such support doubled between 1962 and 1965 (to $6.5 million) and doubled again by 1970. By that time, however, the proportion of total revenues represented by grants and sponsored programs had peaked and begun to decline. In the 1970s Vanderbilt's researchers remained as productive and as highly competitive as ever, but they had to run harder just to stay ahead. As the rate of growth of federal funds fell, the increase in their share fell too. Dollar amounts rose steadily but more gradually, and in the public marketplace research was pressed to compete in terms of social utility as it had not had to do before.[24]

Nationally, one of the most conspicuous trends of the late 1960s and 1970s was the shrinking portion of total medical school operating revenues represented by restricted funds (funds whose use was governed by the conditions of agreements between the school and the donor, public or private), which between 1967 and 1977 fell from 58 to 47 percent. The most notable part of that decrease was in federally sponsored research, which, though the total dollars nearly doubled, dropped from 34 to 20 percent.[25] At Vanderbilt, like other good research-oriented private schools, the proportional reliance on restricted funds was typically much higher (the national averages included public schools that received regular state or municipal appropriations), though the same trend was evident. The numbers increased throughout the 1970s, but the relationships changed. In 1972, sponsored research and other programs at Vanderbilt represented 69 percent of total medical school revenues of $30 million (to the nearest million). In 1978 that fraction had fallen to 45 percent of $38 million.[26] The meaning of such a decline for research generally is not yet clear and probably will not be until the decline stretches across another decade or two, something that seems not unlikely. It is a fair guess, however, that a shrinking portion of medical or health dollars spent on research reflects a general problem of science in a society grown increasingly insistent about its rights and entitlements to medicine's product (that is, health care) and increasingly impatient over why the product is not even better than it is. The nation spent much to make health care better through research in the 1950s, 1960s, and 1970s, and in the history of American public enthusiasms for great causes, thirty years is a long time. How could it be that in the day of such apparent medical miracles as organ transplant and replacement, and technological wonders like CAT scanners and ultrasound, that people still lived in the dark shadow of the great chronic diseases?

It was, simply, because most of the science needed to explain the fundamental biological mechanisms of those diseases, and thus to eliminate the need for organ transplants and renal dialysis, had still not been done yet. It was not for lack of trying or spending. But in the modest results (modest in terms of widely applicable and stunningly effective preventive or therapeutic measures) of that trying and spending was the lesson that science in medicine still took—in addition to money and manpower—time, luck, and patience. It had always been so. With science's public, however, which had also become its chief patron, patience was not always what it might have been. They had seen in a preliminary way what science in medicine could do, and they determined to have more of it. To get it, they invested much talent and treasure, training up and then supporting a whole generation of scientists whose charge it was to find the answers and get the job done. One measure of their confidence that it would be done could be seen in bold—and premature—public declarations of "war" on cancer and other frightful foes.

Such declarations clearly were premature unless the public patrons of science were prepared cheerfully to wait out a long siege. The public had no other choice, but they were not always cheerful about it. There were at least two possible results for those people who actually worked at science. It was possible that, compared with the late 1950s and early 1960s, for example, the conditions of work in science would become less pleasant. There would be less money and to what there was more strings would be attached. There would be constant sniping from nonscientific quarters at activities whose practical purpose seemed unclear. There would be increased insistence on accountability and measures to ensure that it was real and frequent. Scientists would be harried for results by patrons impatient to have what they had paid for. Science would suffer. There was another possibility, contrary to the psychology of halcyon days when money and science seemed so nicely yoked together. It was the old-fashioned notion that hard times brought with them a healthy winnowing of people and ideas. The best people who did the best work would survive, the impulse to real science being hardier than some gave it credit for. There would always be room for excellence and, for the few key leaders destined to have the few original ideas that really lead somewhere, loss of the followers who gathered around the margins of science would matter little. Professional followers unquestionably had gained entry to science during the era of seemingly limitless budgets, and of all the work done then some surely was done for the wrong reasons. The "literature" mushroomed, but it recorded, along with the important ideas, not a little needless replication. Vanderbilt, with its tradition of serious research long antedating large public subsidy, probably sinned in this respect less than most places, though it was not perfectly pure.

Whether harder times augered well or ill for science in medicine, it is clear already that what was once a near-universal national enthusiasm for research has been blunted. The reasons are complex and multiple, but two especially are important and closely related. A diminished sense of national capability, as marked as any in our history, hobbles large collective endeavors as it undermines millions of small private ones. A sluggish economy, persistent high inflation, and the perception of shrinking resources utterly subverted the political and economic orthodoxies of the previous forty years, and in 1980 the nation chose decisively, but largely on faith, for other ways whose virtues were yet unproven. Key to those old orthodoxies was the idea that the United States was a country that primarily dispensed good things and ever more of them. Key to the confusion of the last decade and to what may become the orthodoxy of the foreseeable future is the idea that government in the United States has thrust upon it a new and uncomfortable role as allocator not of good things but of deprivations. Of those people and institutions who had become the employees, clients, or wards of the government—among them medical scientists and medical schools—that new consensus obviously would demand some adjustment. Related to that general cultural problem was the failure of research in medicine quickly to produce widely applicable results. Hard times forced attention to things close at hand whose costs could be justified by clearly apparent benefits. Research is not therefore grinding to a halt, nor is federal support for it about to disappear. But the relative position it has occupied in medicine over the last several decades is changing. For Vanderbilt, a traditionally research-oriented institution but one that long since had lost its independence, that change raised questions about its purpose and function that simply did not have to be asked before. For as the relative position of research changed—and declined—the relative position of other things changed too—and rose.

Ever since its new beginning in 1925, the Vanderbilt Medical School had two purposes in fact, three in rhetoric. It existed to educate, by the best possible reformed standards, the best possible medical doctors. To do so, it relied on a core of full-time scientist-teachers who also were expected to do serious experimental or clinical research to the end of adding to the sum of medical knowledge. The twin functions of education and research were as inseparable in the minds of those first faculty members as they were in the form of Robinson's courts and corridors. Service was something else. The crest of the medical school (not the medical center) bears the words: "Vanderbilt School of Medicine: A Century of Service." There, "service" meant and means the educational service of training doctors. More broadly, service has come to mean something different. Educating excellent physicians and surgeons was obviously a service, especially to the South, which needed them badly and which was where most Vanderbilt doctors stayed. Treating sick people in its clinics and wards, many of whom could not pay, was also a service; there could be no greater service than the personal bedside care given to poor sick patients by Hugh Morgan, Barney Brooks, and others of the great clinicians of that day. It is important to recall, however, that those poor sick people were in the Vanderbilt Hospital because they had been carefully selected by the staff primarily for their value as teaching cases. In conception and in fact, the hospital was a teaching laboratory for the school of medicine with which it was so closely integrated. University officials naturally liked to boast of the benefits to medical care in Nashville of such a hospital, but only secondarily did it actually operate as a community service institution. Initially independent financially, it could do as it pleased.

Since the middle 1970s the Vanderbilt Medical Center has had its own logo: a bold "V" encircled by three broad arrows signifying education, research, and patient care. Patient care, or service, was no longer an ancillary activity; it was in fact a big business, which, as research dollars dwindled, increasingly fueled the whole enterprise. There is no precise watershed that defines at Vanderbilt when medical school became medical center. The phrase crept in during the 1950s (as it did nationally) and by the late 1960s was well established as the umbrella under which was grouped the growing array of medical facilities bunched on the southeast corner of the Vanderbilt campus. It was a "center" literally: an agglomeration of buildings in one place. "Center" also conveyed other meanings: increased size, greater organizational and administrative complexity, and extended function. Size and complexity alone, some said, gave the center of the 1970s a completely different character from the simpler school of the 1920s and 1930s. But it was changing function in the form of a different kind of service that changed things most. In this change, Vanderbilt was responding again to larger national patterns.

Once upon a time, university hospitals had functioned not unlike private charity institutions. They filled their wards with indigents, the cost of whose care was covered by endowment income. It was not pure charity, however, for in return the hospital got something that, as a laboratory for a medical school, was its job to provide: adequate quantity and proper quality of "clinical material." Beds for private patients were limited. At Vanderbilt, that arrangement was disrupted as early as the late 1930s when, as costs rose faster than endowment income, troublesome deficits appeared. By the late 1940s, costs had so outstripped income that the arrangement came in fact wholly unstuck and, as Goodpasture clearly saw, threatened to change the nature of the entire institution. Vanderbilt did not change in the way he recommended, but, muddling through the 1950s, it changed nonetheless. Because it had no other resource, more and more beds were given over to private patients who could pay. A fact bemoaned by many of its older faculty at the time, the hospital took on, for a time, the characteristics simply of a private service institution. Though unlike proprietary institutions it sought no profit, it was pressed to survive by fees paid for services rendered. Though conceived as an academic enterprise governed and financed internally, it was being pushed into the marketplace.

Fortunately, the market was a good one, filled as time went on with more and more people who were able to pay. They were able to pay not because as individuals more Americans were richer and chose to set aside money enough to meet the costs of their hospital care. Rather, Americans collectively over a number of years had decided that it was preferable to pay a part of the costs of everyone's hospital care all of the time than to worry about paying all of their own part of the time. They took out insurance and spread the risks. By the late 1950s private hospital insurance had spread widely to cover the middle class, while in 1965 Medicare and Medicaid extended coverage through public means to the elderly and the poor. Third parties paid the bills, and patient service revenue became the lifeblood of university hospitals. After the passage of Medicare and Medicaid, it seemed that the federal government was destined to become the primary provider of funds for hospitalization and payment of professional fees for much of the population. Although that did not come to pass, the combined coverage of private and public insurers thrust Vanderbilt into a role it had not known before. Wrote dean and director of medical affairs, Randolph Batson, in 1969: "Thus, we shall be compelled to teach on private patients and must adapt our teaching laboratory—the University Hospital—to this concept, attract private patients for teaching, compete in every way with other community hospitals, and seize upon every opportunity to benefit financially. The existence of many proprietary hospitals which flourish by selectively eliminating hospital services which are money losers does not make this adjustment easier. . . . We must take a new look at our responsibilities in health and community services, alter many programs such as the medical school curriculum, find means of maintaining strength in basic research, and construct new competitive hospital facilities. The very nature of our problems argues against orderly progression and easy solutions—yet, we must accommodate."[27] It had not been so long since concern over Vanderbilt's "responsibilities in health and community services" was, in the sense that Batson viewed them, minimal to say the least. Historically, "accommodating" was something Vanderbilt had not done either deliberately or well.

Patients who paid, or who came with the assurance that someone else would pay, were different from indigents wholly beholden to the goodness of Vanderbilt Hospital. No longer passive subjects in a teaching laboratory, patients had become (as the government, hospitals, and economists liked to think of them) active "health care consumers." What they consumed—hospital-based medical care—had become a market commodity to be bought and sold, which for academic Vanderbilt was something new. With insurance money in their pockets and other good hospitals available, patients or their physicians were able to shop around. Vanderbilt's hospital by this time was, to be kind, an aging dowager, the modern additions made to it here and there only seeming to highlight its overall old-fashionedness. Its collegiate Gothic exterior recalled another era, and the linear design inside no longer adapted to the intricacies of modern specialized medicine. There were plans for more additions, but in the end it was replaced by a massive modern structure across the street, itself slated for more expansion and designed to compete.

Back in 1925 at the university's half-century celebration, which also marked the opening of the old hospital, one speaker had referred to it in terms of a "Pullman-car" hospital, which then bespoke everything that was up to date and deluxe. The Pullman cars were all gone by 1980 when the hospital's replacement opened, and no metaphor today connotes quite what that one did then. But the planners of this, the second all-new Vanderbilt Hospital, had designed for comfort and convenience, if not luxury, far more deliberately than had their predecessors half a century before. They had to; tastes had changed. The "health care–consuming public" expected, in addition to first-rate care, certain amenities. The building consisted of three towers; it went up, not out. Long, busy, echoing corridors therefore became a thing of the past. Patient rooms, reached from much shorter hallways, formed quadrants with extensions at the corners and surrounded nursing stations and service areas. Open wards, even in the old hospital, had long been closed in, though four-bed rooms were common. By contrast, of the new hospital's 524 beds, the great majority were private. All had an outside view. There were private baths, telephones, televisions, carpeting, pleasant waiting rooms for the various services. The Vanderbilt Children's Hospital (as in the old building, a hospital within the hospital) boasted on the fifth floor in between the towers a "playground in the sky," a spacious courtyard area that gave children access to outdoor recreation just a few steps from their rooms. Original commissioned artwork decorated public and patient-care areas, while the main hospital lobby welcomed visitors and patients with the atmosphere of a modern luxury hotel.[28]

It was an impressive building that dominated the local landscape. It also dominated many people's notions of what the medical center consisted of: a place where sick people could receive extraordinary and unique clinical services available nowhere else in the region, and generally exemplary medical care. The medical center consisted, of course, of more than that. Its faculty taught young men and women to be doctors, and its scientists worked at uncovering the true mechanisms of disease, just as they had for years. Indeed, Vanderbilt had done all these things for years, long before it was called a center (though for years care was rendered on much different terms than it is today). And the hospital itself was more than a place where sick people could be well looked after. It was still a teaching laboratory where masters and apprentices together taught and learned by doing. But in a time and place as preoccupied with health care as the United States in the 1970s and 1980s, in which virtually all hospitals—including private teaching ones—had become accountable public service institutions, it seems not impossible that their service functions will not overshadow many others. At Vanderbilt, that is and is not happening.

Education, research, and service are the three stated purposes of the medical center. Education and research are purposes of some historical constancy. Harder to define, service over the years has taken on several different meanings. It has been through internal decisions—fierce institutional and individual commitments—that Vanderbilt holds tenaciously to those three purposes and defines its character in terms of them. That much is within its power, as it is in the power of most sound institutions to decide what it is they will be about. It is less clearly in Vanderbilt's power autonomously to control the balance among the three. There never was a balance in the sense that by some measure or other the three could be said to be in perfect equilibrium. It is a difficult thing to measure anyway. But as the institution's independence diminished after World War II, and as it was thrust into the community, the relation of those purposes shifted with the sources and sums of external support available to them—for Vanderbilt could no longer support any of them alone. Thus there appeared, more pronounced at some moments than others, faults between professed purpose and actual behavior. Vanderbilt's source of support reflected the fashions and the commitments of the community by which it lived. Though it is far from perfectly true for this school that where its treasure is there its heart is also, the sources of that treasure have shown little of the constancy proudly associated with its purpose.

Reaping the bounty of the nation's new-found commitment to medical research, for instance, Vanderbilt in the 1950s and 1960s saw the portion of its total revenues derived from grants and other sponsored programs rocket from less than 25 percent to nearly 80 percent. The relative importance of endowment and tuition meanwhile was declining, with endowment declining most sharply. Vanderbilt was not just then alone in seeing the coffers for research overflow, and like other places some of that support spilled over into other uses. Research funds unquestionably subsidized education indirectly. Moreover, large increase in support for one kind of activity does not mean that another kind of activity must necessarily suffer, particularly if the whole institution was experiencing much growth and development, as this one then was. Nevertheless, the complaint generally was not then uncommon that by turning the best medical schools into small versions of NIH their educational responsibility could be slighted. Large grant–supported faculties, many of whose members did not teach, were visible reminders of that possibility. During the 1970s, sponsored research and programs continued to be the single largest source of medical school revenue at Vanderbilt. Though the dollar totals went every year reliably upward, their relative importance went down in 1976, falling to below 50 percent for the first time since the late 1950s.[29] Research was not therefore going away, but something else clearly was crowding the picture. The relative place of endowment income remained low (4 to 5 percent of total revenues); tuition, fees, and gifts hovered between 5 and 6 percent; the recovery of indirect costs on sponsored programs was in the range of 8 to 12 percent. The rest, whose rate of absolute dollar increase was steeper than grants and steeper by far than tuition and endowment, was represented by income from patient care.

Specifically, it was money paid for professional services rendered by the full-time faculty in Vanderbilt's clinics and hospitals, a part of which was harvested for the institution through a professional practice plan. At one time most Vanderbilt clinicians had billed patients only reluctantly. Care, they said, was not their true business and to gain from it only confused their motives in the things that really were their business: teaching and research. In the reluctance to relate charges to costs was an old-fashioned academic attitude destined not to survive a time when the increased third-party funds available to pay for medical care became a beckoning source of income for medical school budgets. Practice, moreover, had become the way most of Vanderbilt's clinicians made their living. The patients they brought into the medical center served teaching needs for sure, but the fees paid by the patients or their insurers served the school's financial needs as well and in an ever-larger way. In the late 1960s income to the school from patient care still limped along at less than 5 percent of total revenues. In the 1970s, however, the practice plan was successful and by the end of the decade brought back to the school over $12.5 million, fully a third of its revenue (1978 figures). At their present rates of increase and decrease (which seem likely to continue if not become steeper), income from patient care will exceed income from sponsored research and programs as the largest single source of revenue before the middle of the 1980s.[30]

With that, a watershed will have been reached. A similar watershed was reached in the middle 1950s when endowment income ceased to be the key to the school's livelihood and was replaced by grants for research and other sponsored programs. That first watershed was the more important in the history of Vanderbilt's devolution from independence to dependence. It meant that henceforth the institution would survive not by the grace bestowed at its own fortuitous origin, but by wits. It had entered that period when every person in the school became a source of revenue for the school, reversing the old Flexnerian formula by which the reformed endowed school ideally provided every person in it the means to teach and investigate—and thus release from the worries of the marketplace. The second watershed marks no change in the fundamental fact of dependence established thirty years before. It marks only a change in the source from which the school will earn a large piece of its daily bread. "Earn" is the key word, for earn it must. To survive and prosper, it must compete in the marketplace, which consists both of the public forum, where its scientists compete for government grants, and of the private one, where its clinicians practice fee-for-service medicine. Its earnings there today constitute between 80 and 90 percent of the school's total annual income. In that simple fact of overwhelming dependence on external support that is either recurring or competitive in nature lies a certain resemblance to pre-Flexner days when the school also lived by the market, albeit a somewhat different one. It then needed above all to compete not for grants but for students whose tuition was the only true income the school had. The faculty (few of whom were scientists then) practiced medicine for at least one of the same reasons as faculty members do today: to support themselves. The resemblance sharpens as the contemporary dependence on practice grows.

The watershed of the 1950s, though marking the end of independence and thus compelling adjustment to new mechanisms of support, only confirmed older, undisputed convictions of what Vanderbilt's function really was. Most of that public money, which so quickly overwhelmed other sources of support, was for research. And in research ever since 1925 the self-image and actual behavior of Vanderbilt's faculty were happily congruent. The watershed of the 1980s raises questions about the relation between the school's sources of support and its functions and is potentially more troubling. Medical care, the source of Vanderbilt's fastest-growing income, was something the institution had always dispensed. But it had earlier been dispensed only to the degree that it was necessary to carry out primary teaching and research functions. Providing medical care as medical care (or, as it is increasingly called, the delivery of health care) today, however, is something for which the public and the private markets are exerting ever-greater pressure. Whether Vanderbilt, which exists solely by the grace of those markets, can resist completely or forever those pressures seems unlikely. That however is for another generation of Vanderbilt faculty to sort out. Things may realign naturally as a new pattern of support becomes established and as a generation of doctors raised under it cease to recall that there ever was any other way. The question is troubling now only because the fact of growing activity in patient care as an autonomous function beclouds that older institutional self-image created by the leaders of Robinson's and Goodpasture's generation and sustained by their first postwar successors. The habit, called a tradition, of research at Vanderbilt is far from spent, just as the coffers to pay for it are far from empty. But it may have to accommodate another activity, which too may become a habit, and whose coffers are even fuller.

How genial will be that new accommodation between science and service will depend both on faculty commitment to the unity of the institution—an imponderable—and on the outside matters and actions that affect the balance among its different functions. Stability and harmony do not require perfect balance and never have. They require only the belief that different functions sensibly relate: merely that they can be defended as belonging in the same house. For most of Vanderbilt's history, sustaining this belief has been small problem. It has become a problem more recently only because the relation of the school to the larger community has changed more than ever it did in the distant past. And from that changed relation has come and will come a changed and changing nature. Robinson, who had an image of what the school should be and then filled in the reality to match it, did his work so well that for years the image truly determined the reality. It was helped, of course, by just the right configuration of outside support. It was also dependent not wholly but in part on that support—the fashion of Flexner's ideas, the power of the foundations, and later abundant public money for research. As that configuration changes, so must Robinson's image. Numbers, however, poorly measure these changes. They leave virtually unaccounted the whole matter of teaching, the other of modern Vanderbilt's three broad arrows. Tuition, the hard money paid by students to be taught medicine, vied with endowment as the smallest source of income to the school. Though it rose precipitously from $690 in 1950 to $5,500 in 1980, the fraction of total revenue represented by tuition fell over those thirty years from over 10 percent to approximately 5 percent. Special grants for teaching and training always trailed far behind grants for research, and even capitation, which could be said to be a direct subsidy for medical teaching, yielded relatively small sums ($290,000 in 1976–77, $477,000 in 1979–80).[31] The irony is that of the three professed aims of the institution, teaching brought in by far the least money but its centrality was hardly disputed.

Teaching became central at Vanderbilt at the same time research did: in the 1920s. Doctors had taught before, some very ably. But only with Robinson and his new staff was introduced the idea that medical teaching like medical research required special skills and commitments distinct from those common to the practice of medicine. Flexner said teaching and research were one, and Robinson's faculty helped prove them so. Even though many of the links between them were broken after the war with the coming of categorical funding for research and the degree of faculty segregation that ensued, enough remain so that there is today still small problem conceiving of the two functions in the same house. Class size may have doubled and the era of the unlimited research budgets may have ended, but the dogma that both belong at Vanderbilt and that one makes little sense without the other is the most enduring product of the school's experience after 1925. Against that history more recent developments in the area of patient care or health care delivery will in time have to fit. The numbers measuring sources of support suggest a return to conditions analogous to those of pre-Flexnerian medical education; the school and its people must once again earn their way in the world, more and more, it would seem, by the practice of medicine. But between them and their predecessors, who in proprietary days also had to earn their way, have intervened fifty fairly momentous years in the history of the union of science and medicine. The medical professors who took care of patients at Vanderbilt in 1980 did so to earn their keep and perhaps because they enjoyed it. But even to get to Vanderbilt they had, more than most doctors, to know and to care about science. If they would be rewarded at Vanderbilt they had, obedient to the orthodoxy of half a century, to do some science as well. Thus the analogy is apt but imperfect. The people's demand for more health care and their impatience with science may in the future carve out new orthodoxies that will change greatly even places like Vanderbilt. For now, the old orthodoxy still reigns there, if not quite as easily as it once did.

The 1960s and 1970s were hard on old orthodoxies generally. Vanderbilt, which by then necessarily and decisively had cast its lot with the community, stood to gain or to lose according to its character and commitments. In the early part of that period, the nation was ambitious for its medical schools among other things, and Vanderbilt like many others changed much in size and form. It grew; it renovated its curriculum; it enjoyed belonging to a group of institutions called upon to do great things. It became large and complex; it changed from a medical school into a medical center. Most important, that change in words signified, above and beyond simple growth and development, a changing relation with the community outside the institution. In spirit, medicine and medical education became public property. The public whose property they were was entertaining new and expanded notions about medicine's proper domain and was establishing an ever-higher level of entitlement to its benefits. Somewhere in the process, "medicine" ceased to be medicine as once understood and became "health care" just as concurrently medical schools were becoming medical centers. Medical centers, by almost any definition, have broader functions than the medical schools from which they came, and they would be hard to imagine within the limited realm once assigned to mere medicine. Health, on the other hand, offers a broad field to run in—and to get lost in. What seems to be the rising star of patient care at Vanderbilt is partly due to economics, but it is also a product of changed public tastes and the public's determination to have what it wants. Medicine turned to health care, indeed, is one of the few public enthusiasms as alive in the 1980s as it was in the early 1960s. "Great societies" dotted with "model cities" spark the same nostalgic curiosity that remnants of Roosevelt's New Deal did twenty years after their beginning, but they do not kindle hot debate, let alone determined action. The debates about medicine and health care have never been hotter, and the action never more determined.

The fate that has befallen Vanderbilt's medical center during these years resembles that of other large complex institutions in recent times. It has grown in size, differentiated in function, and responded because it must to an array of outside pressures. Like universities, corporations, and government, Vanderbilt finds accountability both to its masters and to its customers an ever more pressing reality. Vanderbilt's walls, which once set off its rarefied business from much that went on around it, have become porous, and by the old academic standards espoused by Robinson the institution has become impure. But so has much else, including its parent university, which is also beholden to many masters and is busy doing many things, not all of them purely academic. The university has reaped considerable prestige from the long union (since 1925) with the medical school; the medical school has profited by the proximity of another large body of scholars. So Flexner had said. Neither, however, is what it was when Flexner said it. In the last twenty years, through the activity of the hospital especially, the university has become party to the big business of health care delivery—a "for-hire," essentially noneducational service to the community. No one in the departments of history or English had anything similar to offer. The risks were large, even though the university's policy ever since the frightening financial crisis of the 1940s and 1950s has been not to subsidize the medical center in any way. The single glaring exception to that came in the mid-1970s when, to secure the bond issue needed to build the new Vanderbilt Hospital, there had to be pledged the full good faith and credit of the university. Even assuming that pledge is never called on, the institution as a whole cannot help but worry constantly over the health of its medical parts. The numbers alone had become enormous and have changed the dynamics of the relationship of medical center and university. Too many empty hospital beds could mean deficits as large as the budgets of other whole schools in the university. The public exposure that came with health care delivery in the 1970s and 1980s placed on the university constant pressure of another sort in a consumer culture that every year seemed to grow more adversarial.

Institutional purity was no longer a real issue, however. Opportunity was the issue, and it existed outside, in the mainstream of American public life. The evolution of school to center was a result of the institution's entry into that mainstream. It had and has no other choice. Isolation, once glorious, was long since beyond its means, and no one counseled, for purity's sake, quitting the business. The men and women who run the school, the center, and the university today must among other things be careful pragmatic opportunists, for their margin for error is small. Such a man was Kirkland many years before but with one important difference. Opportunity then had meant taking medicine out of the community and giving it to science, whence would return in time good and useful things. The cost, relatively, was small and could be met through the agency of a few people who controlled a few foundations. Opportunity later meant returning the fruits of science in medicine to the community as service, while maintaining conditions in which science itself still flourished. The cost of that, relatively, was enormous and could be met only through collective action and from the people's own purse.

That the mechanisms for meeting those costs will continue to be collective there is little doubt. How much the people will be willing to pay is less clear. What once seemed, since the 1950s at least, a fairly bottomless exchequer, no longer seems so. The dynamics of national ambition, as apparent in medical or "health" matters as in any area of American life over the last quarter of a century, confront periodically the limits of the nation's productivity. Medicine is no exception. As ambitions are measured against achievements, we are compelled to think again about the expectations that can sensibly be held in medicine and those that cannot. The expansion of this medical school and center in size and function is partly a response to one set of expectations now subject to some scrutiny. What has been true here has been common elsewhere. And although the worlds of academic medicine and of practicing medicine are certainly not identical, they are parts of the same larger national concern over health generally and are subject to some of the same pressures rising from that concern. Academic medical centers like Vanderbilt's have become big businesses in every sense, with whose complex functions have come sophisticated management techniques commonly believed necessary to move large numbers of people doing different things and large sums of money from different places. Practicing medicine in the United States, on the other hand, remains by comparison a cottage industry, with 95 percent of the units in the nonacademic health care industry each employing fewer than twenty people.[32] Practicing medicine consumes far more of the money spent on things medical in this nation than do academic medical centers. Yet to the money spent on both is commonly attached the assumption that there exists a direct, easy-to-see relationship between investment and return.[33] Indeed, unless there has been in recent decades some unnoticed change in the American national character that has made us more patient and far-seeing than historically we once were, the high national investment in health can be explained in only this way.

Science, however, works in other ways, and it is on science that much of the burden of the nation's ambition for health has been placed. The idea of a "crisis in health care," so fashionable in recent years, bespoke considerable discontent with matters of cost, availability, and distribution of the services and personnel associated with the maintenance of health and the treatment of disease. And in that sense, the idea of a crisis was a useful one: around such things energies and resources could be mobilized or remobilized with reasonable hope that from deliberate action results might directly follow. Wanting as it plainly did better access to medical care, the nation was able to move in that direction, though costs remained a problem. The efficacy of will and action was once again demonstrated. But in another sense, the idea of a crisis was not useful at all, for the deeper source of our complaint lay truly not with mere matters of accessibility, distribution, or even of cost but with the limits of our knowledge about how things work: that is, with science. With science, no amount of will and action, expressed in dollars expended, necessarily or even likely assured results. Nowhere was this condition clearer than in the academic medical centers, the chief sites of the union of science and medicine. The problem is not new, and the stresses and pressures that academic medical centers appear to be ever more laboring under are not in this sense a new experience for them.[34] Vanderbilt's medical center has been a stressed institution almost since Kirkland, Flexner, and Robinson rebuilt it: not for long did it stay independent and aloof from the community. When that happened, there surfaced the tension that was implicit in its nature and in the union of science and medicine itself. Medicine as science and medicine as service could never be perfectly mated.

To imagine this difficult relationship as a crisis is either to change the meaning of the word or to suggest that science can be made to move faster and more efficiently toward satisfying our health expectations. Though science, of all the academic disciplines, is the only one that is presumed to "progress," the speed and the efficiency of its progress defy easy measurement, let alone easy manipulation.[35] At Vanderbilt it is impossible yet to say whether science moves faster or more efficiently than it did in the 1930s.[36] Certainly, the social mandate to science and to science in medicine since World War II has been great, but the conditions whereby the individual scientist's intellect was set free—the true engine of science—were established here in 1925, and they may even have deteriorated since then (compare support for research through the fluid research fund with the term grants of NIH). The list of things that science, even after a hundred years of its union with medicine and more than half a century at Vanderbilt, still does not know about health and disease is very long. Not a little of medicine as it is actually practiced remains remarkably empirical; much of it relies on therapies that treat the results of pathological conditions without understanding the mechanisms that cause them. Many of those therapies and "halfway technologies" are very expensive and themselves argue strongly that what is wrong with medicine today is not that its benefits are poorly distributed but that its knowledge is too slight.[37] There is much yet to know, much yet to busy the scientists at a research-oriented institution like Vanderbilt.

Science, then, is one of the problems. Expectations about health are the other. Expectations, or demand, translated to money assigned to research, unquestionably have helped to fuel science. But they have not stopped there. The World Health Organization's famous 1946 definition of health as "a state of complete physical, mental, and social well-being and not merely the absence of disease or infirmity" and similar proclamations from time to time have not brought a health utopia much closer. But they have changed the meaning of the word and, as the meaning broadened, the slippage between the word and the thing increased. If this was health, then with it medicine, as it had evolved since its union with science, had not a lot to do. If the meaning of medicine too was to change, it obviously must entail the vast expansion of medicine's domain and consequently a blurring of the boundaries on the jurisdiction of doctors and other people training in medicine.

Such expansion could be exhilarating—and a little frightening—for implicit in expectations about health thus defined was the right to it. Again, the words slip. The right to health could mean simply a variant on the right to life—that is, the simple fact of existence of which we cannot arbitrarily be deprived by the state or our fellows. Nor can our good health, which is natural, be arbitrarily deprived. Deprived is the key; it is a negative protection. If it means the right to be healthy, however, that is something entirely different. It then entails the right to medical or health care—not simply protection from infringement on a natural condition but the provision of things that supposedly enhance that condition. This is clearly a different sort of "right" from, for instance, those enumerated in the Bill of Rights of the United States Constitution, by which measure it is not a right at all. It is an allocative tool for the securing of certain of society's goods and services, things not preexistent but things produced by people and eminently negotiable. Doing that in a society whose productive capacity is finite requires giving to some while depriving others. Decisions so to allocate resources have been and will continue to be made in health matters, just as they are in education, transportation, housing, and other public policy matters. Perhaps all of those things entail rights. Or perhaps none of them does.

But with rights, one way or the other, science has only slim connection. And it is science that has been the source of greatest achievement in medicine over the last century and likely will remain the source for the century to come. This continued achievement will be in spite of, not because of, rising insistence on the right to health whose immediate visible goal is care and matters of availability and just distribution. Caring, like "health," is broadly comprehensive. Curing, which is what science in medicine has aimed to find ways to do, is not. The distinction is important and real. Seeing it clearly helps to keep some sense of proportion in our view of modern medicine. Within its limited realm, medicine through science still holds untold benefits for humanity. New basic breakthroughs will come, and like others before them they will reduce greatly the sum of physical suffering. It is vital to remember, however, that medicine's realm is limited. Doctors with their vast technological armamentarium better cure our bodies than they care for the rest of us. That is as it should be. They should not be asked for the care best rendered by families, priests, and teachers, and they should not seek those roles for themselves. Society's esteem and their training in science have given doctors greater power than comes to most people. That power can sometimes cure us. It cannot save us. Medicine is not religion, and through it we have not transcended or even greatly transformed our condition.

About the history of Vanderbilt's medical school the same sense of proportion needs to be kept. It is a place where, half a century ago, science and medicine dramatically came together in the form of a physically integrated school and hospital and a faculty of exceptional young scientist-teachers. For a short while, it enjoyed a special kind of freedom to explore and extend that union with little care for the community outside. Later, thanks to its poverty and the growing appeal of the things it represented, it invited outside support and in time intrusion. Physical growth and expanded function followed, eventually bursting Robinson's courts and corridors and raising about the nature of the institution questions that to him and his new leaders had not existed. Throughout, it was a place where some people learned about a certain kind of science from other people who had learned it there or at similar places, and it was a place where scientists themselves worked at extending knowledge about human biology. It rendered service, in the beginning, as it was required to teach and do research. Later, it rendered service for other reasons too. It finds itself today in the mainstream where it must respond to changing fashions and demands. It supports itself increasingly in the market, where it must compete to survive.

Yet even as the medical school competes, there continues among the best of its scientists the quiet work of assembling small pieces of large puzzles. When compared with their successors fifty years later, Robinson's scientists knew little and knew they knew little; today's scientists hold a similar conviction about the knowledge their successors likely will possess. By no means all of what they will know will be useful to medicine. Some of it will be, but inevitably much expensive time and talent will turn out to have been wasted, as it has been in the past. That being so, it is not unthinkable that in research there are limits beyond which for economic or political reasons we ought not to go in the investment of time, talent, and money. There clearly are such limits in health care, and while research is less costly, its dividends are also less apparent. There may also be moral reasons for going so far but no farther: genetic engineering and in vitro fertilization, for example, have raised for some that question of whether there are some things it probably is better not to know. The acknowledgment of limits, if it comes and for whatever reasons, will come gradually. Gradually too, Vanderbilt will then need to seek another justification, another confirming purpose. But in their journey together, science and its public are not nearly there yet, especially not in medicine. And for the moment the character of this place still springs, more than from any other source, from its distinctive origin and early years.

Even so, there is no denying that standards in the world outside are changing. Conceptions of both medicine and health are at once more exalted, more spacious, and less precise than those that had satisfied an earlier, less insistent time. As distinctions have blurred and medicine's domain has expanded, there has been a distraction of the common attention from goals that had once reasonably seemed within reach of talented people with clear and shared ideas. Vanderbilt, at its heart, still belongs to that time. Its history still makes sense as the working out—slowly—of progress through the union of science and medicine, of progress through knowledge. It still echoes with the proud and sober confidence of Kirkland, Flexner, Robinson, and their fellows. The future will judge how well it redeems the promise of that far-off fruitful youth.

Notes

BOT   Vanderbilt University Board of Trust
CMVL   Chancellor's Manuscripts, Vanderbilt University Library
LC   Library of Congress
RAC   General Education Board Files, Rockefeller Archive Center
VL   Vanderbilt University Library
VML   Vanderbilt Medical Library

1. Prologue: Three Men and a Celebration

1. On Cornelius Vanderbilt see: Joshua Wheaton Lane, *Commodore Vanderbilt: An Epic of the Steam Age* (New York: Alfred A. Knopf, 1942); Wayne Andrews, *The Vanderbilt Legend: The Story of the Vanderbilt Family 1794–1940* (New York: Harcourt Brace & Co., 1941). Also, Edwin Mims, *History of Vanderbilt University* (Nashville: Vanderbilt University Press, 1946), and Robert A. McGaw, *The Vanderbilt Campus: A Pictorial History* (Nashville: Vanderbilt University Press, 1978).

2. The word went far. See the *New York Times,* October 16, 1925: "Vanderbilt Expands Its Science Work."

3. The standard source on Kirkland is Edwin Mims, *Chancellor Kirkland of Vanderbilt* (Nashville: Vanderbilt University Press, 1940). Also see Mims, *History of Vanderbilt University.* The best primary sources are the Chancellor's Manuscripts in the Vanderbilt University Library (CMVL). On family matters see the Kirkland-Merritt correspondence in the files of the Vanderbilt Centennial History Project, VL.

4. Mims, *Chancellor Kirkland,* p. 21.

5. Kirkland and his mother, Virginia, corresponded often while he was abroad. See Kirkland-Merritt files, VL.

6. Abraham Flexner, *Medical Education in the United States and Canada* (Bulletin Number Four of the Carnegie Foundation for the Advancement of Teaching, New York, 1910) (hereafter cited as Flexner Report).

7. The autobiography, *I Remember: The Autobiography of Abraham Flexner* (New York: Simon & Schuster) first appeared in 1940. A revised edition was published in 1960 entitled *Abraham Flexner: An Autobiography*. Primary sources include the Flexner Papers, Medical Education Files, Library of Congress (LC); Flexner's correspondence in the files of various of the Rockefeller boards at the Rockefeller Archive Center (RAC); and an oral history interview conducted by Allan Nevins and Saul Benison, *The Reminiscences of Abraham Flexner* (Columbia University, New York: Oral History Research Office, 1959).

8. Flexner, *I Remember*, p. 40.

9. Abraham Flexner, *Abraham Flexner: An Autobiography* (New York: Simon and Schuster, 1960), p. 68.

10. See Daniel M. Fox, "Abraham Flexner's Unpublished Report: Foundations and Medical Education, 1909–1928," *Bulletin of the History of Medicine* 54 (1980): 475–96.

11. Robinson entitled his autobiography *Adventures in Medical Education: A Personal Narrative of the Great Advance of American Medicine* (Cambridge: Harvard University Press, for the Commonwealth Fund, 1957). Also see A. McGehee Harvey, "G. Canby Robinson: Peripatetic Medical Educator," *Johns Hopkins Medical Journal* 143 (1978): 84–101, and C. Sidney Burwell, "George Canby Robinson," *Transactions of the Association of American Physicians* 74 (1959): 40, and Chapters 5–8 below.

12. *Proceedings of the Semi-Centennial of Vanderbilt University, October 15–18, 1925* (Nashville: Vanderbilt University, 1925), pp. 90–91.

2. The True Measure

1. Abraham Flexner, *I Remember* (New York: Simon & Schuster, 1940), pp. 109–12.

2. All prominent medical educators, the other members of the council included John A. Witherspoon from Vanderbilt, William T. Councilman from Harvard, Charles Frazier from the University of Pennsylvania, Victor C. Vaughan from the University of Michigan. The standard history is Herman G. Weiskotten and Victor Johnson, *A History of the Council on Medical Education and Hospitals of the AMA, 1904–1959* (Chicago: American Medical Association, 1959). Witherspoon later became president of the AMA (1913–14), as did Vaughan (1914–15) and Bevan (1918–19).

3. Flexner's own reminiscences of that hectic and exciting time are recorded in his autobiography, *I Remember*, pp. 113–32.

4. Flexner Report, p. x.

5. A number of writers have placed the report in the context of the growing movement for educational reform at the turn of the century. H. D. Banta, "Abraham Flexner—A Reappraisal," *Social Science Medicine* 5 (1971): 655–61; Howard S. Berliner, "A Larger Perspective on the Flexner Report," *International Journal of Health Sciences* 5 (1975): 573–92, and "New Light on the Flexner Report: Notes on the AMA–Carnegie Foundation Background," *Bulletin of the History of*

Medicine 51 (1977): 603–09; Daniel M. Fox, "Abraham Flexner's Unpublished Report: Foundations and Medical Education, 1909–1928," *Bulletin of the History of Medicine* 54 (1980): 475–96; Robert P. Hudson, "Abraham Flexner in Perspective: American Medical Education, 1865–1910," *Bulletin of the History of Medicine* 46 (1972): 545–61; H. Miller, "Fifty Years After Flexner," *Lancet* 2 (1966): 647–54; Saul Jarcho, "Medical Education in the United States, 1910–1956," *Journal of the Mt. Sinai Hospital* 8 (1959): 339–85.

6. Flexner Report, p. 3.
7. Ibid., p. 4. The phrase—"demonstrates the Truth of Theory by Facts"—did not mean quite the same thing in the eighteenth century as it did in the twentieth. To eighteenth-century medicine, theory and system mattered greatly. "Facts" might indeed be summoned to demonstrate "the Truth of Theory," less easily to disprove one, as Flexner seemed to infer from Bond's statement.
8. Ibid., pp. 4–5.
9. Ibid., p. 6.
10. Ibid.
11. One who did succeed despite the old system was pathologist William H. Welch of Johns Hopkins. In defense of the men if not the methods of his own old training ground, the College of Physicians and Surgeons of New York, in the early 1870s, he wrote (and Flexner quoted): "Our teachers were men of fine character, devoted to the duties of their chairs; they inspired us with enthusiasm, interest in our studies and hard work, and they imparted to us sound traditions of our profession; nor did they send us forth so utterly ignorant and unfitted for professional work as those born of the present greatly improved methods of training and opportunities for practical studies are sometimes wont to suppose." Ibid., p. 10.
12. Ibid., p. 12.
13. Ibid., p. 13.
14. Flexner did not, of course, mention why Germany was a poor example socially and politically, however much its laboratories and medical schools made a good example scientifically. Germany in 1910 was a unitary centralized state and not a federated republic. Its people, while not "racially pure," were decidedly less ethnically diverse than the Americans. Its faiths too—Lutheran, Catholic, and Jewish—were less splintered than the babble of American denominations. Like the United States, its greatest historical sectional cleavage was north-south, which was also a religious cleavage. Also like the United States, it industrialized late and exceedingly well. Unlike the United States, it had been a nation only since 1871, and it was a nation whose security could not easily be taken for granted: the United States was hemmed in by oceans and by weak, friendly neighbors; Germany was surrounded by enemies.
15. Flexner Report, p. 20.
16. Ibid., pp. 14, 16.
17. Ibid., p. 156. But Flexner was careful: thus the word "effort." He did not say that "medicine is a discipline in which *knowledge* procured in various ways *is used* in order to effect certain practical ends."
18. Some representative doctor-to-patient ratios in the United States at that time are: in Pennsylvania, 1:636; in Maryland, 1:658; in Nebraska, 1:602; in Colorado, 1:328; in Oregon, 1:646 (Flexner Report, p. 16).
19. Ibid., p. 17.

20. Ibid., p. 26.
21. Ibid., pp. 30, 35.
22. Ibid., p. 43.
23. Ibid., p. 102.
24. Ibid., pp. 110–11.
25. Ibid., pp. 178–79.
26. Ibid., pp. 178–80. See Mary R. Walsh, *Doctors Wanted: No Women Need Apply* (New Haven: Yale University Press, 1977), and James Summerville, *Educating Black Doctors: A History of Meharry Medical College* (University: University of Alabama Press, 1983).
27. Cited in James Morris, *Farewell the Trumpets: An Imperial Retreat* (New York: Harcourt Brace Jovanovich, 1978), p. 122.
28. Such an interpretation of the "scientific" legacy of the Flexner Report is common in medical school histories, most written by doctors. See, for example, Alan M. Chesney, *The Johns Hopkins Hospital and the Johns Hopkins University School of Medicine,* 3 vols. (Baltimore: Johns Hopkins University Press, 1943–63); Thomas B. Turner, *Heritage of Excellence: The Johns Hopkins Medical Institutions, 1914–1947* (Baltimore: Johns Hopkins University Press, 1974); Rudolph H. Kampmeier, *Recollections: The Department of Medicine, Vanderbilt University School of Medicine, 1925–1959* (Nashville: Vanderbilt University Press, 1980); John Romano et al., *To Each His Farthest Star: University of Rochester Medical Center, 1925–1975* (Rochester: University of Rochester Medical Center, 1975).
29. On public health and social service, see Flexner Report, pp. 19, 68, and, on p. 154: "Practically, the medical school is a public service corporation."
30. Ibid., p. 26.
31. The best study of specialism is Rosemary Stevens, *American Medicine and the Public Interest* (New Haven: Yale University Press, 1971). See p. 73.

3. Gathering Substance

1. Flexner later claimed that several hours was all that was really required to find out what he needed to know about most schools (Abraham Flexner, *I Remember* [New York: Simon & Schuster, 1940], p. 121). It is also true that he went deliberately looking for rotten apples and that he found them abundantly. He might have been more thorough had he lingered longer; his conclusions surely would have been the same. Muckraking was his job, and he seemed to enjoy it.
2. Such credentials commonly read:
   "To . . . Dean:
       Sir: I have examined Mr. . . . of . . . , and find his scholastic attainments equal to those requisite for a first-grade teacher's certificate in our public schools, with the equivalent of two years of high school study" (Flexner Report, p. 36).
3. Ibid., p. 88.
4. Flexner, *I Remember,* p. 115. Flexner's notes and summaries, which he sent for checking to the medical school deans and to which he refers in his autobiography, do not survive in his papers in the Library of Congress. Several "questionnaires" do. Flexner Papers, Medical Education Files, LC.
5. Both the seventeen-part questionnaire, headed "Please send answers to the fol-

lowing questions to A. Flexner, Carnegie Foundation, 576 Fifth Ave., New York, N.Y.," and the four-page response from Vanderbilt are undated, but the broad range of questions (compared with more specific things asked in later requests, the first of which is dated five months after Flexner's visit to Vanderbilt) suggests that this, the longest list, came first. Flexner Papers, Medical Education Files, LC.

6. Flexner Report, p. 154.

7. Lucius E. Burch to Flexner, July 21, 1909, Flexner Papers, Medical Education Files, LC.

8. At the council's third annual meeting in 1907 Kirkland spoke pointedly on the subject: "Twenty years ago, Vanderbilt University adopted the policy of . . . placing conditions for entrance that were practically identical with those maintained in the first class institutions of the East. We did that in 1887, and reduced our students with one blow. . . by about one-half. We have sacrificed something for our faith in educational work; and yet, gentlemen, perhaps no one fact can bring before you more forcefully the general condition of things in the southern states than this, that in this year, 1907, twenty years after we have made our fight and twenty years after we have established our standard, the Carnegie Foundation for the Advancement of Teaching issued a bulletin defining the preliminary educational requirements necessary for a high grade college in fourteen units, and the Carnegie Foundation cited our course alone in all the South as meeting those requirements. . . . The Carnegie Foundation for the Advancement of Teaching has caused a shudder to run through all these institutions in the South by the publication of that report. . . . If the council would inspect and tell the truth about all our institutions, point out their defects, point to their equipment and give the facts as regards them, and as regards their manner of teaching, the moral force that would be exerted by such an inspection would be a tremendous power and would have an uplift that could not be calculated or realized. That, sir, would be more efficient in the long run than an attempt by too drastic legislation to secure results that might work disaster to the cause we all have so dearly at heart" (James H. Kirkland, "Controlling General and Medical Education in the South," address to the Third Annual Conference of the Council on Medical Education of the AMA, Chicago, April 29, 1907; cited in Howard S. Berliner, "New Light on the Flexner Report: Notes on the AMA–Carnegie Foundation Background," *Bulletin of the History of Medicine* 51 [1977]: 603).

9. Kirkland, unpublished history of Vanderbilt, p. 301, files of Vanderbilt Centennial History Project, VL.

10. Ibid., pp. 301–02.

11. Ibid., p. 302.

12. Minutes, BOT, March 26, 1873, April 29, 1874, June 19, 1876, June 18, 1877, VL. Cornelius Vanderbilt to Holland N. McTyeire, December 2, 1875, McTyeire-Baskervill Papers, VL.

13. Minutes, BOT, May 24, 1880, May 24, 1881, May 26, 1884; Executive Committee Minutes, BOT, January 16, 1886; and Statement of the Financial Condition of Vanderbilt University, June 4, 1892, VL.

14. During his lifetime, Frederick W. Vanderbilt gave about $500,000, comprising two gifts for the endowment of the college of arts and science ($100,000 in 1917–18 and $250,000 in 1926–29) and one for the endowment of the school of religion

($150,000 in 1935). At his death in 1938, the university's share of his estate exceeded $4.5 million, which was first put into general endowment and later transferred to provide endowment for particular schools (arts and science, $2 million; law, $500,000; religion, $600,000; nursing, $200,000). The balance went for brick and mortar: a school of engineering building, $250,000; Memorial Gymnasium, $500,000; Rand Dining Hall, $526,000; and men's dormitories, $249,000. Financial Report of Vanderbilt University, 1945, 1947, 1953, CMVL.

15. William Kissam Vanderbilt's first gift had come at the turn of the century—for a dormitory named Kissam Hall that cost $144,000. After fire destroyed College (later Kirkland) Hall in 1905, he contributed $150,000 to the rebuilding fund. During the college of arts and science fund drive of World War I, he donated $325,000 toward a goal of $1 million, and in 1920 he gave the university railroad stock valued at $460,000 that was used to obtain $250,000 in matching funds from the General Education Board. In his will, the university received another $250,000. *Vanderbilt Quarterly* (July 1907), p. 172; Financial Report of Vanderbilt University, 1918; Executive Committee Minutes, BOT, January 19, 1921; Minutes, BOT, June 11, 1923; and Financial Report of Vanderbilt University, 1922, CMVL.

William K. Vanderbilt's son, Harold Stirling Vanderbilt (the Commodore's great-grandson), was by far the greatest of the university's family patrons. By the middle of the 1970s his gifts had exceeded $50 million. He gave heavily to endowment fund drives during his lifetime and at his death in 1970 bequeathed the university over $17 million. As of June 30, 1973, the university's general endowment included over $8 million from his estate. Approximately $4 million of the Harold Stirling Vanderbilt trust funds was used in the Stevenson Science Center. Large quantities of his money also went to the endowments of the law, medical, and management schools and to the construction of the University Club and the Joe and Howard Werthan wing of the medical center. Financial Report of Vanderbilt University, 1973, CMVL; records in office of director of records, Alumni and Development Office, Vanderbilt University.

16. Minutes, BOT, October 25, 1910, VL.

17. The official and authorized history of the board is Raymond B. Fosdick, *Adventure in Giving: The Story of the General Education Board, A Foundation Established by John D. Rockefeller* (New York: Harper & Row, 1962). Also see Merle Curti and Roderick Nash, *Philanthropy in the Shaping of American Higher Education* (New Brunswick: Rutgers University Press, 1965), pp. 212–19.

18. John D. Rockefeller, *Random Reminiscences of Men and Events* (New York: Doubleday, Page & Co., 1909), pp. 159–65.

19. Cited in Fosdick, *Adventure in Giving*, p. 8.

20. Ibid.

21. Not that there ever was any doubt about whose money it actually was. But just in case, the board's letterhead announced unambiguously: "The General Education Board, Founded By John D. Rockefeller, 1902."

22. In these efforts, the GEB in part worked with and through the Southern Education Board, which had been established at Ogden's 1901 Winston-Salem meeting (with a gift of $30,000 from George Peabody) to promote tax-supported schools in the South. The aim was not to subsidize such schools—a task too mammoth even for the greatest private philanthropy—but through propaganda to instill in

states and localities appreciation for the value of schools and a willingness to support them with public funds. A bureau of information supplied statistics and arguments, and canvassers crossed the region revival-style, educating the people for education. The boards of the two organizations were largely interlocking, and grants (small and experimental at first) were generally made conditional on the recipient's ability to raise like or larger amounts from private or public sources—a policy that characterized the GEB for much of its history and one faithful to the desire of Rockefeller, Sr., to help only those who helped themselves.

23. Cited in Fosdick, *Adventure in Giving,* pp. 127–28.
24. Ibid., p. 129.
25. Ibid., p. 130.
26. Ibid., p. 135.
27. Though it was somewhat clearer what should constitute a true medical school, and easier to measure how far a place had moved on its own in that direction, even in medical education the decision whom to support sometimes rode on less than wholly "objective" or "scientific" considerations. It certainly did at Vanderbilt. Some schools evidently had more promise than others. As of 1920, only twenty schools had received fully 75 percent of the GEB's grants (see Curti and Nash, *Philanthropy in Higher Education,* p. 217).
28. Kirkland to Buttrick, February 24, 1910; Buttrick to Kirkland, March 1, 1910; and Buttrick to Kirkland, March 8, 1910, CMVL.
29. Buttrick to Kirkland, March 8, 1910, CMVL.
30. The single most glaring exception to this congruence of aims was the GEB's policy of making "academic full-time" a condition of its grants to medical schools, something that caused considerable row in the late 1910s and the 1920s among those who said the foundation had no right to dictate the internal policies of universities—neither the right nor the power, as it turned out. "Full-time" as Flexner imagined it did not become the rule in many clinical departments in American medical schools. The carrot did not work and, there being no stick, the GEB eventually relented. See Part Two below.
31. "The Vanderbilt University School of Medicine," *Vanderbilt Quarterly* (October–December 1915), pp. 259–60.
32. None of Carnegie's money had yet found its way to Vanderbilt. Kirkland had tried, however. Early in 1906 he appealed to Carnegie, through Wallace Buttrick as intermediary, for $150,000 to build a library at Vanderbilt (libraries being the object of Carnegie's first organized philanthropic endeavors), but the request never got past the wily Scot's trusted secretary, James Bertram:
    "There are only 391 students on the campus who will really use the Library Building," Bertram wrote Buttrick. "The other students making up the 835 in attendance at the University being scattered through the different professional schools in buildings in the city." It was best to wait, he said, until the proposed affiliation with Peabody should raise to over 500 the number of students actually on the main campus with convenient access to such a library. In the meantime: "Mr. Carnegie would never consider a $150,000 building for about 500 students. Furthermore even if the amalgamation took place, it would be some time before you erected the other buildings necessary to accommodate the 500 students you anticipate, so that at best, by putting up a $150,000 building now, you would be

erecting something which would only be fully used possibly 10 years hence and the use of the large part of that money would be lost till then." Rules were rules. James Bertram to Wallace Buttrick, February 17, 1906, RAC.

33. Cited in Joseph F. Wall, *Andrew Carnegie* (New York: Oxford University Press, 1970), p. 832.
34. Minutes, BOT, June 16, 1913, VL; see Kirkland–Henry Pritchett correspondence, 1910–13, CMVL.
35. Cited in Wall, *Carnegie*, p. 883. With the establishment of the Carnegie Corporation, Carnegie betrayed his long-held belief that wealth should be dispensed by its individual creator.
36. Edwin Mims, *History of Vanderbilt University* (Nashville: Vanderbilt University Press, 1946), pp. 291–320.
37. Kirkland to Andrew Carnegie, May 1, 1913, File of deeds, plats, and miscellany, Kirkland Hall Vault, Vanderbilt. The same day, it was a careful Kirkland who reported to his executive committee that without infusion of new money the medical school would have to be abandoned—but, as result of consultation with Henry S. Pritchett, it was possible that Carnegie would give, "provided all conditions of administration [the seven-member governing board] could be made acceptable to him" (Executive Committee Minutes, BOT, May 1, 1913, VL).
38. Andrew Carnegie to Kirkland, May 20, 1913, Kirkland Hall Vault, Vanderbilt.
39. Minutes, BOT, June 16, 1913, VL.
40. Kirkland to W. H. Askew, Magnolia, Arkansas, May 26, 1913, CMVL.
41. Kirkland to William L. Moore, Little Rock, May 26, 1913, CMVL.
42. Kirkland to Austin B. Fletcher, New York, May 14 and 21, 1913, CMVL.
43. Though negotiations among Kirkland, Pritchett, and Carnegie antedated the Carnegie Corporation and though Carnegie himself became personally involved in them, the grant to Vanderbilt, by the time it was finalized, was carried on the books of the new philanthropic foundation, as future ones would be.
44. *Nashville Banner,* May 31 and June 19, 1913.
45. *Nashville Christian Advocate,* June 18, 1913. Clipping file, VL.
46. *Raleigh Christian Chronicle,* n.d. Clipping file, VL.
47. *Nashville Banner,* May 31, 1913.
48. "The Controversy Over the Carnegie Gift," *Vanderbilt Quarterly* (July–September 1913), p. 209.
49. *Nashville Banner* and *Nashville Tennessean,* June 19, 1913.
50. Minutes, BOT, June 16, 1913, VL.
51. *Nashville Banner* and *Nashville Tennessean,* June 19, 1913.
52. *Vanderbilt Quarterly* (July–September 1913), p. 209.
53. William H. Witt, "The Bishops and the Carnegie Gift," J. T. McGill Papers, VL.
54. Ibid.
55. This arrangement is not without irony. Though it was not remarked at the time, separate administrative apparatus actually ran counter to Flexner's ideal of close integration of medical school and university. By insisting on a separate board, Carnegie hoped to insulate the school from churchly influence and from the meddling of uninformed laymen and too interested practitioners, things the board did accomplish. The arrangement did less for the unity of the university.
56. John A. Witherspoon served as president of the council, and the acting dean as secretary. R. E. McCotter was elected by the governing board, and William H.

Witt and Duncan Eve by the faculty. "The Annual meeting of the Medical Governing Board," *Vanderbilt Quarterly* (October–December 1913), pp. 275–77.

57. *Proceedings of the Semi-Centennial of Vanderbilt University, October 15–18, 1925* (Nashville: Vanderbilt University, 1925), p. 90.

58. Kirkland to GEB, cited in Edwin Mims, *Chancellor Kirkland of Vanderbilt* (Nashville: Vanderbilt University Press, 1940), p. 202.

59. Though he finally gave $300,000, William K. Vanderbilt, who had donated Kissam Hall in 1899, initially rebuffed Kirkland's plea, claiming war conditions mitigated against raising money for education. Frederick W. Vanderbilt was prevailed upon for $100,000, but Alfred Vanderbilt, on whom Kirkland had pinned large hopes, went down with the *Lusitania* in 1915.

60. "I have not troubled you with letters during the last six months," Kirkland wrote to Buttrick on his progress toward finding the match. "Most of the time I have not felt like writing. Often my discouragement has been so great that Arkansas, Tufts, and every other place I ever heard of seemed more attractive to me than Nashville. . . . I am making you this report in full consciousness of the fact that it is not what it ought to be, but trusting that you are prepared to throw the mantle of charity over a suffering friend who has more than once longed for life in the trenches [it was the second summer of World War I] as a relief out of present difficulties" (Kirkland to Buttrick, July 17, 1915, CMVL).

61. Fosdick, *Adventure in Giving*, p. 328.

4. An Alliance

1. The portal is still there, though no longer the scene for many photographs. The court, now filled with large trees and air conditioners, has been closed off by the addition of the A. B. Learned Laboratory and consequently no longer looks out on anything.

2. See G. Canby Robinson, *Adventures in Medical Education* (Cambridge: Harvard University Press, 1957), p. 100.

3. G. Canby Robinson Personal Diary, on loan to author from O. Boise Robinson, Boston.

4. Conversation of author with O. Boise Robinson, Boston, and Mrs. Russell Angell, Paxton, Mass., February 1980.

5. On GEB aid to medical schools in the 1910s, see Raymond B. Fosdick, *Adventure in Giving: The Story of the General Education Board* (New York: Harper & Row, 1962), pp. 150–73.

6. Kirkland to Flexner, April 5, 1917, CMVL; Edwin Mims, *History of Vanderbilt University* (Nashville: Vanderbilt University Press, 1946), pp. 354–55.

7. Cited in Mims, *History of Vanderbilt University*, p. 355; correspondence between Kirkland and Flexner, summer and fall of 1918, CMVL.

8. In a personal note acknowledging Kirkland's thanks for a profitable experience, Buttrick wrote from New York: "I hope that at a convenient time you may find it possible to go to one or two other medical schools. While everything at Hopkins is the very best, they themselves would hardly claim to have all the good things in the world. To be sure they form a sort of mutual admiration association down there, but after all, they are finely critical of one another." The Hopkins spell was not quite perfect. Buttrick to Kirkland, February 13, 1919, CMVL.

9. Confidential Memorandum, February 27, 1919, CMVL.
10. Ibid.
11. Ibid.
12. Ibid.
13. As compiled by Flexner, Vanderbilt's operating expenditures broke down as follows (with his comparative figures for Johns Hopkins and Washington University):

STATEMENT RE BUDGETS OF MEDICAL SCHOOL

	Johns Hopkins Medical School	Washington University Medical School	Vanderbilt University Medical School NOW	Vanderbilt University Medical School PROPOSED
Administration	$ 4,700	$ 5,255	$ 4,670	$ 5,000
General Expenses	22,000	19,745	9,085	20,000
Anatomy	22,000	12,000	9,200	10,000
Library	2,000	7,000	1,370	3,000
Medicine	39,000–47,000	35,000		20,000
Pathology and Bacteriology	35,000	14,000	18,730	20,000
Pediatrics	25,000–30,000	25,000		15,000
				(Under medicine)
Pharmacology	15,000	5,400		7,500
Phys. Chemistry	8,500	9,700	4,400	6,000
Physiology	14,000	10,000	5,250	8,500
Surgery	40,000	29,000	1,735	25,000
	$240,200	$172,100	$54,440	$140,000

Source: Ibid.

14. Ibid.
15. Flexner to Kirkland, June 26, 1919, CMVL. Never quiet for long, Flexner had written earlier, enclosing a clipping of an article from the *Times* of London on the subject of the full-time plan in medical education.
16. Of the old faculty, only Lucius Burch, then dean and professor of obstetrics and gynecology, would join the reorganized faculty under the new regime, though all of the others were invited to serve on the clinical staff. Many did. The faculty resolution of September 22, 1919, read:

We, the undersigned members and officers of the School of Medicine of Vanderbilt University respectfully call the attention of the Board of Trust and the Governing Board of the School of Medicine to the present difficulties that embarrass this department. These difficulties concern the organization of the School and the financial resources available. They have been growing and are now so acute that we believe it will not be possible to operate the School of Medicine much longer on its present basis.

The financial crisis can be met only by securing additional sums for endowment and for hospital work. In this task we are ready to render assistance, but realize that the initiative must fall to others.

In the matter of department organization we can perhaps, with greater force, express ourselves and make suggestions to the Trustees. We believe that in the near future the Vanderbilt School of Medicine should be reorganized. The simplest way in which this can be accomplished is by making a new start. Casual readjustments would be an endless task. We suggest, therefore, to the Trustees that they should make far-reaching plans to secure means to build up a School of Medicine modern in type, facilities, equipment, personnel, and ideas, and that to this end they should act unhampered by any past or present appointments. A clean slate is essential in order that the new writing may be direct and satisfying. We have labored too long in behalf of Medical education in the South and in connection with Vanderbilt University to hesitate now at this critical moment. Without regard to any personal interests we tender our resignations of the positions held by each of us, same to be accepted by the Trustees at their pleasure. Until such acceptance, we pledge our best services to the School of Medicine, and we further pledge our cooperation and assistance in the new organization without regard to any possible appointments that may be offered us. (Minutes, BOT, September 22, 1919)

17. See Robert A. McGaw, *The Vanderbilt Campus: A Pictorial History* (Nashville: Vanderbilt University Press, 1978), pp. 66–67.
18. Kirkland to Buttrick, September 20, 1919, CMVL.
19. Telegram, Buttrick/Flexner to Kirkland, September 22, 1919, CMVL.
20. Flexner to Kirkland, September 25, 1919, CMVL.
21. Flexner to Kirkland, December 27, 1919, CMVL.
22. Flexner too thus left the door open to the possibility that in the future such noble humane goals might best be advanced by things other than or at least in addition to "modern medical schools." Flexner himself so changed horses in 1928 when he left the GEB and turned his talents and energies to fields other than medical education, quite convinced all the while that the race was the same.
23. *Nashville Banner* and *Nashville Tennessean,* November 27, 1919.
24. Kirkland to Flexner, November 27, 1919, CMVL.
25. Kirkland to Buttrick, December 1, 1919; Kirkland to Flexner, December 2, 1919, CMVL.
26. Flexner to Kirkland, December 1, 1919, CMVL.
27. *St. Louis Globe-Democrat,* December 2, 1919; *Charlotte Observer,* November 27, 1919; *Muncie* (Indiana) *Press,* December 2, 1919. Clipping file, Department of Medicine Archives, VML.
28. *Richmond News-Leader,* n.d. Clipping file, Department of Medicine Archives, VML.
29. Characteristically, Flexner put it this way: "The matter of the announcement to the public lies altogether in your hands. It might be well, in order to avoid any crossing of wires, if after you have drafted your announcement, we had a chance to look it over before it is issued. This is only a suggestion and would doubtless have occurred to you in any event" (Flexner to Kirkland, October 29, 1919, CMVL). It had.
30. Memorandum, Kirkland to Board of Trust, November 9, 1919, CMVL.
31. Fosdick, *Adventure in Giving,* app. 1, p. 327.
32. Flexner, "Memorandum: Medical Education in the United States: A Program," June 1919. Flexner Manuscripts, LC.
33. Fosdick, *Adventure in Giving,* p. 161.
34. Flexner, "Confidential Memorandum Regarding Mr. Rockefeller's Gift To Be

Devoted To The Improvement of Medical Education In The United States," December 4, 1919. Flexner Manuscripts, LC.

35. Ibid.

36. Ibid.; Flexner's emphasis.

37. Ibid. Even so, the GEB over the years assisted only seven medical schools in the South other than Vanderbilt: Baylor, Duke, Emory, Meharry, Tulane, and the Universities of Georgia and Virginia. Baylor, Duke, Emory, Georgia, and Virginia received less than $1 million each. Tulane got $3.4 million, and Meharry, one of the two black schools that the GEB supported (Howard University in Washington, D.C., was the other), received $8.6 million (Fosdick, *Adventure in Giving,* p. 328).

38. The story of the conflict appears in Fosdick, *Adventure in Giving,* pp. 166–67. For another version, see E. Richard Brown, *The Rockefeller Medicine Men: Medicine and Capitalism in the Progressive Era* (Berkeley and Los Angeles: University of California Press, 1979), p. 176.

39. Flexner, "Memorandum: Medical Education in the United States"; Flexner's emphasis.

5. The New Man

1. Flexner to Kirkland, October 21, 1919, CMVL.

2. G. Canby Robinson, *Adventures in Medical Education* (Cambridge: Harvard University Press, 1957), p. 145.

3. Kirkland to Flexner, December 27, 1919, CMVL.

4. Robinson, *Adventures in Medical Education,* p. 146.

5. Robinson to Kirkland, December 31, 1919, CMVL.

6. Kirkland to Flexner, December 27, 1919, CMVL.

7. Kirkland to Robinson, January 5, 1920; Robinson to Kirkland, January 7, 1920; Kirkland to Robinson, January 10 and 13, 1920; and Kirkland to Flexner, January 13, 1920, CMVL.

8. Robinson to Kirkland, January 19, 1920, CMVL.

9. Ibid.

10. Ibid.

11. Kirkland to Robinson, January 26, 1920; and Kirkland to Flexner, January 29, 1920, CMVL.

12. Robinson to Kirkland, January 26, 1920, CMVL; Robinson to Flexner, February 11, 1920, and Robinson to Simon Flexner, February 7, 1920, RAC. To Buttrick, Robinson also wrote: "I want to drop you a line to say I am very enthusiastic over the project and shall do my utmost to have the school there attain the high place you hope for it" (February 5, 1920, RAC).

13. Kirkland to Flexner, January 29, 1920, CMVL.

14. Wrote Flexner to Kirkland: "I need not say that Dr. Buttrick and I are deeply gratified to learn that Dr. Robinson has accepted the deanship. We both believe thoroughly in his wisdom, experience, and training. I am sure that you will work together most harmoniously and effectively in carrying out our great undertaking" (February 7, 1920, CMVL). Wrote Kirkland to Robinson: "I am glad that we had the opportunity to talk this matter over in New York. I think that conversation enabled us to see other's position more satisfactorily than any amount of corre-

spondence. I believe as soon as we conclude our business arrangements that we shall both enter into the new enterprise with all the enthusiasm possible and I have not the slightest doubt that we shall find our greatest happiness in working together for the splendid undertaking" (January 28, 1920, CMVL).

15. Kirkland to Robinson, January 29, 1920, CMVL.
16. Robinson to Kirkland, February 5, 1920, CMVL.
17. Kirkland to Robinson, February 7, 1920, CMVL.
18. Kirkland to Flexner, February 6, 1920; and Flexner to Kirkland, February 10, 1920, CMVL.
19. Flexner to Kirkland, February 7, 1920; and Kirkland to Flexner, February 9, 1920, CMVL.
20. So Whitridge Williams told Flexner on his visit to Hopkins in January 1920. See Flexner to Kirkland, February 7, 1920, CMVL.
21. Kirkland to Robinson, February 9, 1920, CMVL; Kirkland to Flexner, May 1, 1920, RAC. Flexner wrote to Kirkland that both he and Buttrick were disappointed to learn that Dandy was leaning toward practice, but "in our judgment the combination of practice and research—no matter how well-arranged—simply will not work. A man must choose between an academic and professional career" (May 3, 1920, RAC).
22. Robinson to Kirkland, February 5 and 10, 1920, CMVL.
23. Flexner to Kirkland, February 7, 1920, CMVL; Buttrick to Robinson, February 9, 1920, RAC. As Buttrick put it: "I was in Baltimore last week and casually made some inquiries about Dr. Dandy. I was told by Dr. Smith, Superintendent of the Hospital, and Dr. Williams, the Dean, that Dr. Dandy was looked upon by them as perhaps the most promising surgeon in the country. They furthermore said that when, last year, there were some fears that Dr. Halsted might be unable to return to his work, members of the surgical staff and other members of the clinical staff came to them and said that they hoped Dr. Dandy would be called for the succession since they would all work with might and main under him. I mention this because of our little conversation at the station in St. Louis, and not at all to urge anyone on your attention."
24. Robinson to Kirkland, February 5, 1920, CMVL.
25. Flexner to Kirkland, February 17, 1920, CMVL. It was good that Robinson never read that his patron included him among the "young fellows." Youth was one of the complaints Robinson had of Dandy: "Dandy is still an untried man, never having been away from Johns Hopkins. He is rather young" (Robinson to Kirkland, February 5, 1920, CMVL).
26. Robinson to Kirkland, February 16, 1920, CMVL.
27. Robinson to Kirkland, February 5, 1920, CMVL.
28. Robinson, *Adventures in Medical Education*, p. 155.
29. Robinson to Kirkland, July 14, 1920, CMVL.
30. Robinson to Kirkland, August 14, 1920, CMVL; Robinson, *Adventures in Medical Education*, p. 160.
31. "Plan for the Proposed Reorganization of the Vanderbilt Medical School," RAC.
32. Robinson to Flexner, September 23, 1920, RAC.
33. Robinson to Kirkland, September 23, 1920, CMVL.
34. Kirkland to Robinson, October 7 and 11, 1920, CMVL.
35. Flexner to Robinson, October 15, 1920, CMVL.

36. Kirkland to Robinson, November 1, 1921, CMVL.
37. "Plan for the Proposed Reorganization."
38. Ibid.
39. Ibid.
40. Nashville was a place that left scientists relatively isolated from the rest of their profession and yet whose central location in the poor South left it singularly well situated (as Flexner had said) to supply medical service to the region. Ironically, central location for purposes of rendering service left the servers who were also supposed to be scientists isolated from the centers of their profession. What scientist, Robinson was asking, could be expected to come to Nashville without regular—and subsidized—opportunity to leave it?
41. "Plan for the Proposed Reorganization."
42. Robinson to Kirkland, September 24, 1920, CMVL.
43. Kirkland to Flexner, October 18, 1920, CMVL.
44. See Robinson-Kirkland correspondence, October through December 1920, CMVL.
45. Kirkland to Robinson, January 25, 1921, CMVL.
46. Robinson to Kirkland, January 29, 1921, CMVL.
47. Robinson to Kirkland, February 9, 1921, CMVL.
48. Robinson neglected to sign his letter of January 29. Kirkland's testy reply of January 31 began: "I have your letter of January 29 to which you forgot to attach your signature." Robinson shot back a handwritten note on February 2 expresssing regret "that I failed to sign my letter of January 29. This letter may serve as a signature to that one." And he signed it. Robinson-Kirkland correspondence, CMVL.
49. Kirkland was sensitive about his relationship with his patrons. His "Condensed Memorandum Regarding Location of Vanderbilt School of Medicine" (CMVL) concluded: "It occurs to me finally to add only these words that in the original negotiations of Vanderbilt University with the officers of the General Education Board no thought was entertained of raising the question of location. It has come up from other sources [Robinson, clearly]. We are not in any way open to criticism as if this were a problem concealed or information withheld."
50. Kirkland to Robinson, January 31, 1921, CMVL.
51. Robinson to Kirkland, February 9, 1921, CMVL.
52. James H. Kirkland, "Vanderbilt University School of Medicine, Memoranda Numbers One, Two, and Three, West and South Campus Plans"; and "Condensed Memorandum Regarding Location of Vanderbilt School of Medicine," CMVL.
53. Kirkland, "Condensed Memorandum."
54. Wrote Flexner to Kirkland: "The Board was deeply interested in your argument on the question of site" (December 4, 1920, CMVL).
55. Charles Cason to Eileen Bishop, November 28, 1952; and Memorandum of Charles Cason to GEB, 1919 or 1920, CMVL. Also see Edwin Mims, *History of Vanderbilt University* (Nashville: Vanderbilt University Press, 1946), pp. 358–59.
56. Flexner to Trevor Arnett, December 27, 1920, RAC.
57. Robinson to Kirkland, March 18, 1921, CMVL.
58. Flexner to Kirkland, April 1, 1921, CMVL.
59. Kirkland to Robinson, May 23 and 27, 1921; and Flexner to Kirkland, May 27, 1921 (letter and telegram), CMVL.
60. Kirkland to Robinson, May 27, 1921, CMVL.

6. Courts and Corridors

1. Robinson's original drawings are in the Vanderbilt Medical Library.

2. Robinson also knew that his theory of coordination, so embodied in a plan that physically linked laboratories and clinics, might have the undesirable result of "distracting both students and staff from engaging in the less spectacular and less practical activities of the laboratories, and to place too near them the allurements of clinical medicine." Clinician that he was, he well understood those allurements and knew their dangers: "There is much more to be said for carrying forward the laboratories into the clinics than there is for carrying the clinics into the laboratories, and it is hoped that a plan which will effect the former may not unduly produce the latter condition" (G. Canby Robinson, "The Relation of Medical Education to Medical Plant," *Journal of the American Medical Association* 81 [July 28, 1923]: 321).

3. For description and drawing of the 1925 medical school and hospital see ibid., pp. 321–23, and G. Canby Robinson, "Vanderbilt University School of Medicine: History and General Description," in *Methods and Problems of Medical Education*, 13th series (New York: Rockefeller Foundation, 1929).

4. The other Gothic portal—the entrance to the university hospital on Twenty-first Avenue—fell victim in the 1970s to the addition of a new wing, as formidable though wholly different in style from what it masked.

5. Flexner to Kirkland, December 8, 1921, CMVL.

6. G. Canby Robinson, *Adventures in Medical Education* (Cambridge: Harvard University Press, 1957), pp. 161–66; *Baltimore Sun*, June 25, 1921.

7. Through the early 1920s Robinson remained a productive investigator. See A. McGehee Harvey, "G. Canby Robinson: Peripatetic Medical Educator," *Johns Hopkins Medical Journal* 143 (1978): 103. He also served as editor in chief of the *Journal of Clinical Investigation* during its first years in the early 1920s.

8. See Chapter 1 above.

9. Robinson to Kirkland, November 4, 1922, CMVL.

10. Robinson to Kirkland, December 18, 1922, and January 7, 1923, CMVL. A similar form of government was used at Washington University (though there Robinson felt the faculty board dallied too much over matters of salary) and at Hopkins. And, as he learned from talks with George Whipple, head of the reorganized medical school at the University of Rochester, so it would be there also.

11. Kirkland to Robinson, December 18, 1922, and January 10, 1923, CMVL.

12. Robinson to Flexner, September, 1923, CMVL.

13. Robinson, *Adventures in Medical Education*, p. 161.

14. Robinson to Kirkland, October 11, 1923, CMVL.

15. Kirkland to Robinson, October 22, 1923, CMVL.

16. Kirkland to Flexner, October 13, 1923, CMVL.

17. Kirkland to Flexner, October 20, 1923, CMVL.

18. Kirkland to Robinson, December 18, 1923, CMVL.

19. Robinson to Kirkland, December 23, 1923, CMVL.

20. Robinson, "Proposed Budget of Vanderbilt University Medical School," October 1923, CMVL.

21. Robinson to Kirkland, November 23, 1923, CMVL.

22. Kirkland to Robinson, November 26, 1923, CMVL.

23. Robinson to Flexner, November 10, 1923, RAC.

24. Flexner to Robinson, November 14, 1923, RAC.
25. Kirkland to Robinson, December 18, 1923, CMVL.
26. Robinson to Kirkland, December 23, 1923, CMVL.
27. Flexner to Kirkland, January 2, 1924, RAC.
28. Robinson to Kirkland, January 15, 1924, CMVL.
29. Robinson to Kirkland, December 23, 1923, CMVL.
30. Robinson to Kirkland, February 7 and March 7, 1924, CMVL.
31. Robinson to Kirkland, February 21, 1924, CMVL.
32. Robinson to Kirkland, May 10, 1924, CMVL; Hugh Morgan curriculum vitae, Hugh Morgan Papers, VML.
33. Robinson to Kirkland, April 22 and May 1, 1924, CMVL.
34. Robinson to Kirkland, May 1 and April 23, 1924, CMVL.
35. Robinson to Kirkland, May 10, 1924, CMVL.
36. Robinson to Kirkland, June 17, 1924, CMVL.
37. Robinson to Kirkland, March 24, 1925, CMVL.
38. Ibid.
39. Robinson to Kirkland, May 21, 1925, CMVL.
40. Robinson to Kirkland, March 24, 1925; and Barney Brooks to Kirkland, April 1, 1925, CMVL.
41. Robinson to Kirkland, July 16, January 3, and May 30, 1925, CMVL.
42. Only the department of obstetrics and gynecology was left to a local (rather than a new) man: Lucius E. Burch, the dean of the old medical school.
43. In the process of trying to entice Goodpasture to come to Vanderbilt, Robinson reported to Kirkland that his salary at the Singer Laboratory was $10,000 (Robinson to Kirkland, March 7, 1924, CMVL).
44. See Charles Rosenberg, "Martin Arrowsmith: The Scientist as Hero," in *No Other Gods: On Science and American Social Thought* (Baltimore: Johns Hopkins University Press, 1976), pp. 123–31.

7. Medicine

1. See G. Canby Robinson, *Adventures in Medical Education* (Cambridge: Harvard University Press, 1957), pp. 186–87, 219.
2. Robinson to Kirkland, April 27, 1928; and Kirkland to Robinson, October 12, 1928, CMVL. Kirkland never was converted. Even in 1929, after the GEB had capitalized its previous grants, he wrote to Robinson (then at Cornell) that "I regard it as much more important to pay debts than to make new appropriations for research in any department. I fear my views are not generally accepted.

"As you meet a good many numbers of our faculty from time to time I hope you will support my position and say to them that they cannot expect Vanderbilt University to invest anything more in medical education until some benefactor not now discovered shall furnish the means in advance. If you will encourage this attitude of mind it will help me very much" (June 17, 1929, CMVL).
3. The new members of the faculty, who truly did owe Robinson much, held back little in their testimonial: "In large measure credit of the remarkable results that have been attained in the building of the new medical school of Vanderbilt University and the reorganization of the faculty must be attributed to the forethought, wisdom and splendid scientific leadership of Doctor Robinson. His un-

tiring effort, fine spirit, cooperative attitude, intelligent interest and inspirational qualities have been the predominant factors in providing at Vanderbilt University a medical school which meets in an admirable way the modern ideals in medical education" (statement adopted by the executive faculty on the occasion of Robinson's departure, June 1928, VML). Their adulation lasted. See testimonial at the presentation of his portrait to the school, at a formal dinner at the Belle Meade Country Club in 1938, VML.

4. Kirkland to Robinson, June 20, 1928, CMVL.

5. In 1934 and 1935 he served as professor of medicine at Peking Union Medical College in China but only on a temporary, one-year appointment.

6. One of those—Rudolph H. Kampmeier, himself a student of Osler's godson, Campbell Palmer Howard, at the University of Iowa in the early 1920s—served as a distinguished member of the Vanderbilt department of medicine from 1936 to 1963 and, faithful to Osler's belief in the importance of the historical perspective in medical education, became its historian. From his account, *Recollections: The Department of Medicine, Vanderbilt University School of Medicine, 1925–1959* (Nashville: Vanderbilt University Press, 1980), much of the factual matter of what follows is drawn.

7. Among American historians, the influence of Frederick Jackson Turner was perhaps comparable, though it has worn less well.

8. William Osler, "The Hospital As A College" (1903), cited in Kampmeier, *Recollections*, p. 54; also see Osler "The Hospital in University Work," *Lancet* 1 (1911): 211–13.

9. Robinson to C. Sidney Burwell, February 19, 1926, Robinson Papers, VML.

10. Recollection of Lloyd Ramsey, cited in Kampmeier, *Recollections*, p. 61.

11. Kampmeier, *Recollections*, p. 61.

12. On Vanderbilt football during its "golden age" see Edwin Mims, *History of Vanderbilt University* (Nashville: Vanderbilt University Press, 1946), pp. 275–90.

13. See clipping: "Pershing's Men in France," in Hugh Morgan File, History of Medicine Room, VML.

14. Robinson to Kirkland, April 13, 1928, CMVL.

15. Kampmeier, *Recollections*, pp. 64–66; Robinson, *Adventures in Medical Education*, pp. 182–83.

16. Kampmeier, *Recollections*, pp. 66–67.

17. Ibid., p. 73.

18. Ibid., pp. 67–68.

19. Pediatrics in 1928; psychiatry, 1947; neurology, 1965. Dermatology remains a division within the department of medicine.

20. G. Canby Robinson, "Vanderbilt University School of Medicine: History and General Description," in *Methods and Problems of Medical Education*, 13th series (New York: Rockefeller Foundation, 1929), p. 91.

21. Kampmeier, *Recollections*, pp. 77–78.

22. Ibid., pp. 78–79. Robinson, "Vanderbilt University School of Medicine," p. 89.

23. One student was David Strayhorn, Sr., a third-year student in 1926–27 and later both assistant and senior resident. See Kampmeier, *Recollections*, p. 80.

24. Reminiscence of Addison Scoville, in Kampmeier, *Recollections*, pp. 81–82.

25. John B. Youmans and C. Sidney Burwell, address at meeting of Association of American Medical Colleges, 1934, cited in Kampmeier, *Recollections*, pp. 88–89.

26. John B. Youmans, "Vanderbilt—Yesterday, Today, and Tomorrow," *Journal of the Tennessee Medical Association* 59 (January 1966): 46.

27. A. McGehee Harvey, cited in Kampmeier, *Recollections*, pp. 101–02.

28. Youmans, "Vanderbilt—Yesterday, Today, and Tomorrow," p. 43.

29. Kampmeier, *Recollections*, p. 101.

30. Robinson, *Adventures in Medical Education*, p. 85.

31. For a comprehensive summary see Kampmeier, *Recollections*, pp. 179–214.

32. Ibid., p. 193.

33. Ibid., p. 182.

34. See Chapter 9, below. Even that fund, however, did not remove anxiety over how research in the future would be paid for. Sidney Burwell worried in 1935:

> Much of the research has been made possible through the support of the Fluid Research Fund. Useful and indispensable as this support is, I am a little perturbed by the possible development of a situation where most of the research in the department is financed by special funds. A large proportion of the strictly departmental budget is now devoted to routine diagnostic work and to teaching but little of it to research. This is only important in that if special funds were ever interfered with, the research work in the department would have very little support. There is still need in the department for fellows or full-time assistants who can devote their time to research. There should always be more ideas than machinery to carry them out, but the exhaustion of ideas is still a long way off. (Department of Medicine Annual Report for 1935, Department of Medicine Archives, VML)

35. William Osler, "Teaching and Thinking," in *Aequinemitas* (Philadelphia: T. Blackiston's Son & Co., 1905), p. 124.

36. Osler, "The Leaven of Science," in ibid., pp. 98–99.

37. Osler, "Teaching and Thinking," p. 134.

8. Surgery

1. On Brooks's life see: Rollin A. Daniel, Jr., "Barney Brooks, 1884–1952," *Transactions of the Southern Surgical Association* 63 (1951): 415–16; "Dr. Barney Brooks," Vanderbilt Society of Historical Medicine, Memo Number Three, February 26, 1968, VML; Bryan E. Green, Jr., "Doctor Barney Brooks, 1884–1952" (manuscript in the possession of William Meacham, department of neurosurgery, Vanderbilt).

2. Volkmann's contracture—paralysis and contracture of muscles following application of a constricting bandage—had previously been ascribed to arterial obstruction, nerve damage, and toxic agents. Brooks demonstrated experimentally the concept of occlusion of venous return. (See Green, "Doctor Barney Brooks," p. 6).

3. Ibid., p. 7.

4. G. Canby Robinson, *Adventures in Medical Education* (Cambridge: Harvard University Press, 1957), p. 180.

5. On Halsted see: Alfred Blalock, "William Stewart Halsted and His Influence on Surgery," *Proceedings of the Royal Society of Medicine* 45 (1952): 555, in Mark M. Ravitch, ed., *The Papers of Alfred Blalock* (Baltimore: Johns Hopkins University

Press, 1966); Samuel James Crowe, *Halsted of Johns Hopkins—The Man and His Men* (Springfield, Ill.:Thomas, 1957).

6. Ravitch, *Papers of Blalock,* p. 1658.

7. Ibid., pp. 1659–60.

8. Halsted wrote much on such matters. For a compendium, see: *Surgical Papers by William Stewart Halsted,* 2 vols. (Baltimore: Johns Hopkins University, 1924), especially "The Training of the Surgeon" (1904), 2:512–31.

9. Halsted, "Training of the Surgeon," pp. 513–14.

10. Ibid., p. 515.

11. Ibid., pp. 520–21.

12. Ibid., p. 524.

13. Ibid., p. 522.

14. Halsted was at Hopkins from 1886 to 1922. Brooks was at Vanderbilt from 1925 to 1952.

15. Barney Brooks, "Vanderbilt University School of Medicine: Department of Surgery," in *Methods and Problems of Medical Education,* 13th series (New York: Rockefeller Foundation, 1929), pp. 104–05.

16. Ibid., p. 106.

17. Ibid., pp. 107–08.

18. Ibid.

19. Ibid.

20. Material on the daily routine of the department of surgery is based on author's interviews with Drs. Edmund Benz, Louis Rosenfeld, B. F. Byrd, Jr., Charles Trabue IV, William F. Meacham, Edward Barksdale, Eugene Regen, and Barton McSwain, February 1980.

21. Operating Room Logbooks, Vanderbilt Department of Surgery.

22. For lists of department publications, see Annual Reports, Department of Surgery, in Annual Reports of the Dean to the Chancellor, Robinson and Leathers Papers (1926–40), VML.

23. See curriculum vitae and bibliography in Ravitch, *Papers of Blalock,* 2:1982–92.

24. Cited in Alfred Blalock, "Shock and Hemorrhage," *Bulletin of the New York Academy of Medicine* 12 (November 1936): 610.

25. Ibid.

26. Ibid.

27. And so it went for at least one more round with H. William Scott, Jr., Brooks's successor as chief of surgery at Vanderbilt. Though a Harvard (rather than a Hopkins) M.D., Scott served on the Hopkins house staff and worked there with Blalock.

28. Barney Brooks, "Psychosomatic Surgery," *Annals of Surgery* 119 (March 1944): 291.

29. Ibid.

9. Science

1. Bulletin of Vanderbilt University, Catalogue of the School of Medicine, Announcement for 1930–31, pp. 47–48.

2. The only major exception to this funding in the 1920s was the Department of Preventive Medicine and Public Health, which initially was supported by grants from the Rockefeller Foundation.

3. Abraham Flexner, *Funds and Foundations* (New York: Harper & Row, 1952), p. 91.
4. Raymond B. Fosdick, *The Story of the Rockefeller Foundation* (New York: Harper & Row, 1952), p. 137.
5. Ibid., pp. 140–41.
6. Wickliffe Rose, "Scheme for the Promotion of Education on an International Scale," Memorandum, 1923, cited in Fosdick, *Story of the Rockefeller Foundation;* Annual Report of the General Education Board for 1925–26, cited in ibid., pp. 141, 154.
7. Ibid., p. 142.
8. Flexner, *Funds and Foundations,* pp. 77–100.
9. Ibid., pp. 84, 93–94.
10. Ibid., p. 84.
11. Ibid., pp. 85, 88–89.
12. Fosdick, *Story of the Rockefeller Foundation,* pp. 143–44.
13. For the year May 1932–April 1933, the range of budgets was:

Anatomy	$30,688	Pediatrics	$19,380
Biochemistry	22,040	Pharmacology	21,170
Medicine	48,012	Physiology	24,042
Ob-Gyn (not full-time)	6,620	Preventive Medicine	21,624
Pathology	41,600	Surgery	46,000

Source: Budgets, School of medicine, 1931, 1932, 1933, Leathers Papers, VML.

14. Dean's Annual Report, 1930–31, p. 8, Leathers Papers, VML.
15. Ibid.; Leathers to Alan Gregg, November 11, 1931, Leathers Papers, VML.
16. Alan Gregg, *The Furtherance of Medical Research* (New Haven: Yale University Press, 1941), p. 73.
17. Leathers to Alan Gregg, April 6, 1931, Leathers Papers, VML.
18. Norma S. Thompson to Kirkland, December 16, 1931, Leathers Papers, VML. The letter reports formal action of the Rockefeller Foundation to set up the fluid research fund at Vanderbilt.
19. Leathers to Alan Gregg, September 22 and 26, 1931, Leathers Papers, VML.
20. Alan Gregg to Leathers, December 17, 1931, Leathers Papers, VML.
21. Alan Gregg to Leathers, January 22, 1932, Leathers Papers, VML.
22. Dean's Annual Report, 1931–32; and Report of the Meeting January 25, 1932, of the Advisory Committee to the Dean for the Disbursement of the Fluid Research Fund, Leathers Papers, VML.
23. Financial Statements of the Fluid Research Fund, 1932–40; and Dean's Annual Reports, 1932–40, Leathers Papers, VML.
24. Ernest Goodpasture to Leathers, April 24, 1934, Leathers Papers, VML. Hugh Morgan wrote of research in the department of medicine: "I feel that I am correct in making this statement: more than one-half of these papers could never have been published had we not had the grant from the Division of Medical Science. This grant, during the years we have had it, has been a backlog in financing all the investigative work in my Department. As pointed out to you in a recent conversation, it is really unfortunate that every paper published in my Department and representing clinical investigation doesn't carry acknowledgement to the Division of Medical Science" (February 9, 1939, Leathers Papers, VML).

25. Financial Statements of the Fluid Research Fund, 1932–40, Leathers Papers, VML.
26. Dean's Annual Reports, 1935–36, 1938–39, 1939–40, Leathers Papers, VML.
27. Cited in Gregg, *Furtherance of Research*, p. 37. See Walter B. Cannon, *The Way of An Investigator: A Scientist's Experience in Medical Research* (New York: W. W. Norton & Co., 1945).
28. *Nashville Tennessean*, October 16, 1955.
29. J. D. Ratcliff, editor of *Scientific Yearbook of 1944*, clipping entitled "Lifesaver" (otherwise unidentified), Goodpasture File, History of Medicine Room, VML.
30. Ibid.
31. *Nashville Tennessean*, October 16, 1955.
32. Ratcliff, "Lifesaver."
33. Scientific research in medicine could also, of course, have just the opposite result. If by curing disease it made life less hazardous for countless millions, it by definition thus made survival easier—and the "fit" who survived were thus less fit than if they had had a harder time of it. That meant devolution, not evolution, and was something less talked about.
34. See Ernest W. Goodpasture, "Research and Medical Practice," *Science* 104 (November 22, 1946): 473. Address delivered in Baltimore, May 15, 1946, on receiving the award of the Passano Foundation, Inc.
35. In the 1940s, Goodpasture turned down offers from both Hopkins and Harvard to serve as head of pathology. But with others who did leave (Sidney Burwell for one, who went to Harvard as dean in 1935) he remained fast friends. An aficionado of good dinner parties, Burwell soon after his move proudly offered his Boston guests something of the flavor of Tennessee that he had left behind him: a genuine hickory-smoked country ham, sent by farmer Goodpasture with instructions for cooking it. But concerned lest some curious yankee should ask at dinner what really made it taste that way, Burwell wrote his old colleague for the correct response. Goodpasture replied with this telegram:

    > Pack fresh ham in dry salt six months. Hang in smokehouse. Smoke slowly about two months. Sack and hang in smokehouse a year or two.
    > Old well seasoned smokehouse indispensable for best flavor. Hickory wood smoke choice. Age important factor. It's a ham what am. Happy days.
    > Ernest (February 6, 1936, Goodpasture Papers, in possession of Katherine A. Goodpasture, Nashville)

36. Ernest W. Goodpasture, "Some Aspects of Twentieth Century Research on Infectious Diseases," *Washington University Medical Alumni Quarterly* 135 (April 1950): 100–101.
37. Ibid., p. 101.
38. Ernest W. Goodpasture, "Cellular Inclusions and the Etiology of Virus Diseases," *Archives of Pathology* 7 (1929): 114.
39. Already in the 1920s Goodpasture thought that phrase had outlived its usefulness, however. It had become trite, and it invited misuse of the group "as a repository for all sorts of nondescript and ill defined conditions of unknown etiology and indefinite pathology." Better, he felt, "to emphasize other characteristics of such agents which represent their activities and the effects which they induce, rather than to hold tenaciously only to an expression of a single physical characteristic" (Goodpasture, "Cellular Inclusions," pp. 114–32). So his work would prove.

40. Ernest W. Goodpasture, "The Pathology of Certain Virus Diseases," *Southern Medical Journal* 21 (July 1928): 535–39.

41. Ibid.

42. Goodpasture, "Cellular Inclusions"; idem, "Etiological Problems in the Study of Filterable Virus Diseases," *Harvey Lectures* (1931):77–102. Lecture delivered to the Harvey Society of New York, December 19, 1929.

43. Goodpasture, *Harvey Lectures*, pp. 78–79.

44. C. Eugene Woodruff and Ernest W. Goodpasture, "The Infectivity of Isolated Inclusion Bodies of Fowl-Pox," *American Journal of Pathology* 5 (1929): 1–10.

45. Ernest W. Goodpasture, "Virus Diseases of Fowls as Exemplified by Contagious Epithelioma (Fowl-pox) of Chickens and Pigeons," in T. M. Rivers, *Filterable Viruses* (Baltimore: Williams & Wilkins, 1928), p. 235.

46. C. Eugene Woodruff and Ernest W. Goodpasture, "The Relation of the Virus of Fowl-Pox to the Specific Cellular Inclusions of the Disease," *American Journal of Pathology* 6 (November 1930): 713–20.

47. Ibid., p. 719.

48. Goodpasture, *Harvey Lectures*, p. 100; idem, "Cellular Inclusions," p. 2.

49. Claud D. Johnson and Ernest W. Goodpasture, "The Etiology of Mumps," *American Journal of Hygiene* 21 (1935): 46–57; idem, "Experimental Immunity to the Virus of Mumps," *American Journal of Hygiene* 23 (1936): 329–39; idem, "The Histopathology of Experimental Mumps in the Monkey, Macacus Rhesus," *American Journal of Pathology* 12 (1936): 495–510.

50. Ernest W. Goodpasture, "The Pathology and Pathogenesis of Poliomyelitis," in National Foundation for Infantile Paralysis, *Infantile Paralysis: A Symposium Delivered at Vanderbilt University, April 1941* (New York: Foundation for Infantile Paralysis, 1941), pp. 85–125. Goodpasture, "The Pathology of Poliomyelitis," *Journal of the American Medical Association* 117 (July 26, 1941): 273–75.

51. Ernest W. Goodpasture, "The Cell-Parasite Relationship and Virus Infection," *Transactions and Studies of the College of Physicians of Philadelphia* 9 (April 1941): 23.

52. E. Paschen (Hamburg) to Goodpasture, August 8 and October 20, 1932, Goodpasture Papers, in possession of Katherine A. Goodpasture, Nashville.

53. Simon Flexner to Goodpasture, February 13, 1924; and Abraham Flexner to Goodpasture, April 30, 1937, Goodpasture Papers, in possession of Katherine A. Goodpasture, Nashville.

54. Goodpasture, "Some Aspects of Research on Infectious Diseases," pp. 98, 102.

55. Ibid., pp. 104–05.

56. Ibid., p. 99; Goodpasture, "Research and Medical Practice," pp. 473–76.

10. Dependence

1. See John Morton Blum, *V Was For Victory* (New York: Harcourt, Brace, Jovanovich, 1977), pp. 115, 140–46.

2. The feeling of those times as remembered by one who lived through them is well recorded in Rudolph H. Kampmeier's *Recollections: The Department of Medicine, Vanderbilt University School of Medicine, 1925–1959* (Nashville: Vanderbilt University Press, 1980), chap. 5.

3. Chancellor's Report, 1944–45, p. 4, CMVL.

4. On wartime stress, see Dean's Annual Reports, January 1942 (mid-year), 1941–42, January 1943 (mid-year), 1942–43, 1943–44, January 1945 (mid-year), Leathers Papers, VML.

5. C. S. Robinson to Goodpasture, March 26, 1945, and April 2, 1946, Goodpasture Papers, VML.

6. Dean's Annual Report, 1945–46, Goodpasture Papers, VML.

7. See Richard Polenburg, *War and Society: The United States, 1941–1945* (New York: Harper & Row, 1972), p. 241.

8. Blum, *Victory*, p. 144.

9. Ibid.; Polenburg, *War and Society*, p. 241.

10. See OSRD-cmr contract #76: "A study of the chemotherapy of craniocerebral wounds," and contract #462: "The clinical value of penicillin in various infectious conditions," Leathers Papers, VML.

11. See OSRD-cmr contract #11: "Carbohydrate metabolism in shock with special reference to anesthetics," and contract #277: "The determination of degradation products of atabrine in the body (animals and man)," Leathers Papers, VML.

12. See OSRD-cmr contract #505: "The effectiveness of penicillin in the treatment of syphilis," Leathers Papers, VML.

13. A. N. Richards (chairman, Committee on Medical Research, OSRD) to Charles M. Sarratt (vice-chancellor, Vanderbilt), July 27, 1946, Goodpasture Papers, VML.

14. OSRD Administrative Circular 13.12, March 22, 1945, Leathers Papers, VML.

15. See Irwin Stewart (executive secretary, Committee on Medical Research, OSRD) to Leathers, December 2, 1941, Leathers Papers, VML.

16. Andrew B. Benedict to Leathers, with attachments, August 8, 1944, Leathers Papers, VML.

17. OSRD contract # OEM-cmr-11; OSRD Circulars 5.03 (November 18, 1941) and 4.02; and Cobb Pilcher to Leathers, December 10, 1942, Leathers Papers, VML.

18. Dean's Annual Report, 1943–44, Leathers Papers, VML.

19. Dean's Annual Report, February 1945 (mid-year), Leathers Papers, VML.

20. Walter W. Palmer (chairman, Medical Advisory Committee) to Leathers, March 7, 1945, Leathers Papers, VML.

21. Committee on Medical Research (Office of Emergency Management, OSRD), "Confidential Memorandum on a National Foundation for Medical Research," March 1945, Leathers Papers, VML.

22. Ibid.

23. Ibid.

24. The NIH has its origins in the late nineteenth century when a bacteriological laboratory was established within the Public Health Service. It began to assume modern form in the 1930s and after the war it blossomed into fourteen research institutes and divisions plus the National Library of Medicine and five divisions dealing with research and training of health personnel. Its responsibilities are discharged both through direct on-site research and training and through grants to individuals and institutions.

25. Sam Clark to Leathers, March 27, 1945; C. S. Robinson to Leathers, March 27, 1945; Rudolph H. Kampmeier to Leathers, March 27, 1945; Lucius E. Burch to Leathers, April 4, 1945; Amos Christie to Leathers, March 26, 1945; Paul Lamson to Leathers, March 31, 1945; C. E. King to Leathers, April 2, 1945; and Barney Brooks to Leathers, March 30, 1945, Leathers Papers, VML.

26. Committee on Medical Research, "Confidential Memorandum on a National Foundation for Medical Research."

27. See Rosemary Stevens, *American Medicine and the Public Interest* (New Haven: Yale University Press, 1971), pp. 359–60.

28. In addition to Vanderbilt, the following universities were represented: the University of California, Columbia, Cornell, Duke, Harvard, State University of Iowa, Johns Hopkins, University of Michigan, University of Minnesota, New York University, Northwestern, University of Pennsylvania, University of Rochester, Stanford, Tulane, Washington University, Western Reserve, and Yale. See "Statement on Medical Education Made Jointly by Presidents of 19 Universities, March 15, 1947," Goodpasture Manuscripts, VML.

29. Dean's Annual Report, 1945–46, Goodpasture Papers, VML.

30. Dean's Report, January 30, 1946 (mid-year), Goodpasture Papers, VML.

31. Chancellor's Report, December 15, 1948, CMVL.

32. Basil C. MacLean et al., consultants, "A Study of Vanderbilt University Hospital," 1946, VML.

33. Ibid., p. 18.

34. Ibid., pp. 9–10, 14–15, 24.

35. Ibid., pp. 66, 70.

36. Ibid., p. 46.

37. Goodpasture to Harvie Branscomb, January 7, 1949, Goodpasture Papers, VML.

38. Ibid.

39. For Goodpasture's elaboration of his plan, see Goodpasture to Harvie Branscomb, January 22, 1949, Goodpasture Papers, VML.

40. Ibid.

41. Goodpasture to Harvie Branscomb, January 7, 1949, Goodpasture Papers, VML.

42. Ibid.

43. See handwritten note on letter from Goodpasture to Branscomb, January 7, 1949. This was obviously the copy that Goodpasture sent to Clark for review. Also, Clark to Goodpasture, January 19, 1949, Goodpasture Papers, VML.

44. Paul Lamson to Goodpasture, January 25, 1949, Goodpasture Papers, VML.

45. Frank Luton to Goodpasture, February 17, 1949; and Cobb Pilcher to Goodpasture, January 26, 1949, Goodpasture Papers, VML.

46. "Report of the Committee on the Financial Crisis of Vanderbilt University School of Medicine and Hospital" (the Christie committee), December 30, 1948; and Pilcher to Goodpasture, January 26, 1949, Goodpasture Papers, VML.

47. See Harvie Branscomb to Goodpasture, February 8, 1949, Goodpasture Papers, VML.

48. Goodpasture to Branscomb, November 17, 1949, Goodpasture Papers, VML.

49. See Alan Gregg, *The Furtherance of Medical Research* (New Haven: Yale University Press, 1941), pp. 19–20.

50. Youmans to Branscomb, May 6, 1950, Youmans Papers, VML.

51. Lamson to Goodpasture, January 25, 1949, Goodpasture Papers, VML.

52. For yearly budgets from the 1940s and 1950s see Leathers and Goodpasture Papers, VML. They are hand-typed carbon copies, usually less than fifty pages, bound together with string.

53. Dean's Annual Reports, 1950–51, 1954–55, Youmans Papers, VML.

54. See Stevens, *American Medicine and the Public Interest*, chap. 16: "Professionalism and the Medical School."

55. Wrote Branscomb later: "Youmans was an internist who was a recognized specialist in the field of nutrition. I often wanted to ascertain his diet and feed it to the other deans." *Purely Academic* (Nashville: Vanderbilt University, 1978), p. 178.
56. Such transfers were not without problems. See Kampmeier, *Recollections,* pp. 237–38.
57. Dean's Annual Reports, 1951–52, 1952–53, 1953–54, Youmans Papers, VML.
58. Kampmeier, *Recollections,* p. 144.
59. Dean's Annual Report, 1954–55; and H. William Scott, Jr., Annual Report, Department of Surgery, 1954–55, Youmans Papers, VML.
60. Dean's Annual Report, 1954–55, Youmans Papers, VML.

11. Service and Science

1. See *Journal of the American Medical Association (JAMA)* 178 (November 11, 1961): 584–86.
2. Annual Report, Department of Medicine, 1964, Conference Room, Dean's Office; School of Medicine, *Bulletin,* February 1981.
3. School of Medicine, *Bulletin,* February 1981.
4. *JAMA* 202 (November 20, 1967): 726.
5. One of the most comprehensive of the special reports was *The Doctor Shortage: An Economic Analysis* by Rashi Fein of the Brookings Institution, highlights of which appeared in the Brookings Research Report Number 64, "Medical Manpower for the 1970s."
6. Ibid. On continued manpower crisis, also see *JAMA* 210 (November 24, 1969): 1456; 214 (November 23, 1970): 1484; and 226 (November 19, 1973): 894.
7. Dean's Annual Report, 1963–64, Conference Room, Dean's Office.
8. Annual Report, Vanderbilt University Medical School, 1968–69, Conference Room, Dean's Office.
9. See Rosemary Stevens, *American Medicine and the Public Interest* (New Haven: Yale University Press, 1971), pp. 366–67.
10. *JAMA* 222 (November 20, 1972): 963.
11. Ibid.
12. The School of Nursing is not administratively a part of the medical school, but much of its training occurs within the medical center.
13. Dean's Annual Report, 1964, Conference Room, Dean's Office.
14. Liaison Committee on Medical Education (hereafter cited as LCME), Annual Medical School Questionnaire (Vanderbilt University), p. 2, 1979–80, VML.
15. Dean's Annual Report, 1965, Conference Room, Dean's Office.
16. LCME, p. 2, 1979–80.
17. Vanderbilt University Medical Center *Annual Report,* 1977–78, VML.
18. In 1947 the federal government spent $27 million on medical research, or 31 percent of the total national expenditure. NIH's share was $8.3 million, 10 percent of the total. In 1966 the government spent $1.4 billion, 68 percent of the total; NIH's share was $800 million or 40 percent of the total. James A. Shannon, "The Advancement of Medical Research: A Twenty-Year View of the Role of the NIH," *Journal of Medical Education* 42 (February 1967): 97–108.
19. *JAMA* 186 (November 16, 1963): 658.
20. Vanderbilt University Medical Center *Annual Report,* 1976–77, VML.
21. The research centers included: Neuromuscular Disease Research Center, Center

for Population and Reproductive Biology Research, Psychopharmacology Research Center, Research Center for Pharmacology and Drug Toxicology, Clinical Research Center, Diabetes Endocrinology, Center in Environmental Toxicology, Specialized Center for Research in Hypertension, Neonatal Lung Specialized Center of Research, Center for Health Services, Mental Health Center, Pulmonary Specialized Research Center, and Cancer Center.

22. On the growth of that science establishment, see Daniel Greenberg, *The Politics of Pure Science* (New York: New American Library, 1967).

23. See Shannon, "Advancement of Medical Research"; and "Federal Support of Biomedical Sciences Development and Academic Impact," *Journal of Medical Education* 51 (July 1976): 1–98.

24. Dean's Annual Reports, 1964–65, 1968–69, Conference Room, Dean's Office; "Challenge or Crisis—Phase III: For Vanderbilt School of Medicine," report by Leon W. Cunningham, 1981.

25. *JAMA* 238 (December 26, 1977): 2780.

26. Vanderbilt University Medical Center *Annual Reports*, 1975–76, 1977–78; and Supplement to Financial Report of Vanderbilt University, VML.

27. Dean's Annual Report, 1968–69, Conference Room, Dean's Office.

28. "Vanderbilt University Hospital," a brochure published by Vanderbilt University Medical Center, 1980.

29. In 1977 the revenue for sponsored research and programs rose again to 53 percent of the university's total revenue; however, in 1978 the figures resumed their downward trend. Vanderbilt University Medical Center *Annual Reports*, 1975–76, 1976–77, 1977–78; and Supplement to Financial Report of Vanderbilt University, VML.

30. Vanderbilt University Medical Center *Annual Report*, 1977–78; and Supplement to Financial Report of Vanderbilt University, VML; Cunningham, "Challenge or Crisis."

31. LCME, 1976–77, 1979–80; Cunningham, "Challenge or Crisis."

32. David E. Rogers, *American Medicine: Challenges for the 1980s* (Cambridge, Mass.: Ballinger, 1978), p. 83, n. 17.

33. Edward J. Berger, "The Nation's Health and Expenditures for Health: Thoughts on National Policy," *Journal of Medical Education* 49 (October 1974): 927–35.

34. See David E. Rogers, "The Academic Medical Center: A Stressed American Institution," *New England Journal of Medicine* 298 (April 27, 1978): 940–50; idem, "On Preparing Academic Health Centers for the Very Different 1980s" (Alan Gregg Memorial Lecture, 1979), *Journal of Medical Education* 55 (January 1980): 1–12.

35. On the presumption of progress in science generally, see Thomas S. Kuhn, *The Structure of Scientific Revolutions,* 2d ed., rev. (Chicago: University of Chicago Press, 1970), p. 160.

36. However, it is possible to say that science moved faster and more efficiently in either the 1930s or the 1970s than it did in the 1910s, before any of the conditions for science had been met and before, at Vanderbilt, there was any mandate at all. Still, the meaning of "efficiency" in research is hard to pin down. C. P. Snow argued that the efficiency of science probably is related to the clarity of the objectives conceived for it. Thus he saw "a certain grim family resemblance" between military science and medical science ("trying to accelerate people's deaths

or alternatively to delay them"). Clear-cut objectives give "edge and sharpness to the deployment of medical research. For it is not the nature of the objective that makes for speedy action, whether it is destructive or on the side of life. All that matters is that there should be an objective at all" (*Science and Government* [Cambridge: Harvard University Press, 1961], pp. 77–78). If Snow was right, then as medicine's mandate broadens (as without doubt it has)—and blurs—its efficiency will decline.

37. See Lewis Thomas, "The Future of Science in the Art of Healing," *Journal of Medical Education* 51 (January 1976): 23–29.

Suggestions for Further Reading

The primary documentary sources for this book are the extensive archives of Vanderbilt University and its medical center. These include the records of the board of trust, the Chancellor's Manuscripts, the manuscript collections of the Vanderbilt University Library, the Vanderbilt Medical Library, and departmental libraries. Ernest Goodpasture's private papers are held by his widow, Katherine Goodpasture, who freely opened them to the author. The Barney Brooks Papers have recently been acquired by the Vanderbilt Medical Library. The John Youmans Papers are held by the National Library of Medicine in Betheseda, Maryland. Two other collections vital to research in this field are the General Education Board files at the Rockefeller Archive Center in Tarrytown, New York, and the Abraham Flexner Papers in the Library of Congress.

The secondary literature bearing on this particular subject is voluminous, and specific sources are cited in the notes. For the reader interested in further reading the following suggestions may prove helpful. They are not comprehensive.

In the general field of the history of medicine and medical practice in the United States, see Richard Shryock, *Medicine and Society in America* (Baltimore: Johns Hopkins University Press, 1966) and *Medical Licensing in America* (Baltimore: Johns Hopkins University Press, 1967); Robert P. Hudson, *Disease and Its Control* (Westport, Conn.: Greenwood, 1983); Lester S. King, *Medical Thinking: A Historical Perspective* (Princeton: Princeton University Press, 1982); James O. Breeden, *Joseph Jones, M.D.: Scientist of the Old South* (Lexington: University Press of Kentucky, 1975); Charles Rosenberg, ed., *Healing and History: Essays for George Rosen* (New York: Science Library, 1979); Owsei Temkin, *The Double Face of Janus and Other Essays in the History of Medicine* (Baltimore: Johns Hopkins University Press, 1977); Joseph Kett, *The Formation of the American Medical Profession: The Role of Institutions, 1780–1860* (New Haven: Yale University Press, 1968); John S. Haller, *American Medicine in Transition, 1840–1910* (Urbana: University of Illinois Press, 1981); George Rosen, *The Structure of American Medical Practice, 1875–1941* (Philadelphia: University of Pennsylvania Press, 1983); William G. Rothstein, *American Physicians in the Nineteenth Century: From Sects to*

Science (Baltimore: Johns Hopkins University Press, 1972); James G. Burrow, *Organized Medicine in the Progressive Era: The Move Toward Monopoly* (Baltimore: Johns Hopkins University Press, 1977); Morris J. Vogel, *The Invention of the Modern Hospital, 1870–1930* (Chicago: University of Chicago Press, 1980); Albert S. Cowdrey, *This Land, This South: An Environmental History* (Lexington: University Press of Kentucky, 1983); Irving Loudon, "The Concept of the Family Doctor," *Bulletin of the History of Medicine* 58 (Fall 1984): 347–62; Mary R. Walsh, *Doctors Wanted: No Women Need Apply* (New Haven: Yale University Press, 1977); Elizabeth W. Etheridge, *The Butterfly Caste: A Social History of Pellagra in the South* (Westport, Conn.: Greenwood, 1972); John Duffy, *The Healers* (New York: McGraw Hill, 1976).

On medical education and reform, including institutional histories, see Martin Kaufman, *American Medical Education* (Westport, Conn.: Greenwood, 1976); James Summerville, *Educating Black Doctors: A History of Meharry Medical College* (University: University of Alabama Press, 1983); James F. Gifford, Jr., *The Evolution of a Medical Center: The History of Medicine at Duke to 1941* (Durham: Duke University Press, 1972); John Duffy, *The Tulane University Medical Center: 150 Years of Medical Education* (Baton Rouge: Louisiana State University Press, 1984); Thomas B. Turner, *Heritage of Excellence: The Johns Hopkins Medical Institutions, 1914–1947* (Baltimore: Johns Hopkins University Press, 1974); Henry K. Beecher and Mark D. Altschule, *Medicine at Harvard: The First 300 Years* (Hanover: University Press of New England, 1977); George W. Corner, *A History of the Rockefeller Institute* (New York: Rockefeller Institute Press, 1964); John S. Chapman, *The University of Texas Southwestern Medical School* (Dallas: Southern Methodist University Press, 1977); Carleton B. Chapman, *Dartmouth Medical School* (Hanover: University Press of New England, 1973); Ronald Numbers, *The Education of American Physicians* (Berkeley and Los Angeles: University of California Press, 1980); Robert K. Merton, *The Student Physician* (New York: Commonwealth Fund, 1965); Ellen C. Congi, "Abraham Flexner's Philanthropy: The Full-Time System in the Department of Surgery at the University of Cincinnati, 1910–1930," *Bulletin of the History of Medicine* 56 (Summer 1982): 160–74; Kenneth M. Ludmerer, "Reform at Harvard Medical School, 1869–1909," *Bulletin of the History of Medicine* 55 (Fall 1981): 341–70; idem, "Reform of Medical Education at Washington University," *Journal of the History of Medicine and Allied Sciences* 35 (April 1980): 149–73; idem, "The Rise of the Teaching Hospital in America," *Journal of the History of Medicine and Allied Sciences* 38 (October 1983): 389–414; idem, "The Plight of Clinical Teaching in America," *Bulletin of the History of Medicine* 57 (Summer 1983): 218–29; Daniel M. Fox, "Abraham Flexner's Unpublished Report: Foundations and Medical Education, 1909–1928," *Bulletin of the History of Medicine* 54 (Winter 1980): 475–96; Gert Brieger, "Fit to Study Medicine: Notes for a History of Pre-Medical Education in America," *Bulletin of the History of Medicine* 57 (Summer 1983): 1–21; John Harley Warner, "A Southern Medical Reform: The Meaning of the Antebellum Argument for Southern Medical Education," *Bulletin of the History of Medicine* 57 (Fall 1983): 364–81.

On science and research in medicine, see Charles Rosenberg, *No Other Gods: On Science and American Social Thought* (Baltimore: Johns Hopkins University Press, 1976), *The Cholera Years* (Chicago: University of Chicago Press, 1968); Thomas S. Kuhn, *The Structure of Scientific Revolutions*, 2d ed., rev. (Chicago: University of Chicago Press, 1970); Warren Weaver, *Science and Imagination, Selected Papers* (New York: Basic Books, 1967); Walter B. Cannon, *The Way of an Investigator: A Scientist's Experience in Medical Research* (New York: W. W. Norton & Co., 1945); Rene J. Dubos,

The Professor, The Institute, and DNA (New York: Rockefeller University Press, 1976); Anne Sayre, *Rosalind Franklin and DNA* (New York: W. W. Norton & Co., 1975); David Wilson, *In Search of Penicillin* (New York: Alfred A. Knopf, 1976); Harry F. Dowling, *Fighting Infection: Conquests of the Twentieth Century* (Cambridge: Harvard University Press, 1977); Sally Smith Hughes, *The Virus: A History of A Concept* (New York: Science History Publications, 1977); Saul Benison, "Poliomyelitis and the Rockefeller Institute: Social Effects and Institutional Response," *Journal of the History of Medicine and Allied Sciences* 29 (January 1974): 74–92; Robert E. Kohler, *From Medical Chemistry to Biochemistry* (Cambridge: Cambridge University Press, 1982); A. McGehee Harvey, *Science at the Bedside: Clinical Research in American Medicine, 1905–1945* (Baltimore: Johns Hopkins University Press, 1981); Peter C. English, *Shock, Physiological Surgery, and George Washington Crile: Medical Innovation in the Progressive Era* (Westport, Conn.: Greenwood, 1980); Mark M. Ravitch, ed., *The Papers of Alfred Blalock* (Baltimore: Johns Hopkins University Press, 1966).

   On the history of medicine and philanthropy, see Abraham Flexner, *I Remember: The Autobiography of Abraham Flexner* (New York: Simon & Schuster, 1940); idem, *Henry S. Pritchett: A Biography* (New York: Columbia University Press, 1943); Frederick T. Gates, *Chapters in My Life* (New York: Free Press, 1977); Raymond B. Fosdick, *The Story of the Rockefeller Foundation* (New York: Harper & Row, 1952); idem, *Adventure in Giving: The Story of the General Education Board* (New York: Harper & Row, 1962); Joseph F. Wall, *Andrew Carnegie* (New York: Oxford University Press, 1970); David Freeman Hawke, *John D.: The Founding Father of the Rockefellers* (New York: Harper & Row, 1980); Merle Curti and Roderick Nash, *Philanthropy in the Shaping of American Higher Education* (New Brunswick: Rutgers University Press, 1965); Robert Bremner, *American Philanthropy* (Chicago: University of Chicago Press, 1982); E. Richard Brown, *The Rockefeller Medicine Men: Medicine and Capitalism in the Progressive Era* (Berkeley and Los Angeles: University of California Press, 1979).

   On medicine and public policy, see Paul Starr, *The Social Transformation of American Medicine* (New York: Basic Books, 1982); Rosemary Stevens, *American Medicine and the Public Interest* (New Haven: Yale University Press, 1971); Morris Vogel and Charles Rosenberg, eds., *The Therapeutic Revolution: Essays in the Social History of American Medicine* (Philadelphia: University of Pennsylvania Press, 1979); Ronald Numbers, *Almost Persuaded: American Physicians and Compulsory Health Insurance, 1912–1920* (Baltimore: Johns Hopkins University Press, 1978); John B. McKinlay, ed., *Politics and Health Care* (Cambridge: MIT Press, 1981); Martin Marty and Kenneth Vaux, eds., *Health/Medicine and the Faith Traditions: An Inquiry into Religion and Medicine* (Philadelphia: Fortress Press, 1982); H. Wayne Morgan, *Drugs in America* (Syracuse: Syracuse University Press, 1981); John C. Burnham "Change in the Popularization of Health in the United States," *Bulletin of the History of Medicine* 58 (Summer 1984): 182–197; Daniel M. Fox, "The Decline of Historicism: The Case of Compulsory Health Insurance in the United States," *Bulletin of the History of Medicine* 57 (Winter 1983): 596–610; Milton Silverman and Philip R. Lee, *Pills, Profits, & Politics* (Berkeley and Los Angeles: University of California Press, 1976); Aaron E. Klein, *Trial by Fury: The Polio Vaccine Controversy* (New York: Charles Scribner's Sons, 1972); Renee C. Fox and Judith P. Swazey, *The Courage to Fail: A Social View of Organ Transplants and Dialysis* (Chicago: University of Chicago Press, 1974); Stanley Joel Reiser, *Medicine and the Reign of Technology* (Cambridge: Cambridge University Press, 1978); Ivan Illich, *Medical Nemesis* (New York: Pantheon, 1976); C. P. Snow, *Science and Government* (Cambridge: Harvard University Press, 1961).

Index

Haggard, W. D., 190
Haldane, J. B. S., 26
Halifax Medical School, 54
Halsted, William S., 36, 175–82, 185, 197,
   202, 205
   and Brooks, 136, 174–75
   at Hopkins, 20, 106, 188, 190
   and Robinson, 24–25
Hamburger, Louis P., 149
Hamman, Louis, 154
Hampton Institute (Va.), 59
Harris, Seale, Jr., 154, 158
Harrison, Tinsley R., 137, 154, **157**, 158–59,
   167–68, 221
Harvard University, 210, 245
   medical school, 38, 39
      Burwell at, 127, 136, 150, 152, 167
      Councilman at, 177
      and curriculum reform, 282
      Flexner at, 32
      Goodpasture at, 226
      Kirkland at, 20–21
      Lamson at, 136
   school of public health, 207
Harvey, William, 178, 180, 197
Harvey Lecture, 234
Health, and medicine, 276–77, 304–05
Health manpower shortage, 282–88
Health Professions Educational Assistance
   Act (1963), 284
Heart disease, research on, 167–68
Hegeman and Harris Co., 129
Hematology, research on, 168
Hill, James J., 10
Hoss, E. E., 71
Howard, Campbell Palmer, 147, 149, 154
Howard University, 49
Howell, William H., 24, 36, 73–74
Howland, John, 136
Hughes (Howard) Medical Institute, 288
Hunter, John, 177–78, 180, 197
Huxley, Thomas, 28

Illinois
   medical education in, 34, 38
   University of, medical school, 154, 267
Immunochemistry, research in, 292
Infectious diseases, research in, 168, 227–37,
   291–93
Internal medicine, 143–71
International Cancer Research Foundation,
   216

International Congress of Medicine (London,
   1881), 227
International Education Board, 207–08
Iowa, University of, medical school, 47,
   154

Jameson, J. Franklin, 19
Jesup, Morris, 60
Jobling, James, 106–08
Johns Hopkins, xi, 60, 73, 93–94, 99, 166,
   173, 191, 195, 261
   Blalock at, 201, 202
   Brooks at, 136, 174–75
   Burwell at, 127, 136
   Casparis at, 136
   Chesney at, 127
   Cunningham at, 136
   and curriculum reform, 279
   Dandy at, 106–07
   DeLamar Lecture at, 234
   as educational model, 16
   entrance requirements at, 44
   Flexner at, 18–21, 25, 34
   Flexner (Simon) at, 32
   and Flexner's report, 36, 47
   founding of, 39
   GEB funding of medical education at, 78,
      84, 95–96
   Gilman at, 18–20
   Goodpasture at, 136, 226
   Grollman at, 168
   Halsted at, 106, 176–82, 182
   Harris at, 154
   Harrison at, 167
   and Kirkland, 86–87
   Lamson at, 213
   Morgan at, 136, 153
   Osler at, 146–71
   and Robinson, 149
   Robinson at, 24–26, 81–82, 127–28, 145,
      153, 167
   school of public health, 105, 207
   Thomas at, 162
   Tinsley at, 154
   and Vanderbilt medical school, 92
   Wilmer Ophthalmological Institute, 264
   Youmans at, 154
Johnson, Hollis, 163, 168
Johnson, Lyndon, 282
Jones, Edgar, 162, 168
Jordan, Edwin O., 73–74
Journal of Experimental Medicine, 18